AF815415

Physeo

We would like to extend a special thanks to the following individuals who have spent countless hours and support to make Physeo possible.

Ajay Davidson, MD

Alexandra Galel, MD

Alexandra Harding

Anissa Laine Bayabos Amilhamja

Anne-Sophie van Wingerden
Medical Student
Columbia Vagelos College of Physicians and Surgeons

Antonio Acevedo

Ayan Agarwal
MBBS Student
Vardhman Mahavir Medical College and Safdarjung Hospital
New Delhi, India

Brianna Cocuzzo, MsC

Brooke Walsh, MS

Camelita Thrift

Christopher A. Price, MS

Genevieve Saliuk
MD Candidate 2024
UTMB School of Medicine

George Myo Win, BS
University of Missouri-Columbia School of Medicine

Ghadeer Magdy Elshafey, MD

H. Robert Cannon, DO

Dr. Jabran Wasti, House Officer
Dr. Ruth K.M. Pfau Civil Hospital
Karachi, Pakistan

Jae Cheol Bae

Dr. James Nunn

Jennifer M. Locke, BA
MD Candidate

Justin Wong, DO

Kurestin Miller, BA
MD Candidate

Lauren S. Faber, MD

Lauren Schwartz

Lee Azolai

Leslie Jewett, MD

Logan B. Carlyle, OMS-II

Marisol Cárdenas Calderón, MD

Mark Parry, MD, Resident Physician
Department of Obstetrics and Gynecology
OhioHealth – Riverside Methodist
Columbus, Ohio

Mason T. Bennet

Mateo Betancourt Escobar
Universidad Autónoma de San Luis
Potosí, Mexico

Mohamed Elshennawy

Natalia Kerr, MD

Nijat Aliyev, MD

Nikoloz Karazanashvili

Nirupamaa Sivanushanthan
Medical Student

Ostapenko Karolina

Dr. Rahil Patel, Medical Officer
Sharda Hospital
New Delhi, India

Mr. Rishabh Goyal

Roaa Zayat, MD

Rojin Arefi, MD

Ryan Zia

Salikh Murtaliev, MD

Sarah Jaber, D.O.
Internal Medicine Physician

Sergio R. Ortiz, MD, MPH

Shawna-Kay Young
MD Student

Shelia Chandrahas

Soomal Zukhruf Memon

Sumit Raut

Syed Ali Haider

Syed Awais Ahmed, MD

Tori Walsh

Tamari Papidze

Telyn Peterson, OMS-III
Rocky Vista University
Southern Utah

Trey Edwards, DO

Warda Hameed, MD

Yasmeen Abdulrahman, MD

Yomna Dean, MS-4

Zurabi Zaalishvili, MD

TABLE OF CONTENTS

OBESTETRICS

Obstetrics | Section 1: Pregnancy dating, Physiologic Adaptations, Nutrition and Prenatal Care

I. Dating of Pregnancy
  A. LMP known
    1. Naegele's rule: add 7 days to LMP, subtract 3 months, add 1 year
  B. LMP unknown
    1. Ultrasound to estimate gestational age and due date

II. Physiologic Adaptations
  A. Cardiovascular adaptations
    1. Increased blood volume to perfuse the uterus and placenta
    2. Decreased systemic vascular resistance
    3. Increased heart rate and cardiac output
  B. Pulmonary adaptations
    1. Increased central respiratory drive
    2. Significantly increased tidal volume and mildly increased respiratory rate
    3. Mild respiratory alkalosis (low $PaCO_2$)
  C. Renal adaptations
    1. Increased RBF and GFR
    2. Decreased BUN and creatinine
    3. Increased urine output
    4. Mild glucosuria
    5. Hyponatremia (increased ADH)
  D. Hematologic adaptations
    1. Increased prothrombotic coagulation factors
    2. Increased risk for DVT/PE
    3. Dilutional anemia (plasma volume > RBC mass)

III. Nutrition
  A. Normal weight gain (prepregnancy BMI)
    1. 12.7 - 18 kg (< 18.5 kg/m^2)
    2. 11.4 - 15.9 kg (18.5 - 24.9 kg/m^2)
    3. 6.8 - 11.4 kg (25 - 29.9 kg/m^2)
    4. 5 - 9 kg (≥ 30 kg/m^2)
  B. Complications of excessive gestational weight gain
    1. Gestational diabetes mellitus
    2. Macrosomia
    3. Cesarean delivery
  C. Complications of insufficient gestational weight gain
    1. Fetal growth restriction
    2. Preterm delivery
  D. Daily prenatal vitamins
  E. Substance abuse counseling
  F. Avoid
    1. Fish with high mercury levels (swordfish, shark, tilefish)
    2. Unpasteurized dairy products
  G. Clean raw fruits and vegetables

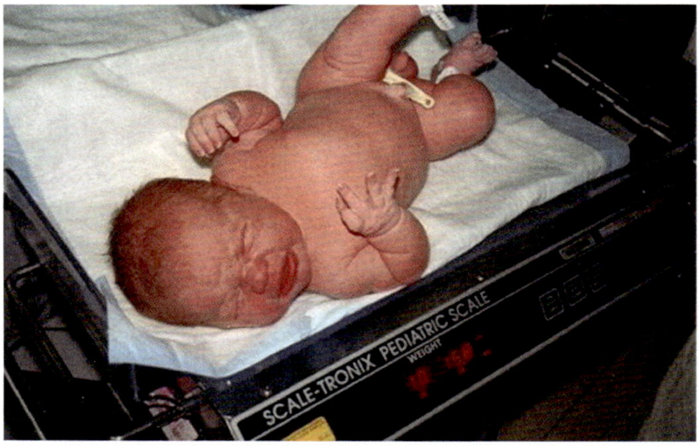

FIGURE 17.1.1 - Macrosomic Baby

IV. Prenatal Care
  A. On initial visit order
    1. CBC, blood type, and Rh status
    2. Rh-antibody screen (if Rh negative)
    3. Urinalysis with culture
    4. Gonorrhea and chlamydia PCR
    5. VDRL and HIV testing
    6. HbsAg
  B. At 10 - 14 weeks perform
    1. Ultrasound to check for size of nuchal translucency
    2. 1st trimester aneuploidy screen OR
    3. Cell free fetal DNA
  C. At 15 - 19 weeks perform
    1. 2nd trimester aneuploidy screen (Quad screen)
    2. Offer amniocentesis to patients with abnormal Quad screen
  D. At 18 - 21 weeks perform
    1. Ultrasound to survey fetal anatomy, placenta, and amniotic fluid
  E. At 24 - 28 weeks perform
    1. 1-hour glucose challenge test
    2. 3-hour glucose challenge test if 1-hour glucose ≥ 140 mg/dL
    3. Administer RhoGAM to Rh negative patients
  F. At 35 - 37 weeks perform
    1. Rectovaginal swab for GBS
    2. Treat with intrapartum penicillin/ampicillin if positive
    3. Repeat Hgb/Hct

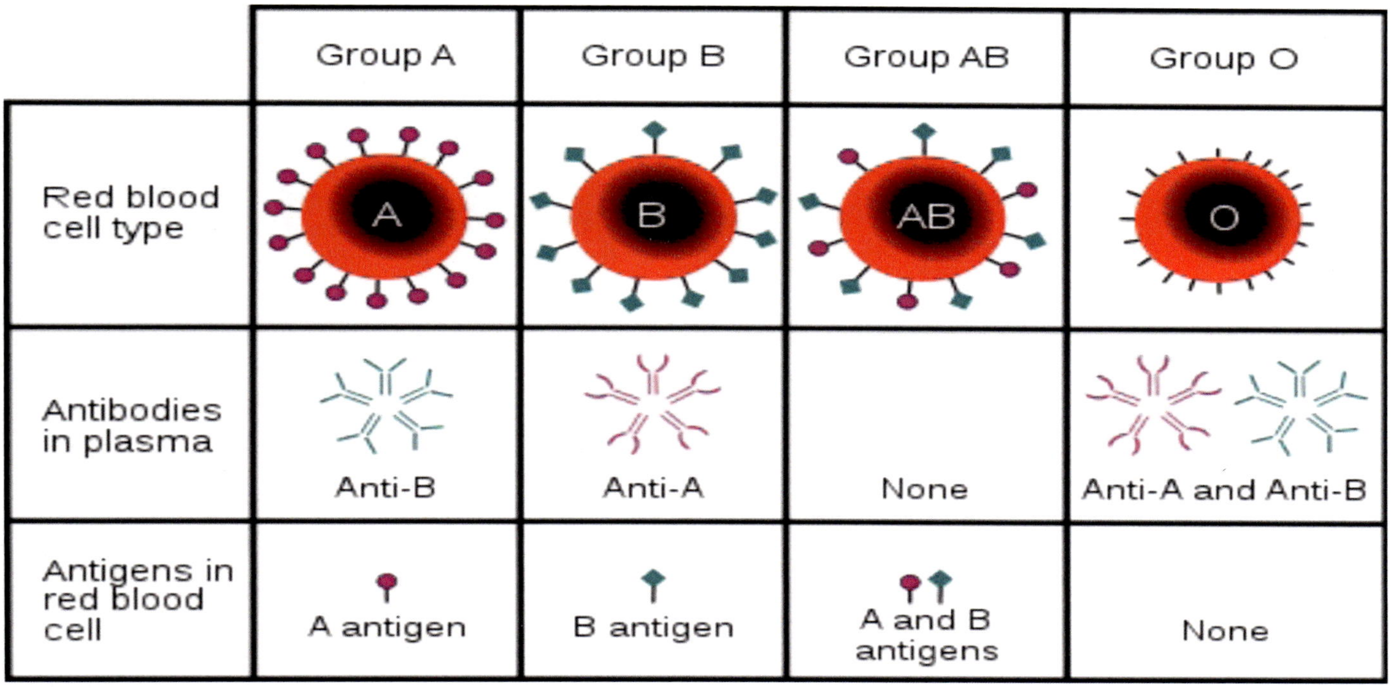

FIGURE 17.1.2 - Blood Groups (ABO Classification System)

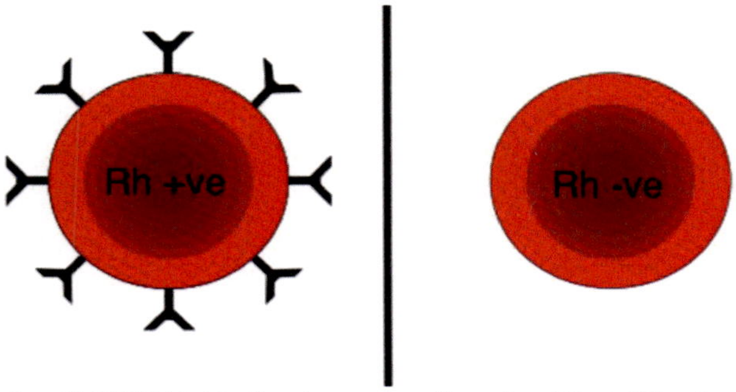

FIGURE 17.1.3 - Blood Groups (Rh Classification System)

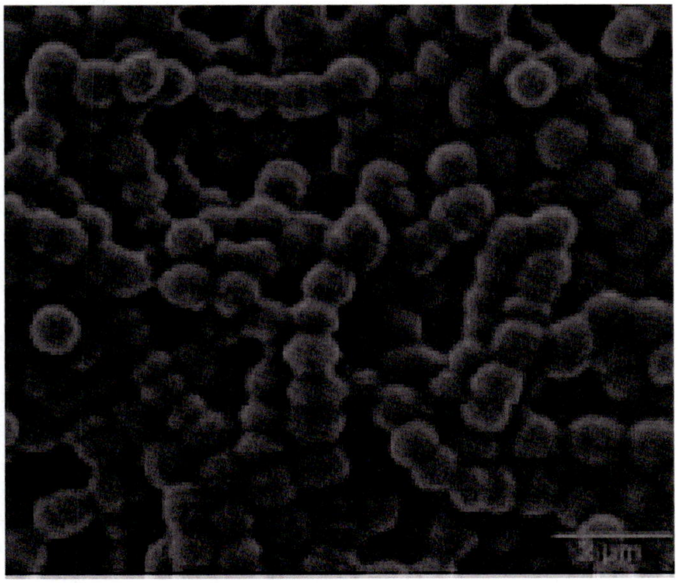

FIGURE 17.1.4 - Microscopy: Colonies of *Group B Streptococcus*

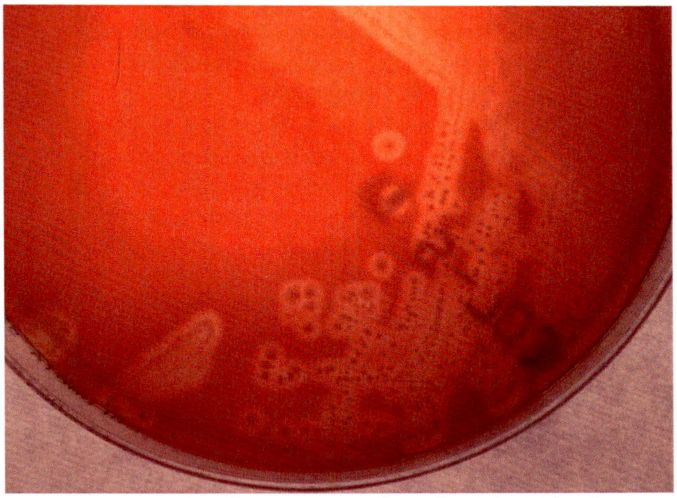

FIGURE 17.1.5 - Blood Agar: Colonies of *Group B Streptococcus*

REVIEW QUESTIONS

4. A 23-year-old woman comes to her primary care physician because of a positive home pregnancy test. Her last menstrual period was on February 9, 2021. What is her estimated date of delivery?

   - **Her estimated date of delivery is November 16, 2022.**
   - Naegele's rule is used to calculate this woman's estimated date of delivery.
   - Add 7 days to her last menstrual period which will be February 16, 2021. Then subtract 3 months, and we will receive November 16, 2021. Then add 1 year which will give us November 16, 2022.

5. A 25-year-old woman comes to her primary care physician because of a positive home pregnancy test. The physician orders all of the necessary tests including a urinalysis with culture. What is the purpose of ordering a urinalysis with culture in this asymptomatic patient?

   - **The purpose of ordering a urinalysis with culture is to screen for asymptomatic bacteriuria.**
   - All pregnant women should be screened for asymptomatic bacteriuria.
   - Asymptomatic bacteriuria is the presence of ≥ 100,000 colony-forming units/mL of urine. Unlike in nonpregnant women, asymptomatic bacteriuria, will be treated in pregnant women because of the increased risk for acute pyelonephritis and preterm delivery.

6. A 27-year-old G1P0 woman comes to her primary care physician at 34 weeks gestation for a routine prenatal visit. She has no specific complaints. Her history is significant for diabetes mellitus in her mother and father. Vital signs include temperature of 96.8° F (37° C), blood pressure of 120/80 mmHg, heart rate of 95 beats/min, and respiratory rate of 18 breaths/min. Physical examination shows a fundal height of 34 cm. Her prepregnancy BMI was 22 kg/m^2. She has gained 6 kg. Which of the following is most likely to be expected?

   A. Macrosomic baby
   B. Gestational diabetes mellitus
   C. Need for cesarean delivery
   D. Preterm delivery

   - **The correct answer is option D.**
   - This pregnant woman comes for a routine prenatal visit at 34 weeks of gestation.
   - Vital signs are withing normal limits.
   - Her prepregnancy BMI was normal (22 kg/m^2).
   - Women with a normal prepregnancy BMI should gain anywhere from 11.4 to 15.9 kg in total.
   - This woman at 34 weeks of gestation has gained only 6 kg, which is insufficient gestational weight gain.
   - One of the most common complications of insufficient gestational weight gain is preterm delivery because the fetus is not recieving enough nutrients to stay in the uterus for the full term.
   - Options A and B are incorrect because macrosomia and gestational diabetes mellitus are the complications of excessive, rather than insufficient, weight gain.
   - Option C, need for cesarean delivery, is incorrect because insufficient gestational weight gain is usually associated with low birth weight rather than macrosomic baby. Therefore, this patient will likely not need cesarean delivery.

Obstetrics | Section 2: Routine Problems of Pregnancy

I. Routine Problems of Pregnancy: Back Pain
   A. Enlarged uterus causes exaggerated lordosis
   B. Ligament laxity from high progesterone
   C. Decreased lumbar support from weak abdominal muscles
   D. Risk factors: excessive weight gain, chronic back pain
   E. Imaging not indicated
   F. Treatment: heating pads, analgesics

II. Routine Problems of Pregnancy: Constipation
   A. Due to progesterone and relaxin-mediated smooth muscle relaxation
   B. Treated with increased fiber and water intake or laxatives

III. Routine Problems of Pregnancy: GERD
   A. Same mechanism as constipation
   B. Treated with antacids and PPIs

IV. Routine Problems of Pregnancy: Hemorrhoids
   A. Due to increased pressure on anorectal venous system
   B. Treated with increased fiber and water intake, sitz baths, and hemorrhoidectomy only in severe cases

V. Routine Problems of Pregnancy: Pica
   A. Eating nonfood substances (hair, ice, dirt, paint chips)
   B. Treated with psychotherapy, nutritional rehabilitation, and SSRIs

VI. Routine Problems of Pregnancy: Urinary Frequency
   A. Due to increased pressure on bladder by gravid uterus
   B. Supportive treatment with relaxation and distraction techniques
   C. Antimuscarinic agents rarely used during pregnancy

VII. Routine Problems of Pregnancy: Varicose Veins
   A. Due to IVC compression by gravid uterus and backflow of blood
   B. Treated with compression stockings and leg elevation

REVIEW QUESTIONS ?

1. A 31-year-old G2P1 woman comes to her primary care physician at 25 weeks gestation for a routine prenatal visit. Her previous pregnancy was uncomplicated. She complains of a sour taste in her mouth, which worsens when she lies down, disrupting her sleep. What is the most likely mechanism for this woman's complaint?
   - **The mechanism of this woman's complaint is that progesterone and relaxin decrease lower esophageal sphincter tone.**
   - This pregnant woman at 25 weeks gestation complains of a sour taste in her mouth, which is worse with lying down.
   - This description is consistent with gastroesophageal reflux disease (GERD).
   - During pregnancy, progesterone and relaxin decrease lower esophageal sphincter tone, resulting in acid reflux.

Obstetrics | Section 3: Prenatal Fetal Assessment

I. Prenatal Fetal Assessment: Nonstress Test (TST)
   A. External fetal heart rate monitoring for 20 - 40 minutes
   B. Normal result: ≥ 2 accelerations in 20 minutes each rising by ≥ 15 beats/min and lasting ≥ 15 seconds (reactive)
   C. Abnormal result: < 2 accelerations (non-reactive); recurrent variable or late decelerations

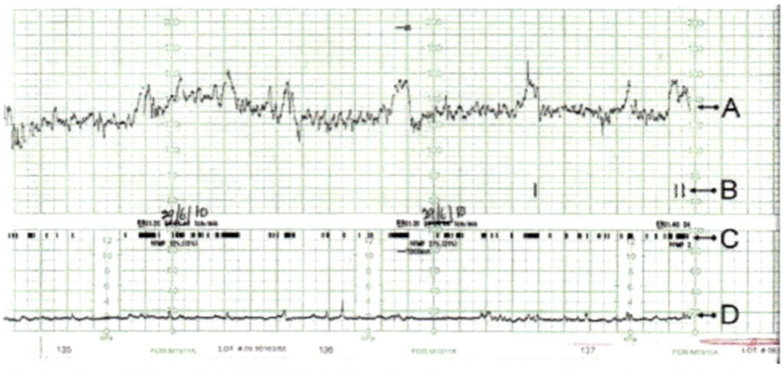

FIGURE 17.1.6 - Nonstress Test: Normal Findings

II. Prenatal Fetal Assessment: Biophysical Profile (BPP)
   A. NST: reactive = 2 points; nonreactive = 0 points
   B. Amniotic fluid volume: ≥ 2 cm deep = 2 points; < 2 cm deep = 0 points; movement: ≥ 3 moves = 2 points; no moves = 0 points
   C. Breathing: ≥ 1 breath lasting ≥ 30 seconds = 2 points; no breathing = 0 points
   D. Tone: ≥ 1 spinal/extremity extension = 2 points; no tone = 0 points

III. Prenatal Fetal Assessment: Contraction Stress Test (CST)
   A. Checks if fetus can tolerate stress of labor
   B. Monitor fetal heart rate during spontaneous or induced uterine contractions
   C. Normal result: no variable or late decelerations
   D. Abnormal result: late decelerations with > 50% of contractions

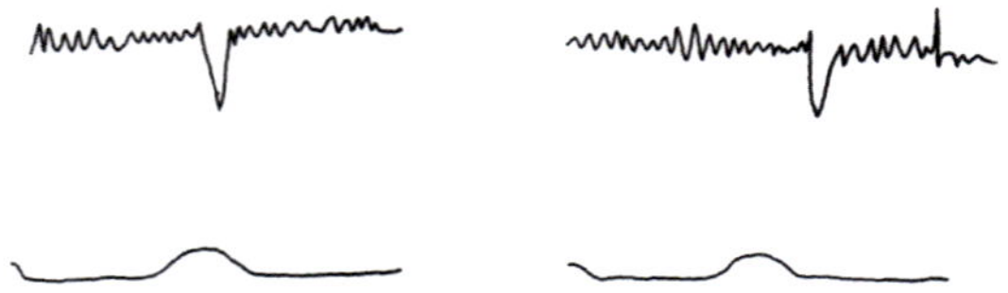

FIGURE 17.1.7 - Contraction Stress Test: Early Deceleration (Left) and Late Deceleration (Right)

IV. Prenatal Fetal Assessment: Doppler Sonography of the Umbilical Artery
   A. Evaluation of umbilical artery blood flow
   B. Normal result: forward end-diastolic blood flow
   C. Abnormal result: decreased, absent, or reversed end-diastolic blood flow
   D. Imminent fetal demise

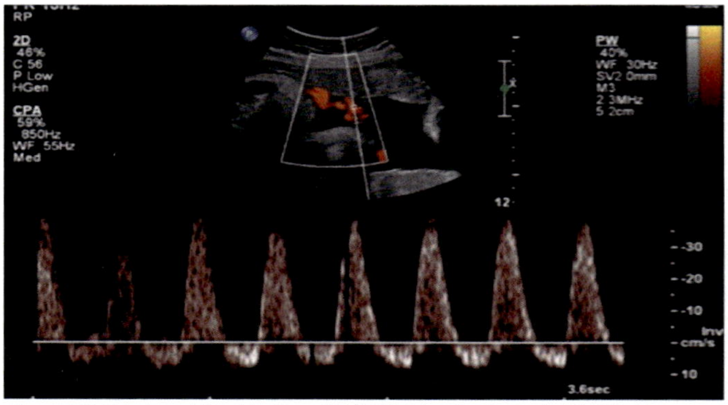

FIGURE 17.1.8 - Umbilical Artery Doppler Ultrasonography: Reversed End-Diastolic Blood Flow

V. Prenatal Fetal Assessment: Percutaneous Umbilical Cord Blood Sampling (PUBS)
   A. Evaluates umbilical venous blood
   B. Can detect low fetal hemoglobin, increased bilirubin
   C. Used to diagnose erythroblastosis fetalis if high index of suspicion
   D. Can be used to transfuse blood to anemic fetus

VI. Prenatal Fetal Assessment: Fetal Lung Maturity Testing
   A. Lecithin : sphingomyelin ratio
      1. 2 - 3 = mature lungs
      2. 1 - 2 = transitional maturity
      3. < 1 = immature lungs (high risk for NRDS)
   B. Surfactant: albumin ratio
   C. Foam stability index

REVIEW QUESTIONS

1. A 26-year-old woman comes to her OBGYN at 30 weeks gestation for a routine prenatal exam. The nonstress test is reactive. Ultrasound shows the deepest amniotic fluid pocket at 4 cm; there are 4 fetal movements and 2 fetal breaths, each lasting 40 seconds. There is no spinal or extremity extension. What is this patient's biophysical profile score?

   - **This patient's biophysical profile score is eight.**
   - A nonstress test is reactive, which is worth 2 points.
   - The deepest amniotic fluid pocket of 4 cm is also worth 2 points.
   - Four fetal movements get 2 points.
   - Two fetal breaths, each lasting 40 seconds, get 2 points.
   - No spinal or extremity extension is worth 0 points.
   - Therefore, this patient's BPP score is 8, which is normal.

Obstetrics | Section 4: Ectopic Pregnancy

I. Ectopic Pregnancy: Introduction
   A. Fertilized egg implants outside uterine cavity
   B. Fertilization takes place in the ampulla
   C. Sites
      1. Fallopian tube: ampulla (most common), isthmus, fimbriae
      2. Others: ovary, cervix, previous cesarean scar

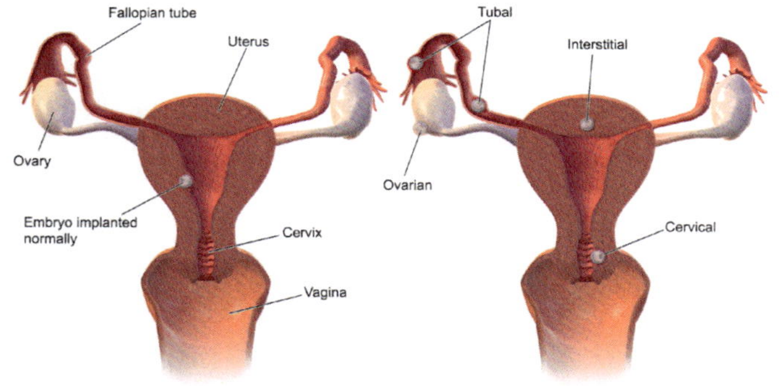

FIGURE 17.1.9 - Normal Pregnancy vs. Ectopic Pregnancy

II. Ectopic Pregnancy: Risk Factors
   A. Previous ectopic pregnancy
   B. Prior tubal surgery
   C. Pelvic inflammatory disease
   D. Endometriosis
   E. Contraceptives: intrauterine devices, oral contraceptive pills
   F. Smoking

III. Ectopic Pregnancy: Clinical Presentation
   A. Usually after 6 to 8 weeks
   B. Lower abdominal pain and tenderness
   C. Vaginal bleeding
   D. Pelvic exam: cervical motion tenderness, closed cervical ostium
   E. Ruptured tubal ectopic pregnancy
      1. Hemorrhagic shock: hypotension, tachycardia, unresponsiveness
      2. Signs of peritonitis: rebound tenderness, guarding

IV. Ectopic Pregnancy: Diagnosis
   A. History and clinical examination
   B. Complete blood count: decreased hemoglobin levels
   C. Transvaginal ultrasound (TVUS)
      1. Gestational sac outside uterine cavity
      2. Tubal pregnancy: blob sign
   D. Exploratory laparoscopy

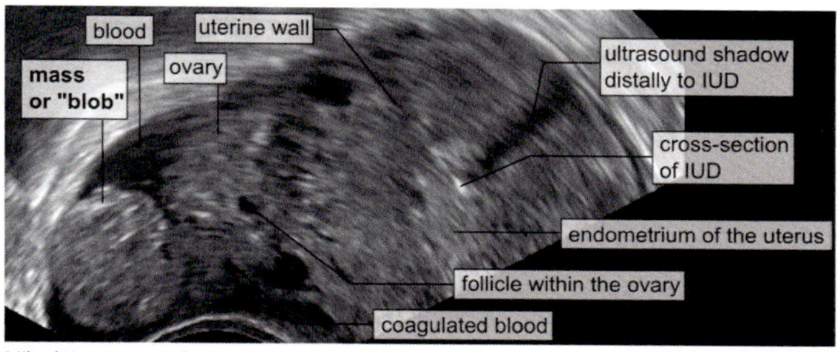

FIGURE 17.1.10 - Transvaginal Ultrasound: "Blob" Sign in Tubal Ectopic Pregnancy

V. Ectopic Pregnancy: Management
   A. Unruptured ectopic pregnancy
      1. Medical: methotrexate
      2. Surgical: laparoscopic (salpingostomy, salpingectomy)
   B. Ruptured ectopic pregnancy
      1. Resuscitation: IV fluids, blood transfusion
      2. Exploratory laparotomy
   C. In Rh-ve women: anti-D immune globulin (to prevent alloimmunization)

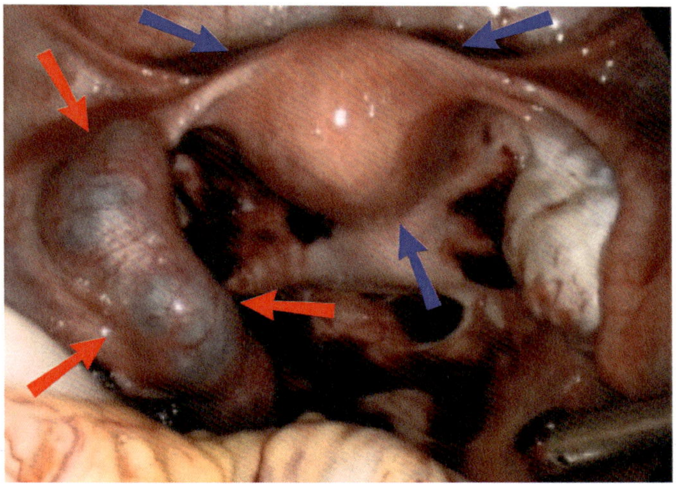

FIGURE 17.1.11 - Laparoscopy: Tubal Ectopic Pregnancy and Hematosalpinx

REVIEW QUESTIONS

1. A 28-year-old G1P0 woman comes to the emergency department because of severe lower abdominal pain for the past 3 hours. She is at 5 weeks gestation. She prefers to lie still on the stretcher because even a slight movement exacerbates her pain. She has a history of pelvic inflammatory disease. She is Rh negative, while her husband is Rh positive. Transabdominal ultrasound shows an enlarged right fallopian tube and blood in the pouch of Douglas. She undergoes exploratory laparotomy for presumed ruptured ectopic pregnancy. What additional intervention should be performed?
   - **The intervention that should be performed is the administration of anti-D immune globulin.**
   - This woman, at 5 weeks of gestation, has severe lower abdominal pain, with US findings showing an enlarged right fallopian tube as well as blood in the pouch of Douglas.
   - This is very concerning for a ruptured ectopic pregnancy.
   - Ruptured ectopic pregnancies increase the risk of fetomaternal blood mixing.
   - Since she is Rh negative and her husband is Rh positive, she needs to receive anti-D immune globulin to prevent alloimmunization against fetal Rh antigen.

Obstetrics | Section 5: Spontaneous Abortion and Fetal Demise

I. Spontaneous Abortion: Introduction
   A. Spontaneous loss of pregnancy up to 20 weeks of gestation
   B. Abortus refers to an embryo or a fetus expelled from the uterus before 20 weeks of gestation or weighs less than 500 g

II. Spontaneous Abortion: Risk Factors
   A. Chromosomal abnormalities (most common during first trimester)
   B. Uterine abnormalities (e.g. septate uterus, adhesions, fibroids)
   C. Maternal diseases (e.g. diabetes mellitus, thyroid disease, antiphospholipid syndrome)
   D. Previous pregnancy loss
   E. Trauma (e.g. chorionic villus sampling, amniocentesis)

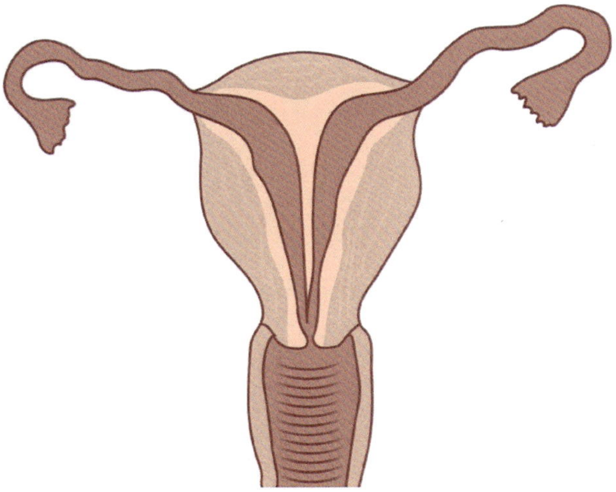

FIGURE 17.1.12 - Septate Uterus

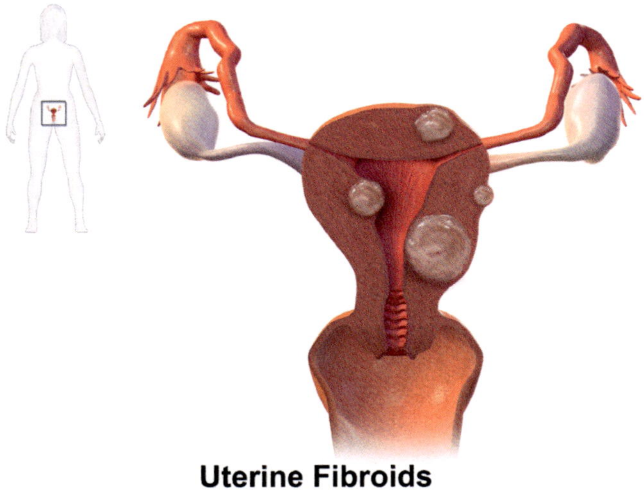

FIGURE 17.1.13 - Uterine Fibroids

III. Spontaneous Abortion: Types
   A. Complete abortion
      1. Complete expulsion of products of conception (POC)
      2. Features: vaginal bleeding, passage of clots or fleshy mass, pain subsides after passage of POC
      3. Pelvic exam: closed cervical os
   B. Incomplete abortion
      1. Partial expulsion of products of conception (POC)
      2. Features: vaginal bleeding, abdominal pain, passage of clots/POC
      3. Pelvic exam: open cervical os, POC may protrude through os
   C. Threatened abortion
      1. Process of abortion has started but is reversible
      2. May proceed to inevitable abortion
      3. Features: vaginal bleeding, mild abdominal pain, fetal cardiac activity is present
      4. Pelvic exam: closed cervical os, no POC
   D. Inevitable abortion
      1. Inevitable abortion
      2. Process of expulsion is unavoidable
      3. Features: vaginal bleeding, abdominal pain
      4. Pelvic exam: open cervical os, POC lies at cervical canal or lower uterine segment
   E. Missed abortion
      1. Non-viable embryo or fetus retained inside the uterus
      2. Features: asymptomatic, absent fetal cardiac activity
      3. Pelvic exam: closed cervical os
   F. Septic abortion
      1. Infection of the retained products of conception
      2. Commonly after unsafe abortions, missed/incomplete abortion
      3. Features: vaginal bleeding, abdominal pain, signs of sepsis (fever, chills, hypotension, tachycardia)
      4. Pelvic exam: cervical os close/open, cervical motion tenderness, foul-smelling vaginal discharge/bleeding

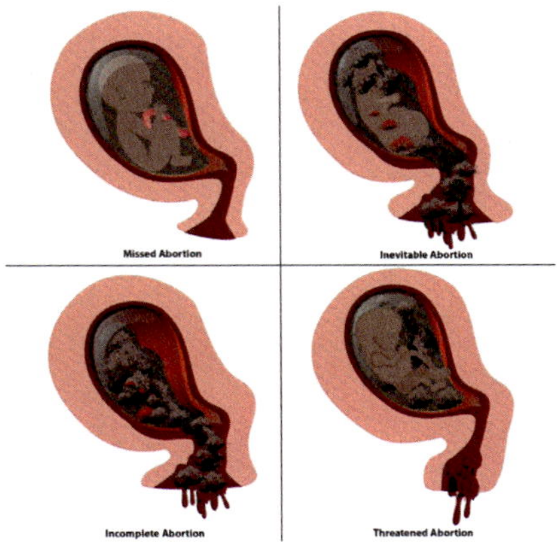

FIGURE 17.1.14 - Types of Abortion

IV. Spontaneous Abortion: Diagnosis
   A. History and clinical findings
   B. Transabdominal/transvaginal ultrasound
      1. Threatened abortion: viable fetus, fetal cardiac activity present
      2. Inevitable abortion: fetal cardiac activity present/absent
      3. Complete abortion: empty uterine cavity
      4. Incomplete/missed/septic abortions: presence of retained products of conception, fetal cardiac activity absent
   C. Laboratory findings
      1. Serial serum β-hCG: decreasing pattern
      2. CBC: ↓ hemoglobin, increased WBC count (septic abortion)
      3. Blood cultures (signs of sepsis)

V. Spontaneous Abortion: Management
   A. General management
      1. Patient stabilization (IV fluids)
      2. Blood transfusion (hemoglobin < 8 mg/dL)
      3. In Rh negative women: anti-D immune globulin (to prevent alloimmunization)
   B. Threatened abortion
      1. Adequate rest
      2. Routine ultrasonography to assess fetal viability
      3. May progress to inevitable/incomplete/complete abortion
   C. Incomplete/inevitable/missed abortion
      1. Stable patients: expectant management
      2. Unstable patients: emergency surgical intervention
      3. Surgical: manual uterine aspiration, dilation and curettage (D&C) for first trimester, dilation and evacuation (D&E) for second trimester
      4. Medications: misoprostol, mifepristone
   D. Complete abortion
      1. Observation for bleeding
   E. Septic abortion
      1. Broad-spectrum antibiotics
      2. Surgical: manual uterine aspiration, dilation and curettage (D&C)

VI. Spontaneous Abortion: Complications
   A. Disseminated intravascular coagulation (DIC)
      1. Characterized by intravascular activation of coagulation
      2. Consumption of clotting factors and platelets → intravascular thrombosis and bleeding
   B. Uterine adhesions (Asherman's syndrome)
   C. Uterine perforation, bleeding, infection

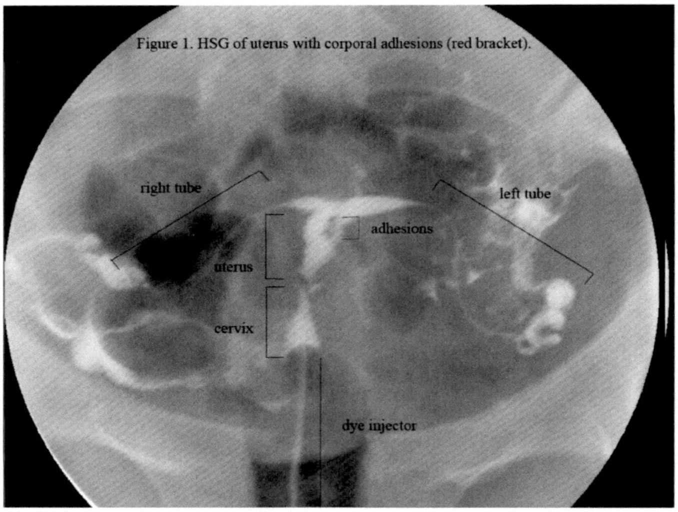

FIGURE 17.1.15 - Hysterosalpingography: Intrauterine Adhesions in Asherman's Syndrome

VII. Fetal Demise
   A. Fetal death at ≥ 20 weeks
   B. Absent cardiac activity on ultrasound
   C. Management
      1. 20 - 23 weeks: dilation and evacuation or vaginal delivery
      2. ≥ 24 weeks: vaginal delivery
   D. Complication
      1. Maternal coagulopathy in case of prolonged retention

REVIEW QUESTIONS

1. A 37-year-old G4P3 woman comes to her OBGYN at 35 weeks gestation because of decreased fetal movements for the past day. All of her previous pregnancies were uncomplicated. Ultrasound shows absent fetal cardiac activity. A cervical exam shows a closed cervical os. What is the best next step in the management?

   - **The best next step in the management is vaginal delivery within the next several days.**
   - This woman, at 35 weeks gestation, has decreased fetal movements and the US showing absent fetal cardiac activity consistent with fetal demise.
   - The management of fetal demise depends on the gestational age of the patient.
   - If stillbirth occurs from 20 to 23 weeks of gestation, the woman can undergo either dilation and evacuation or vaginal delivery.
   - In contrast, if stillbirth occurs at ≥ 24 weeks of gestation, the woman has to undergo vaginal delivery within the next several days. Prolonged retention of the fetus in the uterus can cause coagulopathy, such as disseminated intravascular coagulation.

2. A 22-year-old G1P0 woman comes to her OBGYN at 15 weeks gestation due to vaginal bleeding and pelvic cramps. She started having symptoms five hours ago. She smokes one pack of cigarettes per day. Vital signs include temperature of 98.6° F (37° C), blood pressure of 118/80 mmHg, heart rate of 94 beats/min, and respiratory rate of 16 breaths/min. Physical examination shows an open cervical os with products of conception palpable at the external os. Transabdominal ultrasound shows retained products of conception and absent fetal cardiac activity. Which of the following is the most likely diagnosis in this patient?

   A. Threatened abortion
   B. Inevitable abortion
   C. Incomplete abortion
   D. Complete abortion

   - **The correct answer is option B.**
   - This patient presents with vaginal bleeding and pelvic cramps.
   - Physical examination shows an open cervical os with products of conception palpable at the external os.
   - Transabdominal ultrasound reveals retained products of conception and absent fetal cardiac activity.
   - All of these findings are consistent with inevitable abortion.
   - Option A is incorrect because threatened abortion is characterized by vaginal bleeding, closed cervical os, and the presence of fetal cardiac activity on transabdominal ultrasound. This patient, on the other hand, has an open cervical os and absent fetal cardiac activity.
   - Option C is incorrect because incomplete abortion is characterized by vaginal bleeding, open cervical os, and incomplete expulsion of products of conception. This patient's products of conception are still palpable at the external os.
   - Option D is incorrect because complete abortion is associated with a closed cervical os and complete expulsion of products of conception.

Obstetrics | Section 6: Cervical Insufficiency

I. Cervical Insufficiency: Introduction
   A. Painless dilation of cervix during second trimester of pregnancy
   B. Absent uterine contractions
   C. Bulging of fetal membranes through open cervix
   D. Risk of preterm delivery

II. Cervical Insufficiency: Risk Factors
   A. Surgical procedures (e.g. cervical biopsy, dilation and curettage)
   B. Trauma: cervical lacerations during previous pregnancy
   C. Exposure to diethylstilbestrol in utero

III. Cervical Insufficiency: Clinical Presentation
   A. Mostly asymptomatic
   B. Mild pelvic and back pain
   C. Vaginal discharge
   D. History of prior pregnancy loss
   E. Preterm birth

IV. Cervical Insufficiency: Diagnosis
   A. Clinical diagnosis
   B. History of ≥ 2 prior mid-trimester pregnancy loss before 24 WOG
   C. Transvaginal ultrasound: cervical length < 25 mm

V. Cervical Insufficiency: Management
   A. Cervical cerclage
      1. Procedure that uses sutures for cervical reinforcement during pregnancy
      2. At cervical-vaginal junction or the level of internal os
      3. At 12 to 14 weeks of gestation

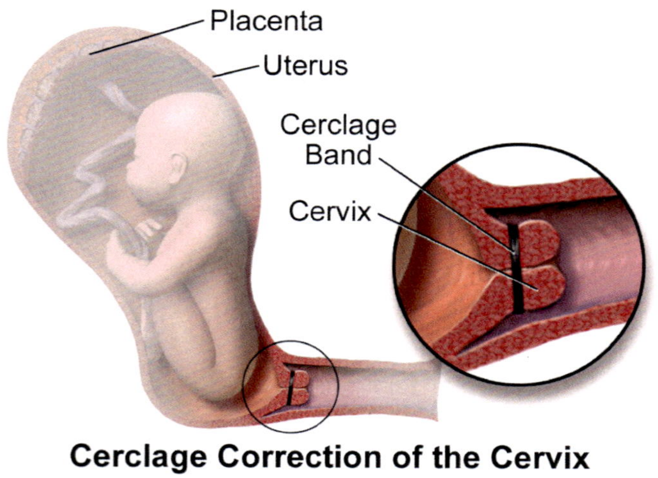

FIGURE 17.1.16 - Cervical Cerclage

REVIEW QUESTIONS

1. A 33-year-old G3P0 woman at 13 weeks gestation comes to her OBGYN for a routine prenatal visit. She has a history of spontaneous abortion in her first two pregnancies at 14 and 16 weeks. Her vital signs are unremarkable. Physical examination shows a dilated cervix. What is the best next step in the management?

   - **The best next step in management is cervical cerclage placement.**
   - This woman at 13 weeks gestation, presents for a routine prenatal visit.
   - She had two prior spontaneous abortions.
   - Physical examination shows a dilated cervix concerning for cervical insufficiency.
   - The next best step in the management of cervical insufficiency is cervical cerclage placement, which stabilizes the cervix with sutures.

Obstetrics | Section 7: Recurrent Pregnancy Loss

I. Recurrent Pregnancy Loss: Introduction
   A. Three or more consecutive loss of pregnancies before 20 weeks of gestation

II. Recurrent Pregnancy Loss: Risk Factors
   A. History of prior pregnancy loss
   B. Uterine defects: septate uterus, uterine fibroids, polyps, adhesions
   C. Cervical insufficiency
   D. Endocrine disorders: thyroid disorders, hyperprolactinemia (decrease GnRH), luteal phase defect (inadequate progesterone)
   E. Antiphospholipid syndrome: autoimmune disorder characterized by thrombotic events and recurrent pregnancy loss

III. Recurrent Pregnancy Loss: Diagnosis
   A. History
   B. Karyotyping: chromosomal abnormalities
   C. Hysterosalpingography
      1. To evaluate uterine and tubal anomalies
   D. Hysteroscopy and laparoscopic evaluation
   E. Ultrasound
      1. To differentiate between septate and bicornuate uterus
   F. Laboratory
      1. Antiphospholipid antibodies (anticardiolipin, lupus anticoagulant)
      2. Thyroid function test, blood sugar levels

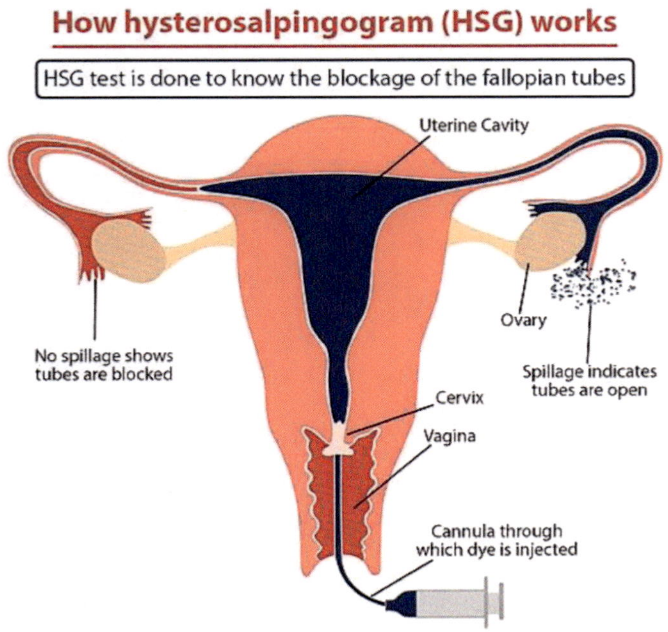

FIGURE 17.1.17 - Hysterosalpingogram

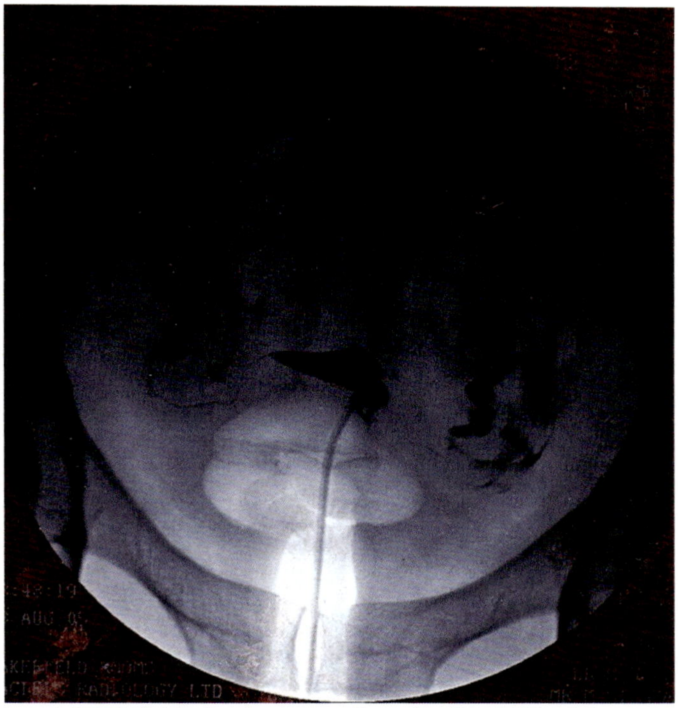

FIGURE 17.1.18 - Hysterosalpingography

IV. Recurrent Pregnancy Loss: Management
   A. Depends on the underlying pathology
   B. Parental karyotype abnormality: IVF using donor sperm or egg
   C. Medical treatment
      1. Luteal phase defect: progesterone
      2. Antiphospholipid syndrome: low molecular weight heparin (LMWH), low dose aspirin; avoid warfarin during pregnancy due to teratogenic effects
   D. Surgical treatment
      1. Uterine anomalies: surgical repair of bicornuate uterus, septate uterus
      2. Cervical insufficiency: cervical cerclage
   E. Others: treat diabetes mellitus, thyroid disorders

REVIEW QUESTIONS

1. A 25-year-old woman comes to her primary care physician for a follow-up visit after having a spontaneous abortion 2 weeks ago. She has had 3 pregnancy losses, all before 20 weeks of gestation. Abnormalities of her reproductive tract, thyroid disorders, and hyperprolactinemia are all excluded. She has a history of two episodes of deep vein thrombosis. She has never taken oral contraceptive pills. Laboratory findings are significant for a partial thromboplastin time of 50 seconds (25 - 40 seconds). The presence of which antibody best explains this patient's recurrent pregnancy loss?

   - **The presence of lupus anticoagulant best explains this patient's recurrent pregnancy loss.**
   - This patient has recurrent pregnancy loss and two occurrences of deep vein thrombosis with no history of taking oral contraceptive pills.
   - Her partial thromboplastin time is elevated.
   - All of these findings point towards the diagnosis of antiphospholipid syndrome.
   - Falsely elevated partial thromboplastin time (PTT) is explained by the presence of lupus anticoagulant in this patient.
   - Lupus anticoagulant impairs fixation of the clotting factors in the test tube and results in high PTT.
   - It is an antibody against phospholipids on the cell membranes, so it can damage endothelium predisposing to thrombus formation.
   - Hence, even though antiphospholipid syndrome is characterized by a prolonged partial thromboplastin time, it actually induces a hypercoagulable state, which can lead to recurrent pregnancy loss.

Obstetrics | Section 8: Trisomy 21, 18 & 13

I. Down Syndrome (Trisomy 21)
   A. Trisomy 21 (Down syndrome)
   B. Most cases due to meiotic nondisjunction
   C. Minority of cases due to Robertsonian translocation
   D. Most common cause of genetic intellectual disability
   E. Risk factors
      1. Advanced maternal age > 35 years
      2. Carrier of Robertsonian translocation
   F. Signs and symptoms
      1. Intellectual disability
      2. Flat facies
      3. Prominent epicanthal folds
      4. Single transverse palmar crease
      5. Curved 5th finger (clinodactyly) and "sandal toe"
      6. Brushfield spots (white spots on iris)
   G. Complications
      1. Duodenal atresia ("double bubble")
      2. Hirschsprung disease (aganglionic segment, proximal dilation)
      3. AV septal defects (most common congenital cardiac defect in Down syndrome patients)
      4. Acute myelogenous or acute lymphoblastic leukemia
      5. Early onset Alzheimer disease

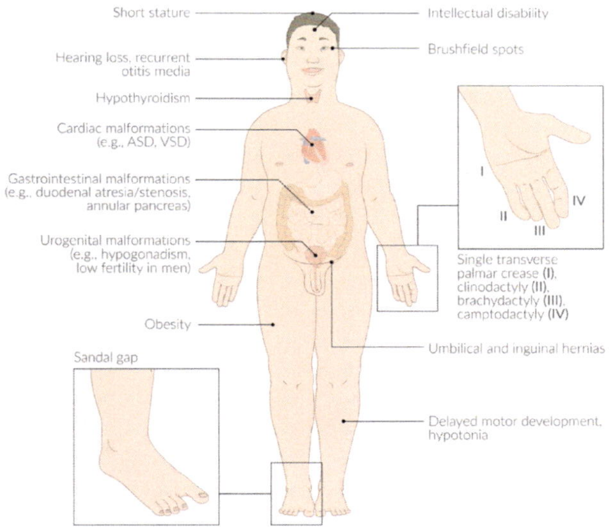

FIGURE 17.1.19 - Down Syndrome

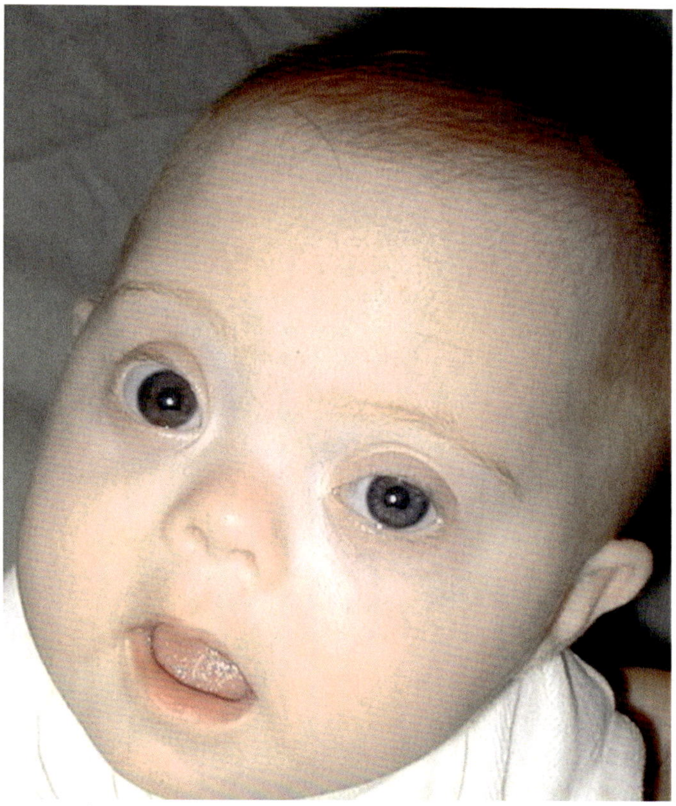

FIGURE 17.1.20 - Brushfield Spots

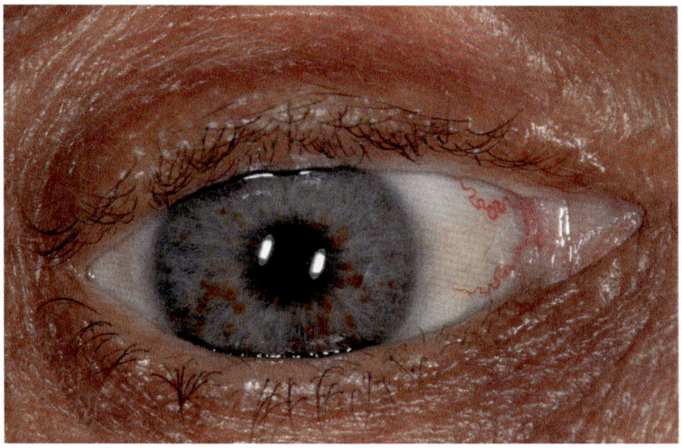

FIGURE 17.1.21 - Lisch Nodules

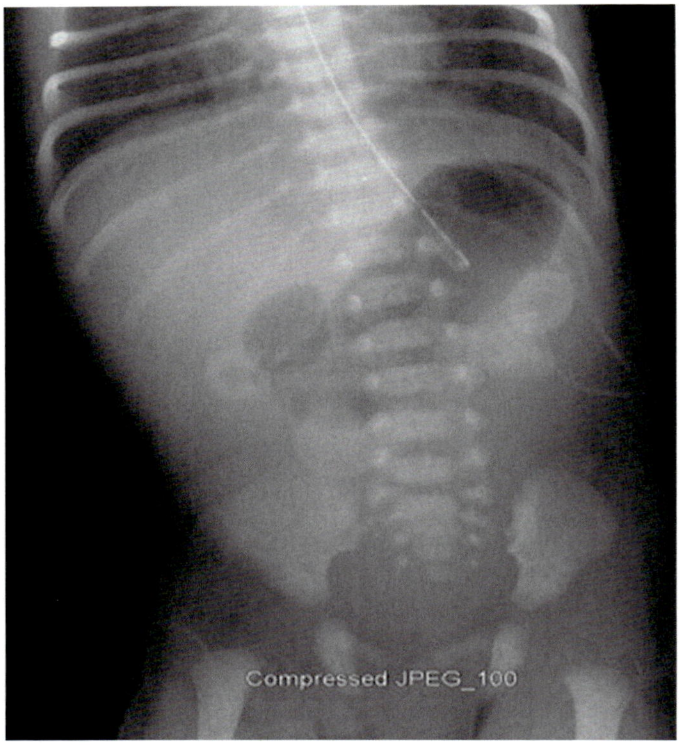

FIGURE 17.1.22 - Abdominal X-ray: "Double-Bubble" Sign in Duodenal Atresia

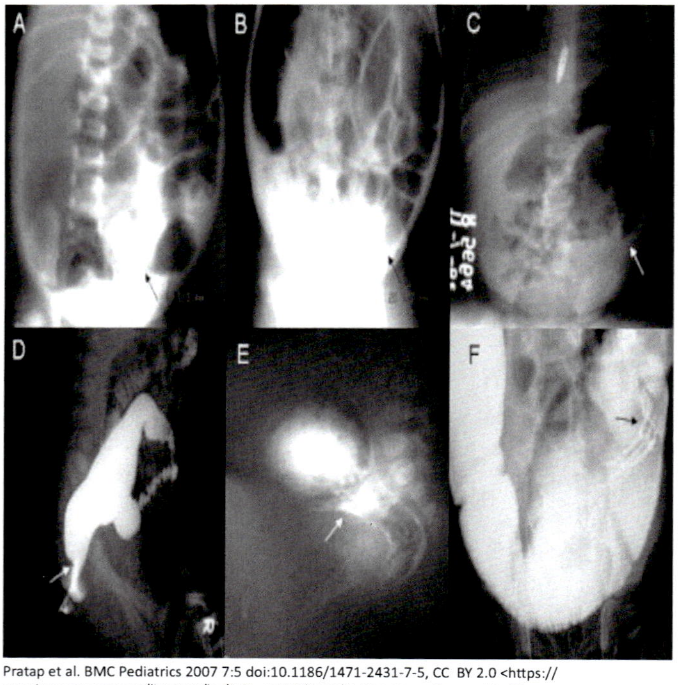

FIGURE 17.1.23 - Abdominal X-ray: Transitional Zone in Hirschsprung Disease

II. Edwards Syndrome (Trisomy 18)
    A. Trisomy 18 (Edwards syndrome)
    B. Most cases due to meiotic nondisjunction
    C. 2nd most common autosomal trisomy resulting in live birth
    D. Risk factors
        1. Advanced maternal age > 35 years
    E. Signs and symptoms
        1. Intellectual disability
        2. Prominent occiput
        3. Clenched fists with overlapping fingers
        4. Rocker-bottom feet
        5. Small jaw (micrognathia)
        6. Low-set ears
    F. Complications
        1. Congenital heart disease (ASD, VSD)
        2. Omphalocele
        3. Myelomeningocele
        4. Death usually by 1 year

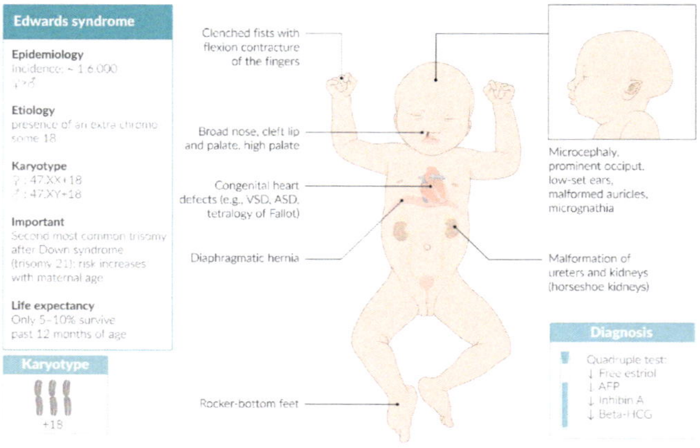

FIGURE 17.1.24 - Edward's Syndrome

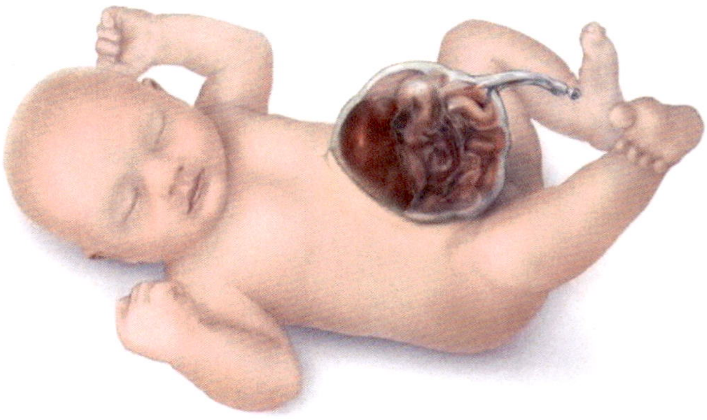

FIGURE 17.1.25 - Omphalocele

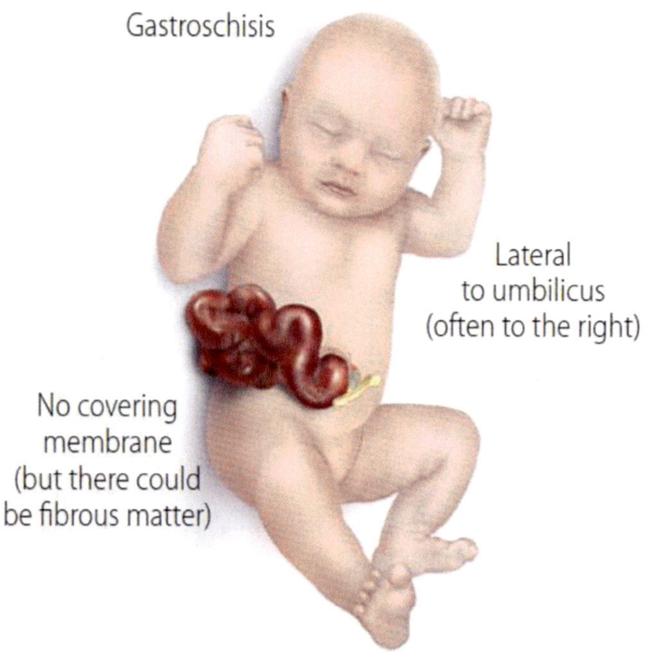

ATTRIBUTION

FIGURE 17.1.26 - Gastroschisis

III. Patau Syndrome (Trisomy 13)
   A. Trisomy 13 (Patau syndrome)
   B. Most cases due to meiotic nondisjunction
   C. 3rd most common autosomal trisomy resulting in live birth
   D. Risk factors
      1. Advanced maternal age > 35 years
   E. Signs and symptoms
      1. Midline defects (e.g. hypotelorism) due to failure of fusion of prechordal mesoderm
      2. Severe intellectual disability
      3. Microphthalmia
      4. Microcephaly
      5. Cleft lip/palate, cutis aplasia, and polydactyly
   F. Complications
      1. Congenital heart disease (ASD, VSD)
      2. Holoprosencephaly
      3. Polycystic kidney disease
      4. Death usually before 1 year

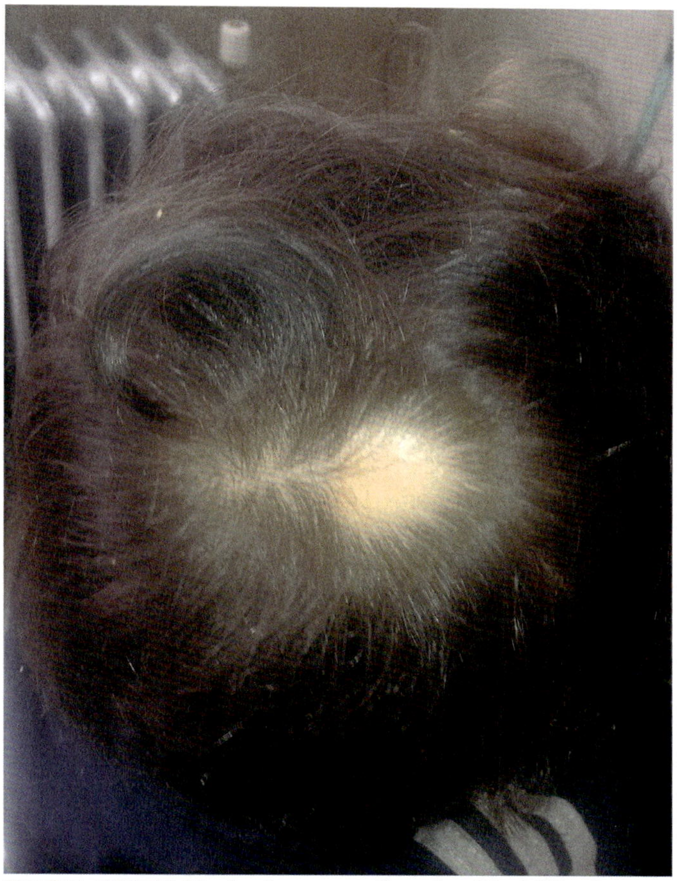

FIGURE 17.1.27 - Cutis Aplasia

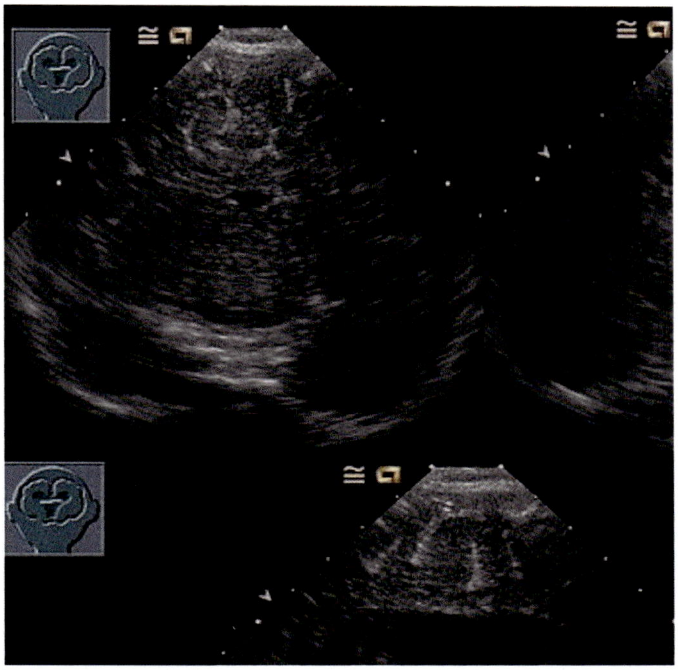

FIGURE 17.1.28 - Ultrasonography: Holoprosencephaly

REVIEW QUESTIONS

1. A 38-year-old man is brought to his primary care physician by his parents because of memory changes. Family members first noticed these changes 4 years ago. He commonly forgets his parents' names and has been lost in his neighborhood several times during the past year. He was diagnosed with Down syndrome as a child. What is the best explanation for his early-onset memory changes?

   - **The best explanation for this patient's early-onset memory changes is faster accumulation of beta-amyloid.**
   - This patient with Down syndrome has had memory changes for the last 4 years.
   - He commonly forgets his parents' names and has been lost several times in his neighborhood.
   - This presentation is consistent with early-onset Alzheimer's disease.
   - The reason why Down syndrome patients usually have early-onset Alzheimer's disease is that the gene for amyloid precursor protein is located on chromosome 21. They have an extra copy of chromosome 21, so amyloid beta accumulates in the brain faster.

2. A 2-month-old boy is brought to his primary care physician by his parents for a well-child visit. He was born at 38 weeks gestation via vaginal delivery to a 39-year-old woman. Physical examination shows closed fists with index and little fingers overlapping the other fingers, a large occipital protuberance, bilateral convexity of the feet, and a small jaw. What is the most likely genetic mechanism of this patient's condition?

   - **The most likely genetic mechanism of this patient's condition is meiotic nondisjunction.**
   - This infant has closed fists with overlapping fingers, a large occipital protuberance, bilateral convexity of the feet, and a small jaw.
   - His mother has an advanced age of > 35 years.
   - All these clues are consistent with the diagnosis of Edwards syndrome.
   - Edwards syndrome, just like any other trisomies, is most commonly caused by meiotic nondisjunction.

Obstetrics | Section 9: Sex Chromosome Abnormalities

I. Klinefelter Syndrome
   A. 47, XXY (Klinefelter syndrome)
   B. Tall stature
   C. Testicular atrophy
   D. Gynecomastia and increased risk for breast cancer
   E. Female pattern hair distribution
   F. Learning disabilities
   G. Presence of one inactivated X chromosome (Barr body)
   H. Laboratory findings
      1. Primary (hypergonadotropic) hypogonadism
      2. Low testosterone
      3. Low inhibin B
      4. High estrogen
      5. High LH and FSH

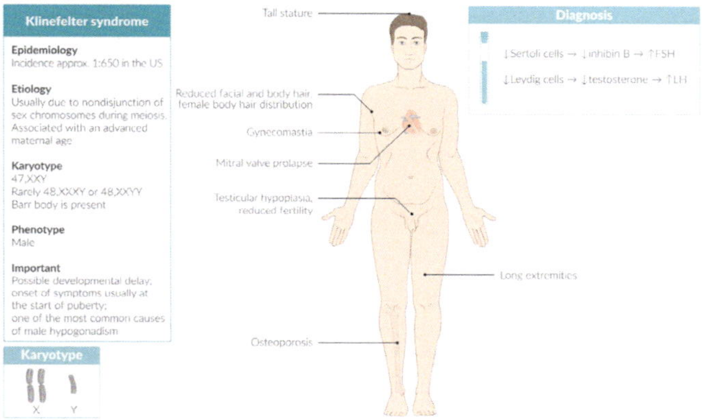

FIGURE 17.1.29 - Klinefelter Syndrome

II. Turner Syndrome
   A. 45, XO (Turner syndrome)
   B. Short stature
   C. Amenorrhea
   D. Shield chest with widely spaced nipples
   E. Bicuspid aortic valve
   F. Aortic coarctation
   G. Lymphatic defects (cystic hygroma, webbed neck)
   H. Laboratory findings:
      1. Primary (hypergonadotropic) hypogonadism
      2. Low estrogen (streak ovaries), high LH and FSH
   I. Treatment:
      1. Growth hormone injections for height
      2. Estrogen and progesterone therapy for puberty
      3. Pregnancy possible via ART (e.g. in vitro fertilization)

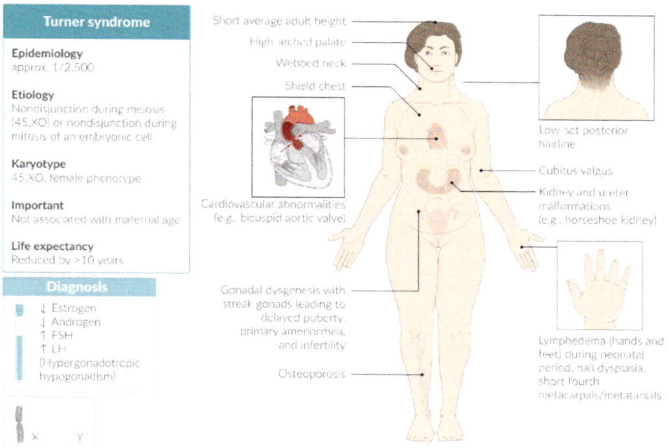

FIGURE 17.1.30 - Turner Syndrome

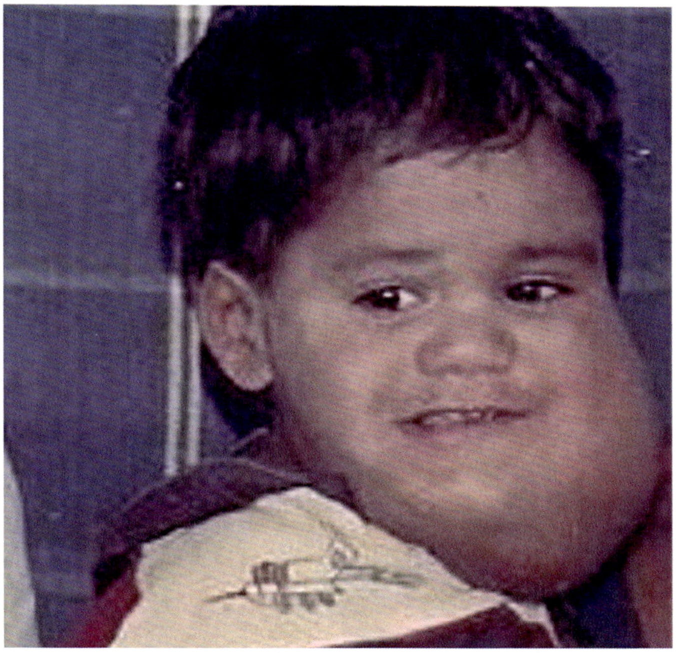

FIGURE 17.1.31 - Cystic Hygroma

III. Double Y Males
   A. 47, XYY (double Y males)
   B. Usually undiagnosed
   C. Tall stature
   D. Severe acne
   E. Learning disabilities
   F. Autism spectrum disorders
   G. Normal fertility

IV. Ovotesticular Disorder of Sex Development
   A. Ovotesticular disorder of sex development
   B. 46, XX > 46, XY
   C. Ovarian and testicular tissue present
   D. Ambiguous genitalia
   E. Previously known as true hermaphroditism

REVIEW QUESTIONS

1. A 15-year-old boy is brought by his parents to his primary care physician because of difficulties at school. He has trouble learning new material in all subjects, which makes him anxious. Physical examination shows a height of 78 in, decreased facial and body hair, and a large pelvis. Genitourinary examination shows testicular atrophy. What is the genetic mechanism accounting for his height?

    - **The genetic mechanism accounting for this patient's height is an extra X chromosome.**
    - This patient has learning difficulties, tall stature, testicular atrophy, decreased facial and body hair, and a large pelvis, characteristic of Klinefelter syndrome.
    - Klinefelter syndrome patients are very tall because they have an extra X chromosome containing *SHOX* genes.
    - *SHOX* genes and several other genes are responsible for an individual's height.

Obstetrics | Section 10: Prenatal Screening for Chromosomal Abnormalities

I. 1st Trimester Aneuploidy Screening
   A. Performed at 12 to 13 weeks of gestation
   B. Ultrasound for size of nuchal translucency
   C. Laboratory markers
      1. Beta-hCG and PAPP-A
      2. Down syndrome: high beta-hCG and low PAPP-A
      3. Edwards and Patau syndromes: low beta-hCG and PAPP-A

II. 2nd Trimester Aneuploidy Screening
   A. Laboratory markers
      1. Beta-hCG, PAPP-A, estriol, inhibin A
      2. Down syndrome: high beta-hCG and inhibin A, low PAPP-A and estriol
      3. Edwards syndrome: all markers are low except for inhibin A
      4. Patau syndrome: all markers are normal

III. Cell-Free Fetal DNA (cffDNA)
   A. Fetal DNA detectable in maternal circulation
   B. Used to screen for aneuploidy
   C. Not used in obese women
   D. Not used before 10 weeks of gestation

IV. Chorionic Villus Sampling (CVS)
   A. Performed at 10 to 13 weeks of gestation
   B. Obtains sample of placental tissue
   C. Used to diagnose aneuploidy and screen for cystic fibrosis, sickle cell anemia, Tay-Sachs disease, thalassemia
   D. Transabdominal or transcervical approach
   E. Might cause maternal bleeding or fetal loss

V. Amniocentesis
   A. Performed at 15 to 20 weeks of gestation
   B. Obtains sample of amniotic fluid
   C. Used to diagnose aneuploidy and screen for cystic fibrosis, sickle cell anemia, Tay-Sachs disease, thalassemia
   D. Transabdominal approach
   E. Might cause maternal bleeding or fetal loss

VI. Percutaneous Umbilical Cord Blood Sampling (PUBS)
   A. Performed when high suspicion for fetal anemia
   B. Used mostly in Rh hemolytic disease of the newborn
   C. Blood taken from umbilical vein
   D. Checks fetal hemoglobin and serum bilirubin
   E. Can be used to transfuse blood to anemic fetus

VII. Fetal Ultrasound
   A. Performed periodically throughout the pregnancy
   B. Used to check for:
      1. Fetal anatomy
      2. Pathologies like right to left or left to right cardiac shunts
      3. Fetal growth
      4. Measured parameters: gestational sac diameter, crown-rump length (CRL), biparietal diameter (BPD), head circumference (HC)

REVIEW QUESTIONS

1. A 37-year-old G2P1 woman comes to her primary care physician at 11 weeks gestation for a routine prenatal visit. She has no specific complaints. Vital signs include temperature of 96.8° F (36° C), blood pressure of 125/70 mmHg, heart rate of 95 beats/min, and respiratory rate of 15 breaths/min. Physical examination is significant for a BMI of 31 kg/m2. Laboratory studies show high levels of beta-hCG and low levels of pregnancy-associated plasma protein A (PAPP-A). She is counseled about the increased risk for fetal aneuploidy, and she is willing to undergo more tests. Which of the following is the best next step in the management?

   A. Quadruple screen
   B. Cell-free fetal DNA
   C. Chorionic villus sampling
   D. Amniocentesis

- **The correct answer is option C.**
- This woman at 11 weeks of gestation presents for a routine prenatal visit.
- She has advanced maternal age, and laboratory studies show elevated beta-hCG and low PAPP-A, consistent with a pattern associated with Down syndrome
- However, beta-hCG and PAPP-A are just screening markers, and they do not confirm any aneuploidy.
- The test that is used to diagnose fetal aneuploidy syndrome from 10 to 13 weeks gestation is the chorionic villus sampling.
- Option A is incorrect because the quadruple screen is a 2nd-trimester screening test. This patient is still in her 1st trimester and needs a confirmatory, rather than a screening, test.
- Option B is incorrect because cell-free fetal DNA is another screening test rather than a confirmatory one. Also, this patient is obese, and cell-free fetal DNA has a low diagnostic yield in obese women.
- Option D is incorrect because amniocentesis is a confirmatory test for fetal aneuploidy that is performed at 15 to 20 weeks gestation when there is sufficient amniotic fluid in the gestational sac.

Obstetrics | Section 11: Neural Tube Defects, Anencephaly, & Potter Sequence

I. Fetal Congenital Anomalies
   A. Neural tube defects (NTDs)
      1. Rostral or caudal neuropores fail to close by 4th week
      2. Associated with diabetes and folate deficiency
   B. Several subtypes
      1. Spina bifida occulta
      2. Spina bifida cystica (meningocele, myelomeningocele)
      3. Myeloschisis and anencephaly
   C. Spina bifida occulta
      1. Failure of vertebral arch to fuse around spinal cord
      2. At the lower back (L5 - S1 vertebral level)
      3. Skin dimple
      4. Tuft of hair
      5. Normal AFP and AChE
   D. Spina bifida cystica
      1. Failure of vertebral arch to fuse around spinal cord
      2. At the lower back (L5 - S1 vertebral level)
      3. Cyst covered with thin skin at the lower back
      4. Meningocele: cyst containing only meninges
      5. Myelomeningocele: cyst containing cauda equina and meninges
      6. High AFP and normal AChE
   E. Myeloschisis
      1. Also known as rachischisis
      2. Failure of neural tube to close
      3. Skin continuous with neural tissue at the lower back
      4. Dermal and meningeal coverings absent
      5. High AFP and AChE
   F. Anencephaly
      1. Failure of rostral neuropore to close
      2. No forebrain
      3. Open calvarium
      4. "Frog-like" appearance of head
      5. Polyhydramnios due to absent fetal swallowing center
      6. High AFP and AChE
   G. Potter sequence
      1. Oligohydramnios with fetal compression against amnion
      2. Associated with ARPKD, bilateral renal agenesis, posterior urethral valves, placental insufficiency
      3. Limb deformities
      4. Facial defects (flattened nose, retrognathia)
      5. Pulmonary hypoplasia (cause of death)

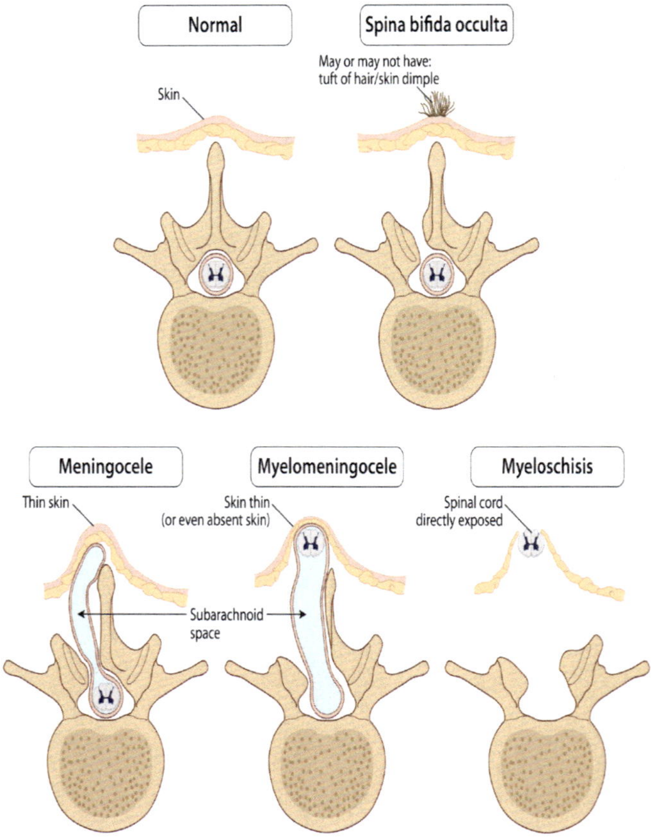

FIGURE 17.1.32 - Spina Bifida Occulta

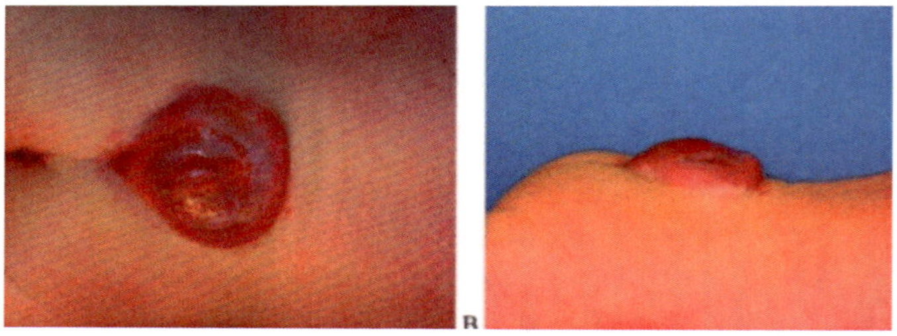

FIGURE 17.1.33 - Spina Bifida Cystica (Myelomeningocele)

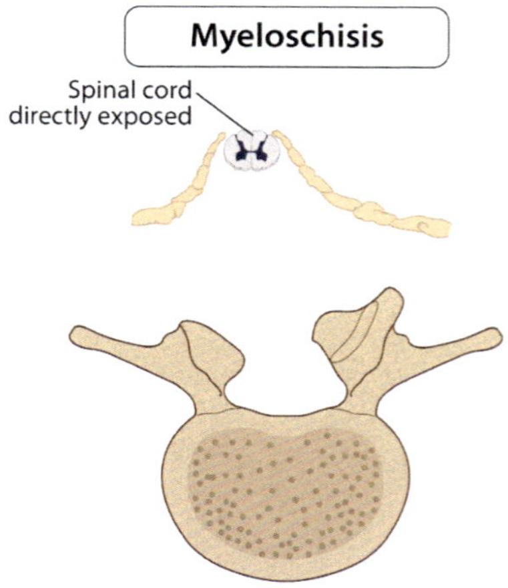

FIGURE 17.1.34 - Myeloschisis

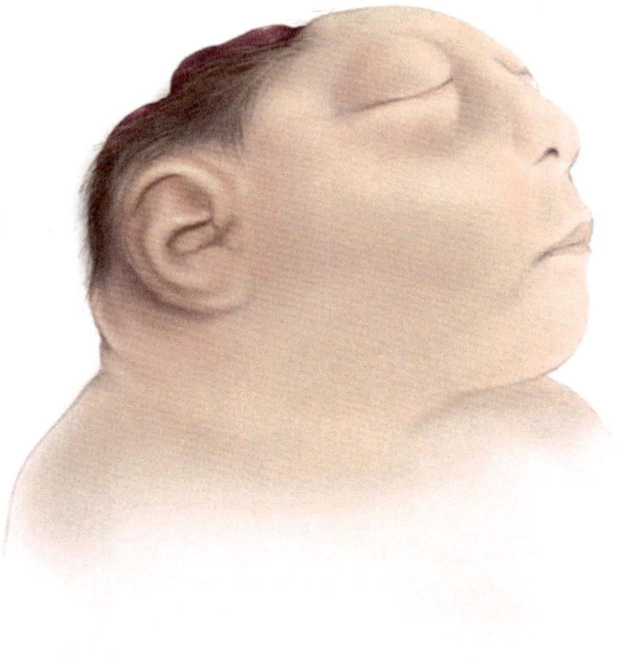

Centers for Disease Control and Prevention, Public domain, via Wikimedia Commons

FIGURE 17.1.35 - Anencephaly

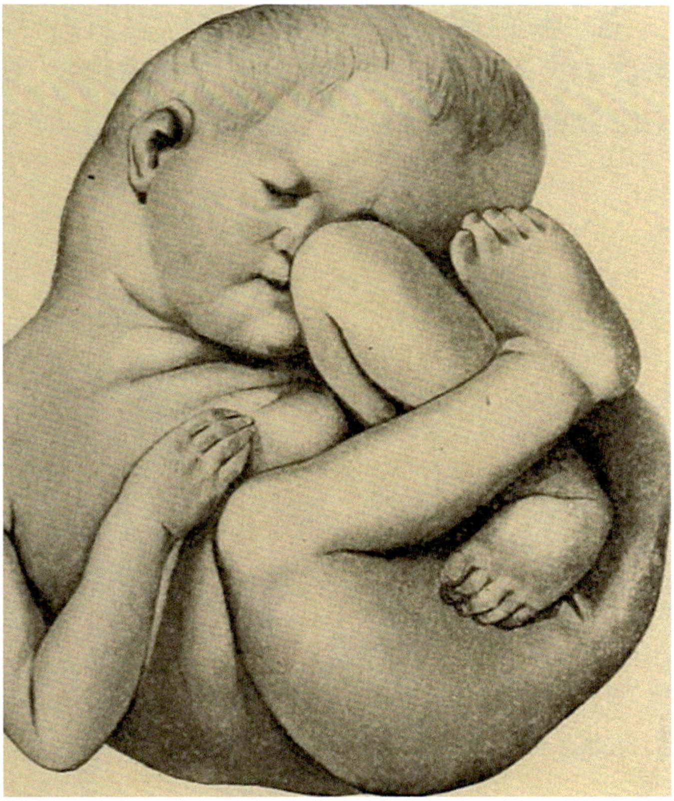

Public Domain

FIGURE 17.1.36 - Potter Sequence

REVIEW QUESTIONS

1. A 28-year-old G1P0 woman comes to her primary care physician at 28 weeks gestation for a routine prenatal exam. Her pregnancy is uncomplicated. She has a history of epilepsy treated with carbamazepine. Transabdominal ultrasound shows a cystic enlargement at the lower back of the fetus. What changes are expected in the levels of AFP and AChE in the amniotic fluid of this patient?

   - **Expected changes in the amniotic fluid of this patient include high AFP and normal AChE.**
   - This woman at 28 weeks gestation comes to the physician for a routine prenatal visit.
   - Transabdominal ultrasound shows a cystic enlargement at the lower back of the fetus concerning for spina bifida
   - Additionally, she has a history of epilepsy treated with carbamazepine which can disrupt folate levels.
   - Spina bifida cystica is characterized by high alpha-fetoprotein (AFP) and the normal acetylcholinesterase (AChE) in the amniotic fluid.

2. A 2-hour-old boy is transferred to the neonatal intensive care unit because of labored breathing. He was born at 39 weeks gestation via vaginal delivery. The mother was told on one of her prenatal visits that both of his kidneys were missing. Physical examination of the newborn shows a flattened nose, retracted jaw, and twisted extremities. Despite resuscitation, the patient dies 3 hours later. What is the most likely cause of his death?

   - **The most likely cause of death is pulmonary hypoplasia.**
   - This newborn presents with a flattened nose, retracted jaw, and twisted extremities and previously noted bilateral renal agenesis.
   - This presentation is classic for Potter sequence, which is caused by oligohydramnios resulting in fetal compression against the amnion.
   - Pulmonary hypoplasia due to oligohydramnios is the most common cause of death in patients with Potter sequence.

Obstetrics | Section 11: Normal Labor and Delivery Part 1

I. Rupture of Membranes
  A. SROM: rupture of membranes after onset of labor
  B. PROM: rupture of membranes before onset of labor
  C. PPROM: preterm rupture of membranes before onset of labor (< 37 weeks of gestation)
  D. AROM: artificial rupture of membranes
  E. "Bloody show": blood-tinged vaginal mucus related to onset of cervical effacement

II. Fetal Lie, Presentation, and Position
  A. Fetal lie
    1. Relationship of fetal longitudinal axis to maternal longitudinal axis
    2. Longitudinal, oblique, and transverse lie
  B. Fetal presentation
    1. Body part of fetus that is deepest in maternal pelvis
    2. Cephalic presentation (most common)
    3. Breech, brow, and face presentations
  C. Fetal position
    1. Position of fetal presenting part relative to maternal pelvis
    2. Occiput anterior: physiologic position with least complications
    3. Cephalic presentation
      a) Occiput anterior; left occiput anterior; right occiput anterior
      b) Occiput posterior; left occiput posterior; right occiput posterior
      c) Left occiput transverse, right occiput transverse

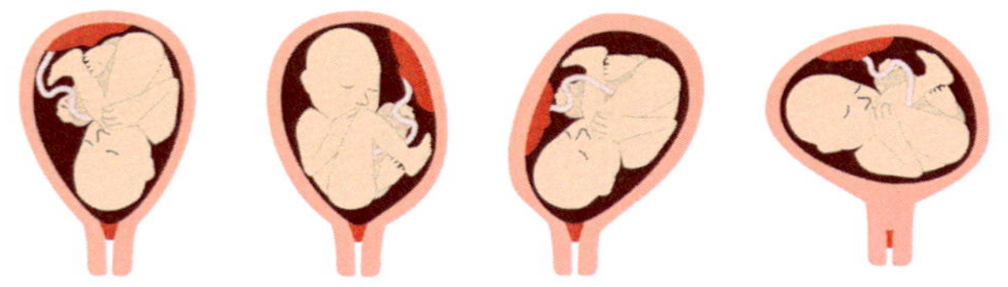

FIGURE 17.1.37 - Longitudinal, Oblique, and Transverse Fetal Lies

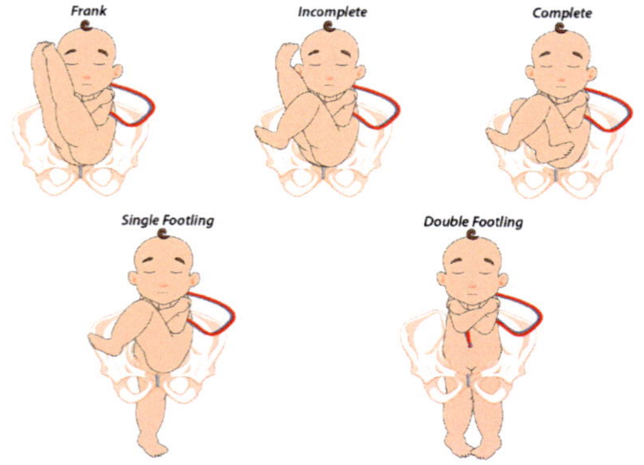

FIGURE 17.1.38 - Breech Presentations

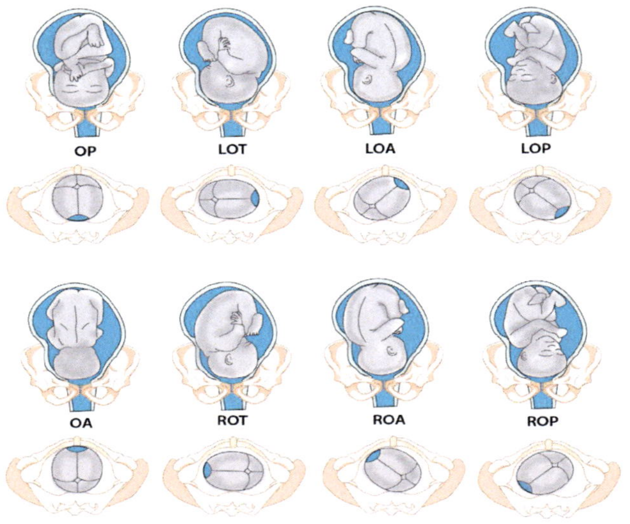

FIGURE 17.1.39 - Cephalic Presentations

III. Fetal Heart Rate Monitoring
  A. Normal fetal heart rate: 110 - 160 beats/min
  B. Fetal bradycardia: fetal heart rate < 110 beats/min
  C. Fetal tachycardia: fetal heart rate > 160 beats/min
  D. Normal fetal heart rate variability: 6 - 25 beats/min
  E. Acceleration: sudden rise in the baseline fetal heart rate > 15 bpm for > 15 seconds
  F. Deceleration: sudden drop in the baseline fetal heart rate > 15 bpm for > 15 seconds
  G. Early, late, and variable decelerations
  H. Distinguished by timing relative to uterine contraction
  I. Etiology ("**VEAL CHOP**")
    1. Variable deceleration: Cord compression
    2. Early deceleration: Head compression
    3. Acceleration: Okay
    4. Late deceleration: Placental insufficiency
  J. Variable decelerations
    1. Umbilical cord compression (oligohydramnios)
    2. No temporal relationship to uterine contractions
    3. Onset-nadir time < 30 seconds
  K. Intermittent variable deceleration: present with < 50% of uterine contractions in 10 minutes (observation)
  L. Recurrent variable deceleration: present with ≥ 50% of contractions
    1. Amnioinfusion and repositioning; C-section in refractory cases
  M. Early decelerations
    1. Fetal head compression due to uterine contraction
    2. Synchronous with uterine contraction
    3. Onset-nadir time > 30 seconds
    4. Due to fetal head compression
  N. Benign finding
  O. No intervention needed
  P. Late decelerations

1. Uteroplacental insufficiency
2. Compromised placental blood flow (e.g. diabetes, hypertension, cocaine)
3. Deceleration starts after the peak of uterine contraction
4. Onset-nadir time > 30 seconds

Q. Ominous finding: needs maternal and fetal evaluation
1. Intermittent late decelerations: present with < 50% of contractions
2. Recurrent late decelerations: present with ≥ 50% of contractions

R. Fluids, repositioning, stop uterotonics, C-section

S. Sinusoidal fetal heart rate pattern
1. Sine waves with regular amplitude and frequency
2. Absent beat-to-beat variability
3. Associated with fetal anemia
   a) Feta anemia thought to cause autonomic nervous system dysfunction and increased serum vasopressin levels

T. Category I fetal heart rate (normal)
1. Rate of 110 - 160 beats/min with accelerations
2. No late or variable decelerations

U. Category II fetal heart rate: does not meet criteria for category I and III

V. Category III fetal heart rate
1. Recurrent late or variable decelerations
2. Fetal bradycardia or sinusoidal pattern

W. Management of category I
1. Observation and expectant management

X. Management of category II
1. Maternal repositioning, IV fluids, oxygen
2. Delivery in refractory cases

Y. Management of category III
1. Urgent delivery

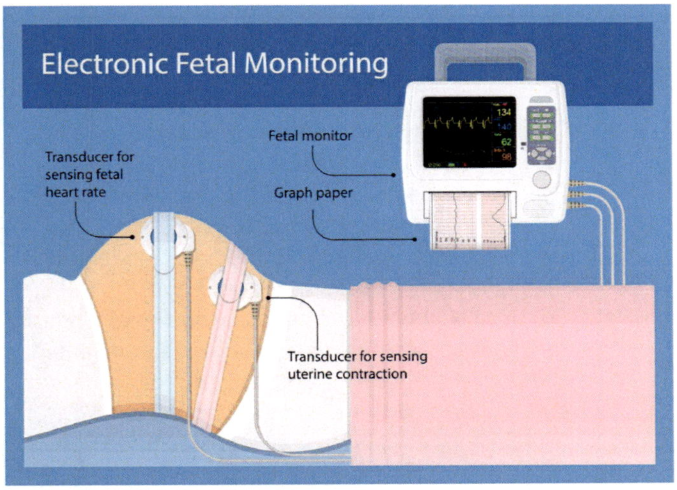

FIGURE 17.1.40 - Electronic Fetal Heart Rate Monitoring

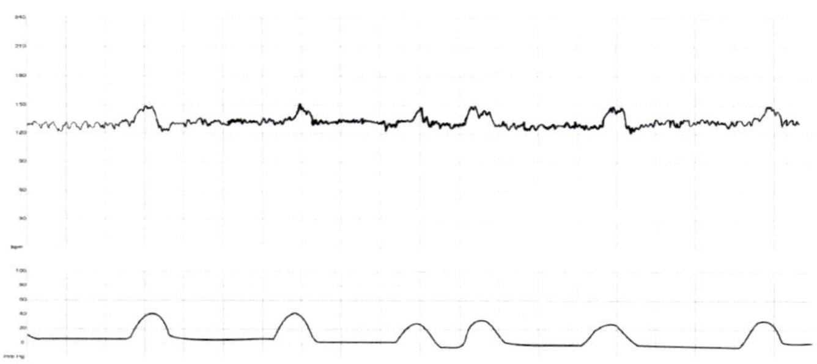

FIGURE 17.1.41 - Cardiotocography: Normal Fetal Heart Rate Tracing

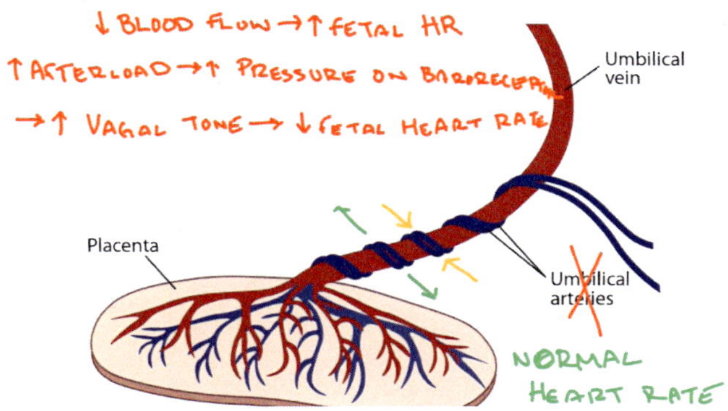

FIGURE 17.1.42 - Pathophysiology of Late Decelerations

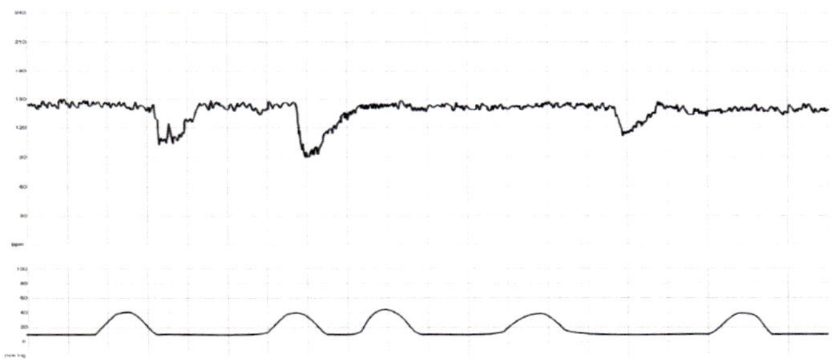

FIGURE 17.1.43 - Cardiotocography: Variable Decelerations

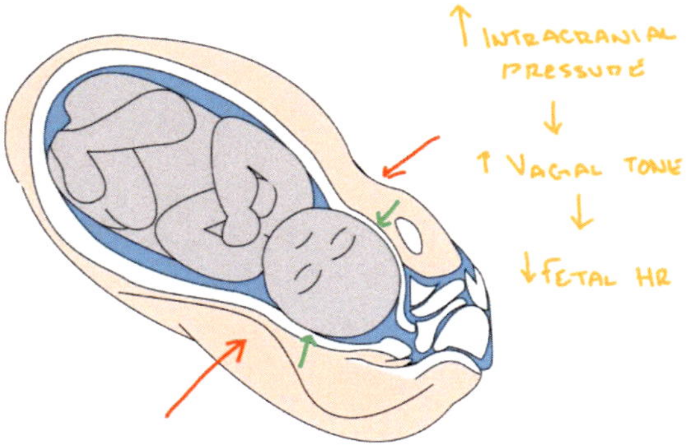

FIGURE 17.1.44 - Early Decelerations Due to Uterine Contractions

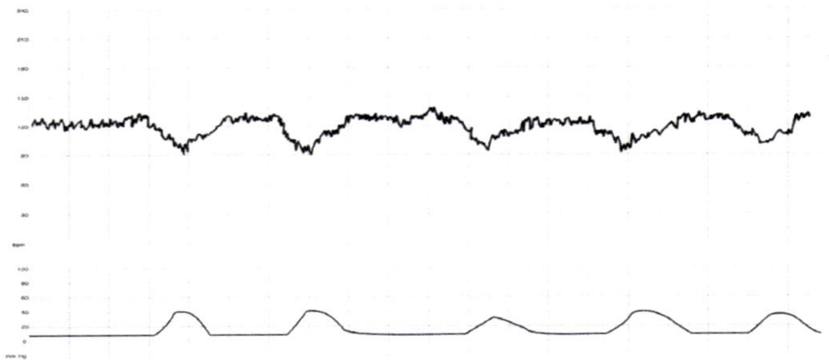

FIGURE 17.1.45 - Cardiotocography: Early Decelerations

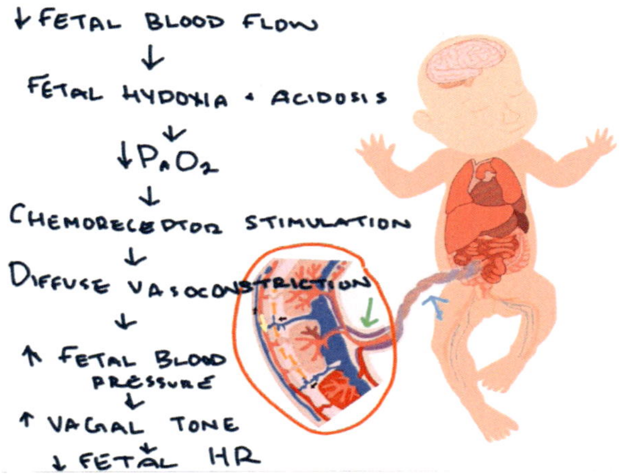

FIGURE 17.1.46 - Uteroplacental Insufficiency

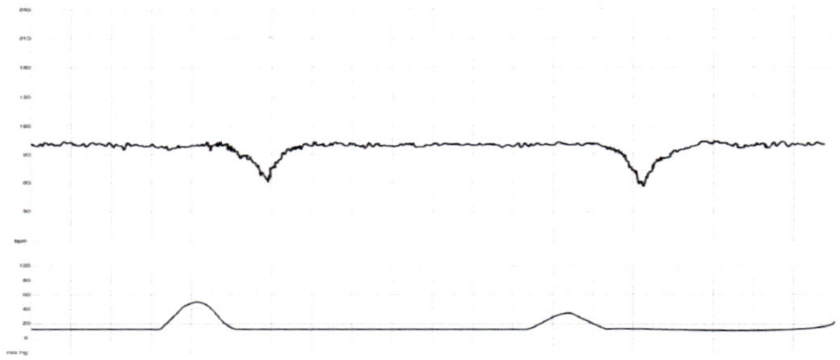

FIGURE 17.1.47 - Cardiotocography: Late Decelerations

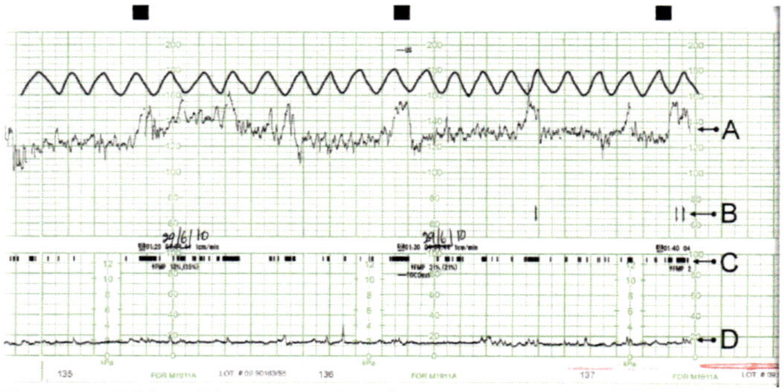

FIGURE 17.1.48 - Cardiotocography: Normal Fetal Heart Rate

REVIEW QUESTIONS

1. A 32-year-old G2P1 woman is brought to the emergency department by her husband because of severe lower abdominal pain for the last 3 hours. She is having regular, strong uterine contractions. The Leopold maneuver is performed and shows that the fetal head is located near the maternal symphysis pubis, and the angle between the fetal and maternal longitudinal axis is from 0 to 90 degrees. The labor progresses, and the physician observes that the fetal occiput is directed toward the maternal symphysis pubis. What are the fetal lie, presentation, and position in this pregnancy?
   - **The fetal lie, presentation, and position in this pregnancy are oblique, cephalic, and occiput anterior, respectively.**
   - The fetal presentation is cephalic since the fetal head is located near the maternal symphysis pubis.
   - The fact that the angle between the fetal and maternal longitudinal axis is from 0 to 90 degrees suggests that the fetus is in an oblique lie.
   - Finally, the fetal occiput is directed towards the maternal symphysis pubis indicating that the presenting part of the fetus has an occiput anterior position.

2. A 34-year-old G3P2 woman comes to her OBGYN at 36 weeks of gestation for a routine prenatal visit. She has a past medical history of type 1 diabetes mellitus, diagnosed 20 years ago. She is on a daily insulin regimen. Her previous two pregnancies were complicated by fetal macrosomia. Cardiotocography at this prenatal visit shows a gradual decline in fetal heart rate with an onset-nadir time > 30 seconds that starts after the peak of uterine contraction. What is the most likely cause of the cardiotocographic findings in this patient?
   - **The most likely cause of uteroplacental insufficiency in this patient is diabetes-induced hyaline arteriolosclerosis of the placental vessels.**
   - This pregnant patient with a 20-year history of type 1 diabetes mellitus has cardiotocographic findings classic for late decelerations.
   - Specifically, there is a gradual decline in fetal heart rate with an onset-nadir time > 30 seconds that starts after the peak of uterine contraction.
   - Late decelerations are due to uteroplacental insufficiency or inadequate placental blood flow.

Obstetrics | Section 13: Normal Labor and Delivery Part 2

I. Stages of Labor
   A. Labor
      1. Regular strong uterine contractions with the cervical changes
      2. Cervical dilation, effacement, and softening
   B. Braxton-Hicks contractions
      1. Irregular weak contractions
      2. No cervical changes
      3. Not a true labor
   C. Cervical effacement
      1. Cervical thinning
      2. Expressed in percentage
   D. Cervical softening
      1. Firm: consistency similar to nose
      2. Medium: consistency similar to lips
      3. Soft: consistency similar to butter
   E. First stage
      1. From onset of uterine contractions to full cervical dilation at 10 cm
   F. Latent phase from onset of uterine contraction to cervical dilation at 6 cm
      1. ~ 10 - 12 hours in nulliparous; ~ 6 - 8 hours in multiparous
   G. Active phase from cervical dilation at 6 cm to 10 cm
      1. ~ 4 - 6 hours in nulliparous; ~ 2 - 3 hours in multiparous
   H. Second stage ("pushing" stage)
      1. From complete cervical dilation to delivery of fetus
      2. Lasts ~ 4 - 6 hours in nulliparous and ~ 2 - 3 hours in multiparous
      3. Prolonged in case of epidural anesthesia
      4. Fetal location in birth canal denoted by fetal stations
      5. Ischial spine: station 0
      6. Negative stations above ischial spine; positive ones below
   I. Third stage
      1. From delivery of fetus to delivery of placenta
      2. Lasts ~ 30 minutes in both nulliparous and multiparous women

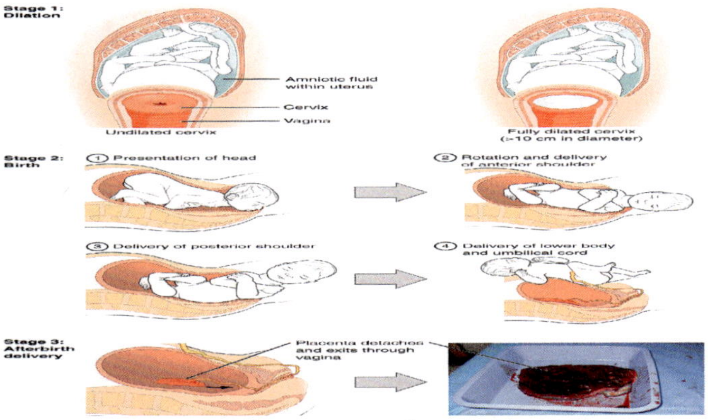

FIGURE 17.1.49 - Cervical Dilation

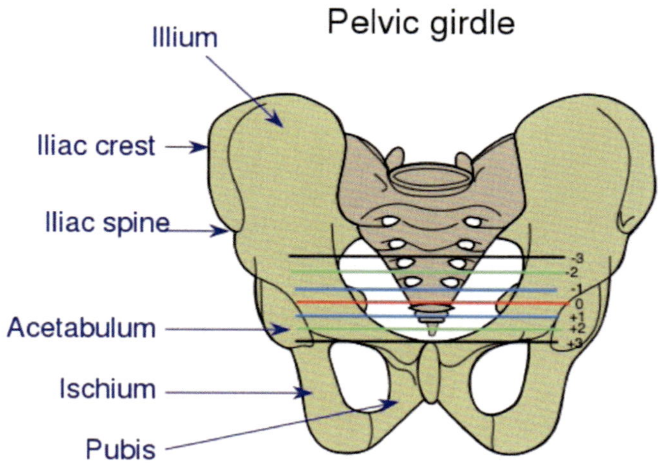

FIGURE 17.1.50 - Fetal Stations

II. Bishop Score
   A. Assesses whether cervix is favorable for vaginal birth
   B. 5 criteria
      1. Cervical effacement, dilation, consistency, position, fetal station
   C. Cervical effacement, dilation, and fetal station are scored from 0 to 3 points
   D. Cervical consistency and position are scored from 0 to 2 points
   E. Cervical dilation
      1. Closed: 0 points
      2. 1 - 2 cm: 1 point; 3 - 4 cm: 2 points; at least 5 - 6 cm: 3 points
   F. Cervical position
      1. Posterior: 0 points; middle: 1 point; anterior: 2 points
   G. Cervical consistency
      1. Firm: 0 points; medium: 1 point; soft: 2 points
   H. Cervical effacement
      1. 0 - 30%: 0 points
      2. 40 - 50%: 1 point; 60 - 70%: 2 points; at least 80%: 3 points
   I. Fetal station
      1. -3: 0 points; -2: 1 point; -1 or 0: 2 points; +1, +2: 3 points
   J. Maximal score: 13
   K. Minimal score: 0
   L. Interpretation
      1. Score ≤ 5: unfavorable cervix; induction likely needed
      2. Score 6 - 7: equivocal; need for induction based on clinical judgment
      3. Score ≥ 8: favorable cervix; induction likely not needed

III. Cardinal Movements of Labor
   A. Performed by fetus in stage II of labor
      1. Engagement: fetal biparietal diameter descends below pelvic inlet
      2. Flexion: fetus flexes the head
      3. Descent: fetus descends further in the birth canal
      4. Internal rotation: fetus internally rotates head
      5. Extension: fetus extends the head
      6. Restitution: fetus externally rotates head; expulsion - fetus is born

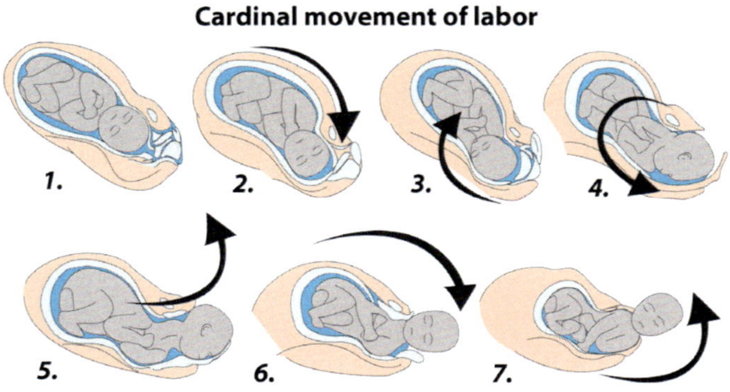

FIGURE 17.1.51 - Cardinal Movements of Labor

IV. Intrapartum Anesthesia
   A. Epidural anesthesia
      1. Most commonly used
      2. Needle inserted between L3 - L4 or L4 - L5 (below L2 vertebra)
      3. Anesthetic injected in the epidural space blocking cauda equina nerve roots
      4. Relatively high dose of anesthetic needed
      5. Relatively slow onset of anesthesia (vs. spinal)
   B. Spinal anesthesia
      1. Less commonly used
      2. Needle inserted between L3 - L4 or L4 - L5
      3. Anesthetic injected in the subarachnoid space
      4. Relatively low dose of anesthetic needed
      5. Relatively fast onset of anesthesia (vs. epidural)
   C. Pudendal nerve block
      1. Local perineal anesthesia
      2. Contractions still felt by woman
      3. Anesthetic injected intravaginally with needle directed towards the ischial spine
      4. Used in case episiotomy or fetal macrosomia

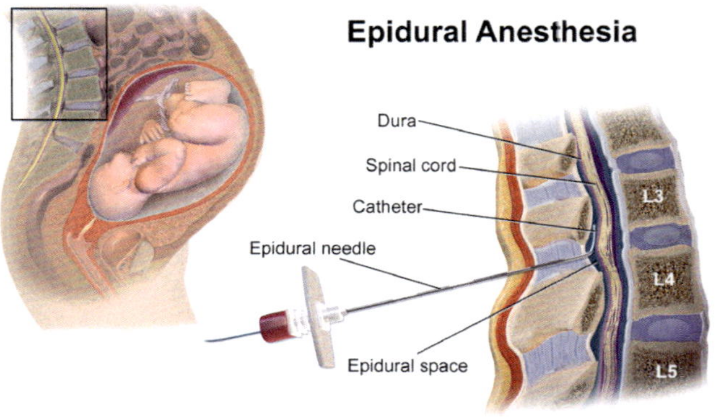

FIGURE 17.1.52 - Epidural Anesthesia

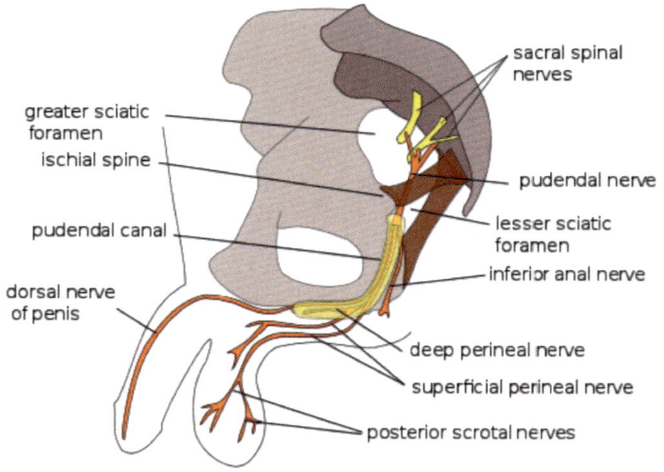

FIGURE 17.1.53 - Pudendal Nerve

REVIEW QUESTIONS

1. A 29-year-old G3P2 woman comes to her primary care physician at 35 weeks of gestation reporting uterine contractions for the past day. Her contractions are mild to moderate and occur irregularly. She has not had rupture of membranes. Vital signs are unremarkable, and the physical examination shows a closed cervix. How does this patient's condition differ from true labor?

    - **This patient has mild, irregular uterine contractions with no cervical changes, differing from true labor.**
    - This pregnant patient at 35 weeks of gestation experiences mild to moderate, irregular uterine contractions with no cervical change.
    - This phenomenon is known as Braxton-Hicks contractions or "false labor."
    - While Braxton-Hicks contractions are characterized by mild, irregular uterine contractions, true labor has strong, regular contractions.
    - Additionally, Braxton-Hicks contractions are not associated with cervical changes, while true labor is.

2. A 25-year-old G1P0 woman at 39 weeks of gestation is brought to the hospital by her partner after her "water broke." She is feeling strong, regular uterine contractions. Physical examination shows a soft anterior cervix dilated at 3 cm and effaced at 60%. The fetal station is -3. What is the correct interpretation of this patient's Bishop score?

    - **This patient's Bishop score is 8, suggesting a favorable cervix and labor induction is likely unnecessary.**
    - This pregnant patient, at 39 weeks of gestation, reports that her "water broke," indicating rupture of membranes, and that she is feeling strong, regular uterine contractions.
    - The physical examination shows a soft anterior cervix dilated at 3 cm and effaced at 60%.
    - Considering these findings, she is likely in true labor.
    - This patient's Bishop score should be calculated.
    - The cervix is soft, giving this patient 2 points.
    - Cervix is in the anterior position, giving her another 2 points.
    - Dilation at 3 cm is scored 2 points, and 60% effacement is scored 2 points.
    - Fetal station of -3 is equivalent to 0 points.
    - Therefore, the Bishop score of this patient is 8.
    - Score ≥ 8 suggests a favorable cervix, and induction or augmentation of the labor is likely not needed.

3. A 36-year-old G2P1 woman with no prenatal care comes to the emergency department at 38 weeks of gestation, reporting severe lower abdominal pain. She is feeling strong uterine contractions every 3 minutes. She has a history of type 2 diabetes mellitus, diagnosed 5 years ago. Her prepregnancy BMI was 28 kg/m^2. Vital signs include a temperature of 96.8° F (36° C), blood pressure of 110/80 mmHg, heart rate of 110 beats/min, and respiratory rate of 17 breaths/min. Several hours after normal labor progression, the fetal station is +2. However, the fetus does not progress further, and it is considered to be macrosomic. Episiotomy is planned to widen the birth canal. Which anatomical landmarks should be used for proper local anesthesia of this patient before episiotomy?

    A. Ischial spine
    B. Ischial tuberosity
    C. Pubic ramus
    D. Coccyx

    - **The correct answer is option A.**
    - This pregnant patient at 38 weeks of gestation presents in active labor.
    - She had no prenatal care.
    - She has a past medical history of type 2 diabetes mellitus, and her prepregnancy BMI was high.
    - Although the fetal station is +2 several hours after the normal labor progression, the fetus does not progress down further. It is considered to be macrosomic, and episiotomy is planned to widen the birth canal.
    - Pudendal nerve block is commonly administered before episiotomy.
    - During pudendal nerve block, the needle should be facing the ischial spine to ensure proper nerve block.
    - Options B, ischial tuberosity, C, pubic ramus, and D, coccyx, are incorrect because although they are part of the pelvic girdle, they are not the closest anatomical landmarks to the pudendal nerve.

Obstetrics | Section 14: Placental Abruption, Placenta Previa & Vasa Previa

I. Placental Abruption: Definition
   A. Premature separation of the placenta from the uterine wall
   B. Could be partial or complete

II. Placental Abruption: Risk Factors
   A. Previous abruption
   B. Maternal hypertension, preeclampsia, and eclampsia
   C. Smoking, cocaine use
   D. Abdominal trauma

III. Placental Abruption: Clinical Features
   A. Sudden-onset 3rd trimester vaginal bleeding
   B. Severe abdominal or back pain

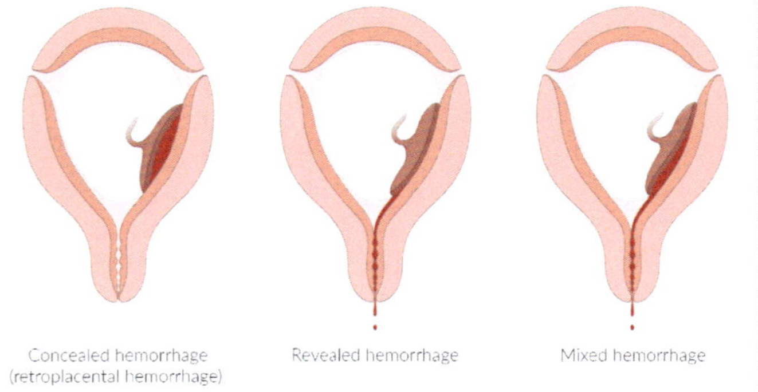

FIGURE 17.1.54 - Types of Hemorrhage in Placental Abruption

IV. Placental Abruption: Complications
   A. Fetal hypoxia
   B. Fetal demise
   C. Preterm delivery
   D. Hypovolemic shock
   E. DIC
   F. Weak uterine wall: risk of future uterine rupture

V. Placental Abruption: Diagnosis
   A. Clinical diagnosis
   B. Physical exam: tender, rigid uterus; vaginal exam is contraindicated
   C. Ultrasound: rule out placenta previa; retroplacental hematoma
   D. Fetal heart monitoring: late decelerations due to placental insufficiency and hypoxia

VI. Placental Abruption: Management
   A. Stabilize the patient
      1. Fluid resuscitation (crystalloids), monitor vitals, maintain airways
      2. Hemorrhagic shock: put patient in lateral decubitus position, blood transfusion
   B. RhD prophylaxis: to Rh- mothers
   C. Mild abruption and premature fetus: manage expectantly
   D. Moderate/severe abruption: immediate delivery
      1. Fetus and mother stable: vaginal delivery
      2. Fetal distress or mother unstable: C-section

VII. Placenta Previa: Definition
   A. Abnormal implantation of the placenta over or in close proximity to the internal cervical os

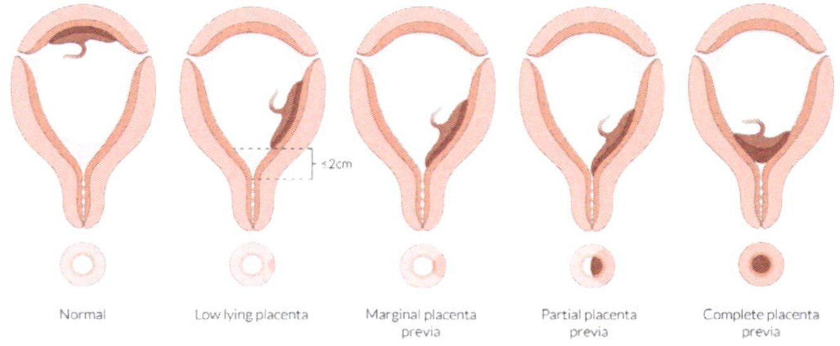

FIGURE 17.1.55 - Types of Placenta Previa

VIII. Placenta Previa: Risk Factors
   A. Previous placenta previa
   B. Uterine scarring: C-section, uterine surgery (e.g. myomectomy)
   C. Multiparity
   D. Advanced maternal age (> 35)

IX. Placenta Previa: Clinical Features
   A. Painless 3rd trimester vaginal bleeding: stops within 1 - 2 hours, recurs during birth
   B. Usually no fetal distress (bleeding is maternal in origin)

X. Placenta Previa: Diagnosis
   A. Digital vaginal exams are contraindicated; speculum examination is safe
   B. Ultrasound: transabdominal followed by transvaginal
      1. Initially diagnosed prenatally
      2. Follow-up ultrasound in the 3rd trimester to see if it has resolved

XI. Placenta Previa: Management
   A. Asymptomatic patients: outpatient management, 'pelvic rest' (avoiding sexual intercourse)
   B. Symptomatic patients: hospitalization, continuous fetal monitoring, IV access
      1. Immediate C-section: in active and unstoppable labor, severe bleeding, or fetal distress
   C. Vaginal birth is contraindicated

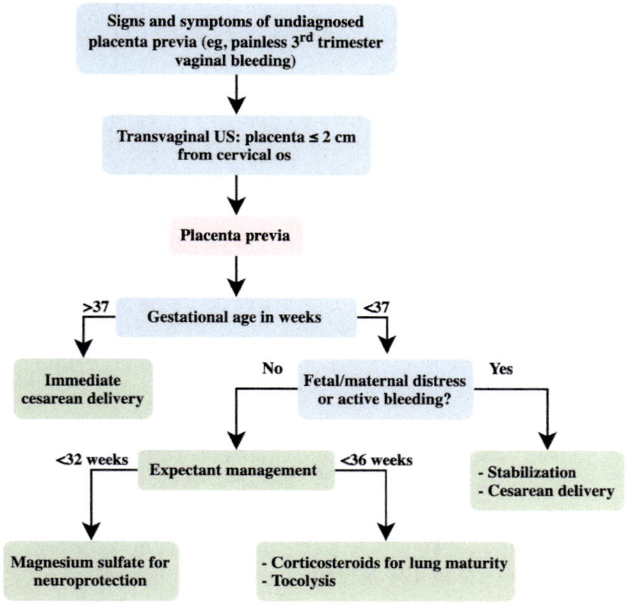

FIGURE 17.1.56 - Management of Placenta Previa

XII. Vasa Previa: Definition

A. Fetal blood vessels cross or pass over the internal cervical os

XIII. Vasa Previa: Pathophysiology

A. Most commonly occurs due to congenital placental anomalies such as velamentous umbilical cord insertion or multiple-lobed placenta leaving vessels unprotected and prone to shearing, laceration, and bleeding

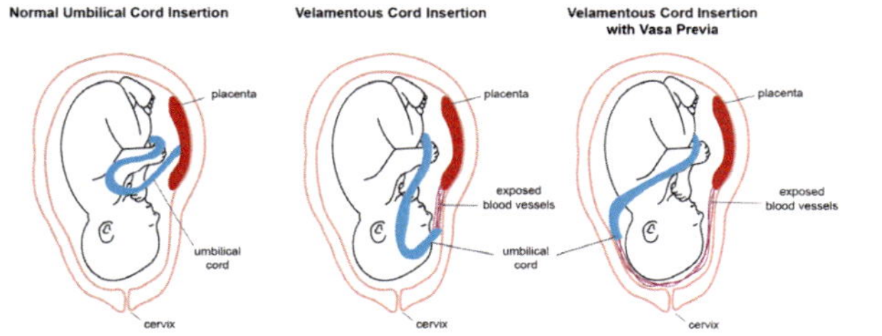

FIGURE 17.1.57 - Velamentous Cord Insertion with/without Vasa Previa

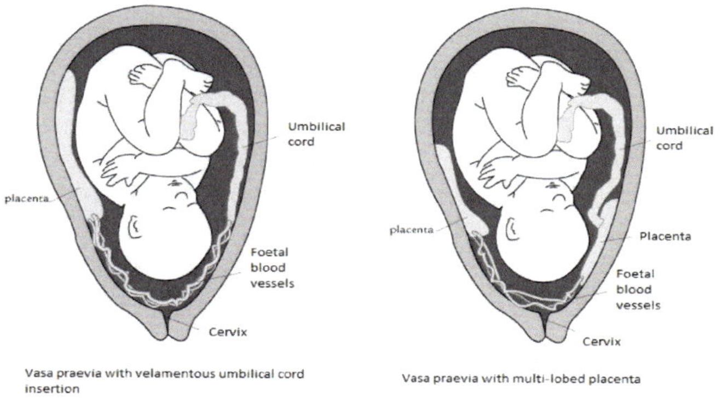

FIGURE 17.1.58 - Multi-Lobed Placenta with Vasa Previa

XIV. Vasa Previa: Risk Factors

A. Placental anomalies (e.g. velamentous umbilical cord insertion, bilobate placenta)
   1. Advanced maternal age, IVF

B. Multiparity

XV. Vasa Previa: Clinical Features

A. Painless vaginal bleeding with rupture of membranes

B. Fetal heart rate variations: decelerations, fetal bradycardia, sinusoidal pattern; fetal distress

C. Complications: severe bleeding may lead to fetal death; fetal asphyxiation

XVI. Vasa Previa: Diagnosis

A. Ideally diagnosed antenatally

B. Doppler ultrasound (gold standard): transabdominal and transvaginal

XVII. Vasa Previa: Management

A. Emergency C-section: in case of acute bleeding and fetal distress

B. If diagnosed antenatally:
   1. < 32 GW: steroids for fetal lung maturity
   2. Hospitalization at 30 - 32 GW for monitoring and scheduled C-section

C. Uncomplicated vasa previa: scheduled delivery can be attempted at 34 - 35 weeks

Condition	Definition	Key Features
Placental abruption	- Premature separation of the placenta from the uterine wall	- Painful 3rd trimester vaginal bleeding; frequent uterine contractions - Fetal distress: late decelerations, fetal bradycardia
Placenta previa	- Abnormal implantation of the placenta over or in close proximity to the internal cervical os	- Painless 3rd trimester vaginal bleeding; stops within 1 - 2 hours, recurs during birth - No fetal distress (bleeding is maternal in origin)
Vasa previa	- Fetal blood vessels overlying the internal cervical os	- Painless vaginal bleeding with rupture of membranes - FHR: decelerations, fetal bradycardia, sinusoidal pattern; fetal distress

TABLE 17.1.1 - Placental Abruption, Placenta Previa, and Vasa Previa

REVIEW QUESTIONS

1. A 29-year-old woman at 34 weeks gestation is brought to the emergency department by her partner because of acute onset abdominal pain and vaginal bleeding for the last few hours. Physical examination shows the uterus is tender to palpation, and there is continuous dark vaginal bleeding. Her extremities are cool to the touch, and vitals are significant for tachycardia. The fetal heart rate shows late decelerations. What is the most likely diagnosis of the patient?
   - **The most likely diagnosis is placental abruption.**
   - Important risk factors for placental abruption include previous abruption, maternal hypertension including preeclampsia and eclampsia, smoking, cocaine use, and abdominal trauma.
   - This 29-year-old woman is presenting with third-trimester vaginal bleeding and acute abdominal pain.
   - Physical examination shows a tender uterus, and her fetus is in distress.
   - There are signs of hypovolemic shock, such as tachycardia and cool extremities.
   - All of these findings are consistent with placental abruption as the most likely diagnosis.
   - Important risk factors for placental abruption include previous abruption, maternal hypertension including preeclampsia and eclampsia, smoking, cocaine use, and abdominal trauma.

2. A 33-year-old G4P3 woman at 35 weeks gestation is brought to the emergency department by her partner because of painless vaginal bleeding for 2 hours. She says she had a previous episode of vaginal bleeding 2 days ago that resolved on its own. Physical examination shows active bright red vaginal bleeding and no uterine tenderness. Her blood pressure is 87/57 mmHg, and her pulse is 120 beats per minute. What would most likely be evident on transvaginal ultrasound? After stabilizing the patient, what is the next best step in managing this patient?
   - **Transvaginal ultrasound will likely show the placenta covering the internal cervical os.**
   - **After stabilizing the patient, the best next step in management is to perform a cesarean section, as there is active bleeding and the mother is unstable.**
   - This 33-year-old multiparous woman presents with active, painless third-trimester vaginal bleeding.
   - She is hemodynamically unstable.
   - The most likely diagnosis is placenta previa because she has acute onset painless vaginal bleeding.
   - If there was no active bleeding and the mother and fetus were both stable, then expectant management would be more appropriate.

3. A 27-year-old woman with known vasa previa is brought to the emergency department by her partner because of profuse painless vaginal bleeding with rupture of membranes. She appears unstable, with tachycardia and hypotension noted on her vitals. Fetal heart rate shows fetal bradycardia. What is the best next step in the management?
   - **The best next step in the management is to administer IV fluids for stabilization.**
   - This patient has vasa previa and presents with profuse painless vaginal bleeding with rupture of membranes.
   - Fetal heart rate typically shows tachycardia followed by bradycardia.
   - Administration of intravenous fluid is the best initial step in the management of all unstable patients with antepartum hemorrhage, regardless of the underlying cause.

Obstetrics | Section 15: Uterine Rupture & Other Etiologies of Antepartum Hemorrhage

I. Uterine rupture: Definition
   A. A life-threatening pregnancy complication where the uterus ruptures
   B. Occurs during the delivery process

II. Uterine rupture: Risk Factors
   A. Uterine scarring or distention
      1. Previous uterine surgeries (e.g. C-section, myomectomy)
      2. Fetal macrosomia
      3. Uterine anomalies
      4. Induction of labor or prolonged labor
   B. Trauma

III. Uterine rupture: Clinical Features
   A. Acute-onset severe abdominal pain
   B. Cessation of uterine contractions (loss of uterine pressure)
   C. Loss of fetal station, palpable fetal parts, fetal distress
   D. Bleeding: hemorrhagic shock
      1. Intra-abdominal bleeding: signs of hemorrhagic shock (tachycardia, hypotension)
      2. Vaginal bleeding: spotting to severe hemorrhage

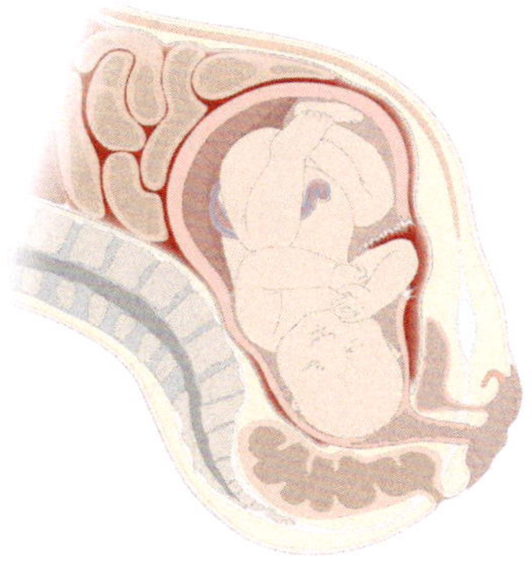

FIGURE 17.1.59 - Complete Uterine Rupture

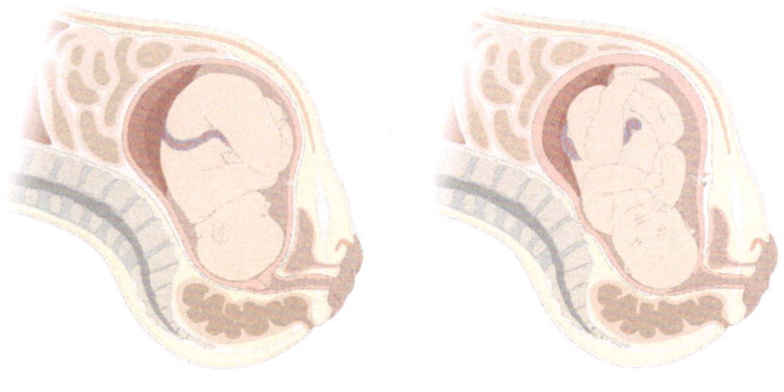

FIGURE 17.1.60 - Image Showing Uterine Scar and Concealed Uterine Rupture

IV. Uterine rupture: Clinical Features
   A. Imminent rupture: maternal agitation, hyperventilation, tachycardia

V. Uterine rupture: Diagnosis
   A. Clinical diagnosis
   B. Fetal heart rate monitoring will reveal fetal distress: decelerations

VI. Uterine rupture: Management
   A. Uterine rupture: emergent laparotomy with C-section
   B. Imminent rupture: IV tocolysis and emergency C-section
   C. Planned C-section prior to onset of labor: uterine dehiscence
   D. Hysterectomy: refractory bleeding

VII. Uterine rupture: Prevention
   A. Patients with history of:
      1. Low transverse C-section or myomectomy without entry to uterine cavity: may attempt vaginal delivery
      2. Classical C-section or myomectomy with entry to uterine cavity: vaginal delivery is contraindicated

VIII. Other Etiologies of Antepartum Hemorrhage
   A. Obstetric: still birth, bloody show
   B. Nonobstetric: cervical trauma

IX. Other Etiologies of Antepartum Hemorrhage
   A. Still-birth: vaginal bleeding with crampy abdominal pain that occurs after the 20th gestational week, with uterine contractions and cervical dilations
   B. Bloody show: bloody mucus vaginal discharge with a dilated cervix; signals the onset of normal labor
      1. Small amount of blood-tinged mucus, regular uterine contractions, no associated pain
   C. Cervical trauma can occur during sexual intercourse or birth; patients have a positive history; tender, bruised cervix without signs of active bleeding

Condition	Definition	Key Features
Uterine rupture	- Life-threatening pregnancy complication where the uterus ruptures	- Severe abdominal pain; cessation of uterine contractions, loss of fetal station, palpable fetal parts, fetal distress - Hemorrhage: intra-abdominal and vaginal
Still-birth	- Birth of a dead fetus after 20th gestational weeks	- Vaginal bleeding with crampy abdominal pain > 20th GW; uterine contractions, cervical dilations
Bloody show	- Blood-tinged mucus discharge at the onset of labor	- Small amount of blood-tinged mucus, regular uterine contractions, no associated pain
Cervical trauma	- Trauma to the cervix during birth or sexual intercourse	- Tender, bruised cervix without signs of active bleeding

TABLE 17.1.2 - Uterine Rupture and Other Etiologies of Antepartum Hemorrhage

REVIEW QUESTIONS

?

1. A 32-year-old woman at 32 weeks gestation comes to her OBGYN for a routine prenatal examination. She has had two previous cesarean sections the past, one of which was an emergency. Her medications include insulin for gestational diabetes. She is a smoker, but she has not smoked since she discovered she was pregnant. Based on her history, what is the most important risk factor for uterine rupture in this patient?

- **The most important risk factor for uterine rupture is a uterine scar after C-section.**
- Risk factors for uterine rupture include factors that cause uterine scarring and/or distention, which include previous uterine surgeries, fetal macrosomia, which can cause uterine stretching, uterine anomalies, prolonged labor, and trauma.

2. A 28-year-old G1P0 woman at 37 weeks gestation is brought to the emergency department by her husband because her water broke. She has progressively intense uterine contractions every 2 minutes. The cervix is dilated at 5 cm. She has a past medical history of poorly controlled type I diabetes mellitus. An abdominal ultrasound shows polyhydramnios. Six hours after the onset of labor, she experiences sudden worsening of abdominal pain. The fetal station returns from +1 to -3. The patients vital signs include blood pressure of 60/40 mmHg, heart rate of 140 beats/min, and respiratory rate of 24 breaths/min. Cardiotocography shows recurrent late decelerations. IV fluids are administered. Which of the following is the best next step in management of this patient?

   A. Emergent C-section
   B. Planned C-section after 24 hours
   C. Emergent vaginal delivery
   D. Planned vaginal delivery after 24 hours

- **The correct answer is option A.**
- This pregnant woman was diagnosed with polyhydramnios, likely because of her poorly controlled type I diabetes mellitus.
- She develops sudden worsening of abdominal pain after 6 hours of labor, and the fetal station returns from +1 to -3.
- Based on her vitals hemodynamically unstable, and the fetus is experiencing hypoxia evidenced by recurrent late decelerations.
- All these findings are concerning for uterine rupture.
- Uterine overdistension by polyhydramnios possibly predisposed this patient to uterine rupture.
- The next best step in management is an emergent C-section.
- Option B, planned C-section after 24 hours, is incorrect because both mother and fetus are hemodynamically unstable, and immediate intervention is warranted.
- Options C and D are incorrect because vaginal delivery is time-consuming and potentially lethal for both the fetus and the mother in case of uterine rupture.

Obstetrics | Section 16: Preterm Labor, Tocolytics, Abnormal Labor Patterns, and Breech Presentation

I. Preterm Labor
   A. Delivery between 24 and 37 weeks of gestation
   B. Management:
      1. 34 - 36 weeks: +/- betamethasone; penicillin if GBS positive or unknown
      2. 32 - 34 weeks: betamethasone, penicillin, nifedipine (tocolytic)
      3. 24 - 32 weeks: betamethasone, penicillin, indomethacin (tocolytic), magnesium sulfate (neuroprotective)

II. Tocolytics
   A. Indomethacin
      1. Cyclooxygenase inhibitor: decreases prostaglandin levels (PGE_1, PGE_2, PGF_{2a})
      2. Used from 24 to 32 weeks of gestation
      3. Beyond 32 weeks: high risk of closing ductus arteriosus
      4. Use for more than 72 hours not recommended: high risk of closing ductus arteriosus
   B. Nifedipine
      1. Dihydropyridine calcium channel blocker
      2. Used beyond 32 weeks or when indomethacin is contraindicated
      3. Side effects: hypotension and flushing (due to vasodilation)
   C. Terbutaline and ritodrine: beta-2 receptor agonists
      1. Rarely used

III. Abnormal Labor Patterns
   A. Protracted latent phase
      1. Latent phase lasts > 20 hours in nulliparous or > 14 hours in multiparous
      2. Management: discharge or inpatient monitoring
   B. Protracted active phase
      1. Cervical dilation progresses by < 1 cm/hour
      2. Management: oxytocin administration
   C. Active phase arrest
      1. No cervical change for ≥ 4 hours with adequate contractions (MVU > 200)
      2. No cervical change for ≥ 6 hours with inadequate contractions (MVU < 200)
      3. Management: cesarean delivery

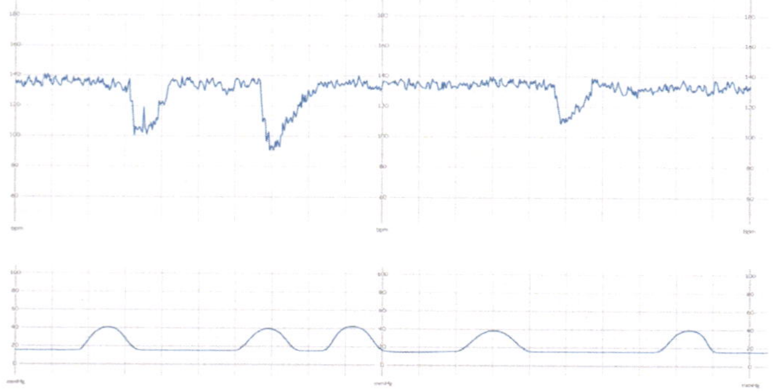

FIGURE 17.1.61 - Montevideo Unit

IV. Breech Presentation
   A. Presenting part is fetal rump
   B. Several types
      1. Frank, incomplete, complete, single footling, and double footling breech
      2. Management: external cephalic version or cesarean delivery
      3. Vaginal delivery usually avoided due to high risk of perinatal asphyxia and fetal death

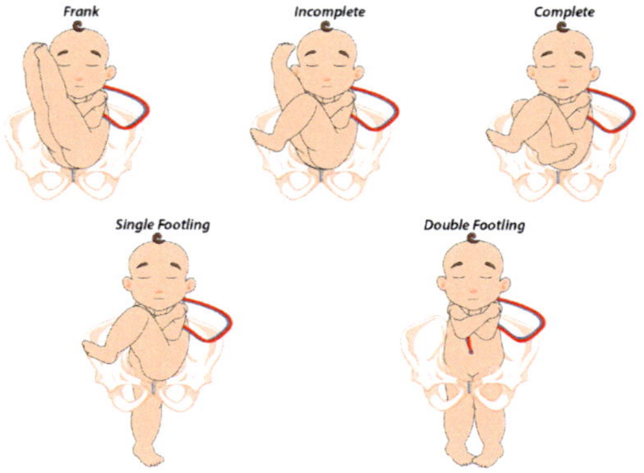

FIGURE 17.1.62 - Different Types of Breech Presentation

REVIEW QUESTIONS

1. A 25-year-old G1P0 woman is brought to the emergency department by her partner due to severe lower abdominal pain for the last hour. She is at 30 weeks gestation. She is feeling regular, progressively strong uterine contractions every two minutes. Vital signs are unremarkable. Physical examination shows cervical dilation at 4 cm and 30% effacement. What are the best treatment options for this patient?
   - **The best treatment options for this patient is the administration of betamethasone to accelerate fetal lung maturity, penicillin for *group B Streptococcus* prophylaxis, indomethacin to delay labor, and magnesium sulfate for neuroprotection**
   - This woman presents at 30 weeks of gestation due to severe lower abdominal pain and regular, progressively strong uterine contractions every two minutes.
   - The cervix is 4 cm dilated and 30% effaced, indicating preterm labor
   - In case of preterm labor from 24 to 32 weeks gestation, betamethasone is administered to accelerate fetal lung maturity; penicillin for *group B Streptococcus* prophylaxis; indomethacin to delay labor, and magnesium sulfate for neuroprotection

2. A 31-year-old G3P2 woman at 38 weeks gestation comes to her OBGYN for a routine prenatal visit. All of her pregnancies were uncomplicated. Physical examination shows fundal height at 38 cm. A transabdominal ultrasound shows the fetal rump is closest to the maternal symphysis pubis, and both hips and knees are flexed. What is the best mode of delivery for this patient?
   - **The best mode of delivery is cesarean section.**
   - This patient presents at 38 weeks of gestation.
   - Transabdominal ultrasound shows the fetal rump closest to the maternal symphysis pubis.
   - In other words, the fetal rump is the presenting part.
   - Additionally, both hips and knees are flexed.
   - This is a classic description of a complete breech presentation.
   - Since this patient is already at term, the baby will likely not change to cephalic presentation.

Obstetrics | Section 17: PROM, PPROM, Operative Delivery and Shoulder Dystocia

I. PROM and PPROM
   A. Premature (prelabor) rupture of membranes
      1. Rupture of chorion and amnion at term before the onset of regular uterine contractions ("gush of fluid")
   B. Diagnosis: blue discoloration on nitrazine paper and ferning pattern of vaginal fluid under microscopy; no digital vaginal exam
   C. Management: expectant (wait for onset of natural labor), active (induction by oxytocin)
   D. Preterm prelabor rupture of membranes
      1. Rupture of chorion and amnion at < 37 weeks of gestation before onset of regular uterine contractions
   E. Risk factors
      1. Prior PPROM
      2. Antepartum bleeding
      3. Genitourinary infections (e.g. asymptomatic bacteriuria, BV)
   F. Diagnosis
   G. Sterile speculum exam, nitrazine paper test, and ferning pattern on microscopy
   H. Treatment
   I. < 34 weeks (reassuring): latency antibiotics, betamethasone
   J. < 34 weeks (non-reassuring): magnesium sulfate (< 32); delivery
   K. ≥ 34 weeks: delivery

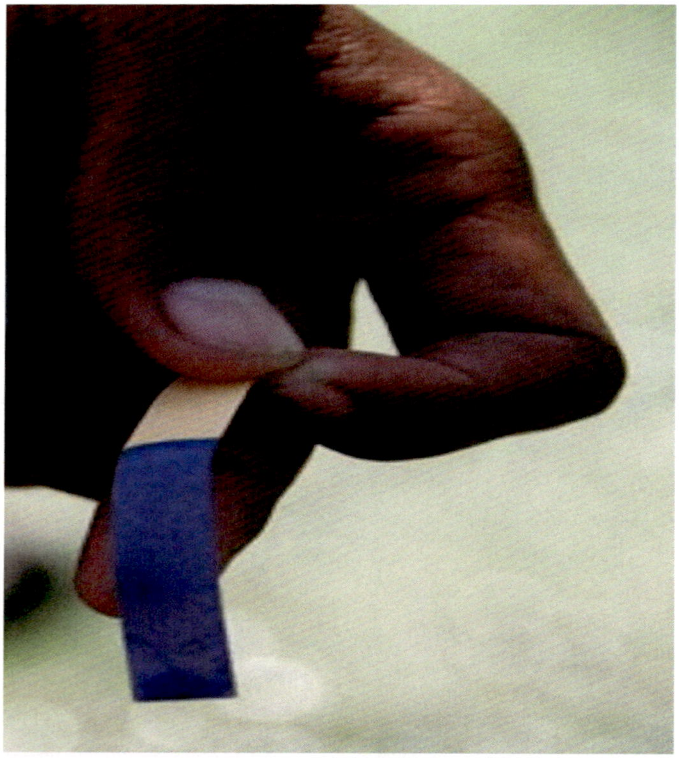

FIGURE 17.1.63 - Blue Discoloration of the Nitrazine Paper

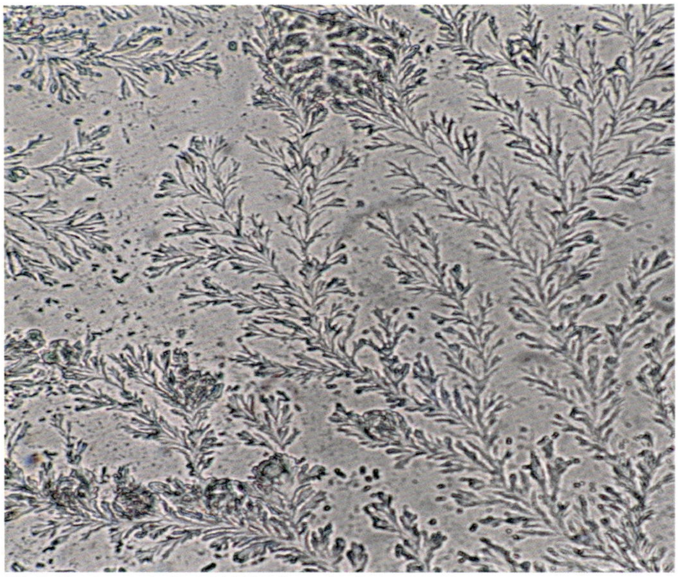

FIGURE 17.1.64 - Photomicrograph Showing the Ferning Pattern of Amniotic Fluid Under Microscopy

II. Operative Delivery
   A. Cesarean section: surgery to deliver baby
   B. Indications: fetal distress, active phase arrest, macrosomia, multiple gestation pregnancy
   C. Most commonly performed via lower transverse uterine incision
   D. TOLAC permitted in case of lower transverse incision
   E. Classical C-section: vertical uterine incision
   F. TOLAC is avoided in classical C-section due to risk for uterine rupture
   G. Complications
      1. Forceps: fetal scalp hematoma, vaginal lacerations
      2. Vacuum: fetal scalp hematoma, vulvar and vaginal hematoma
   H. Indications
      1. Maternal exhaustion and inability to push
      2. Maternal cardiac disease
      3. Prolonged second stage of labor

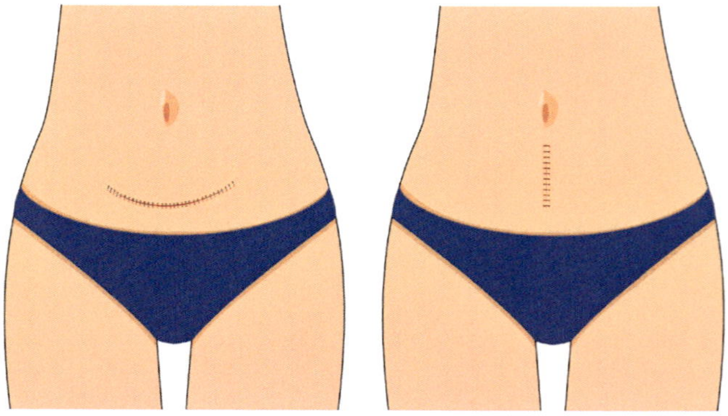

FIGURE 17.1.65 - Comparison Between Lower Transverse and Classic C-Section

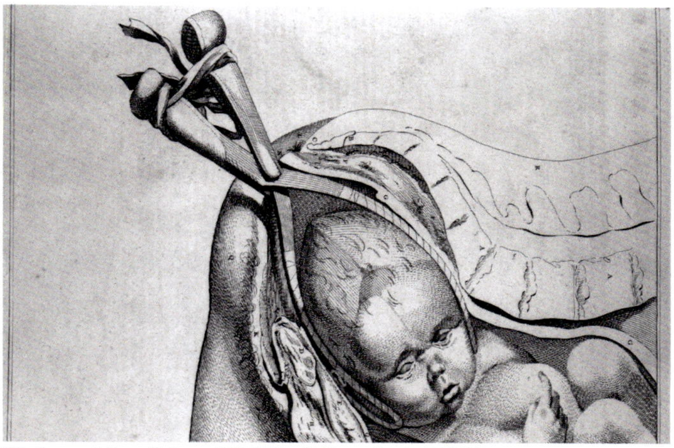

FIGURE 17.1.66 - Forceps Delivery

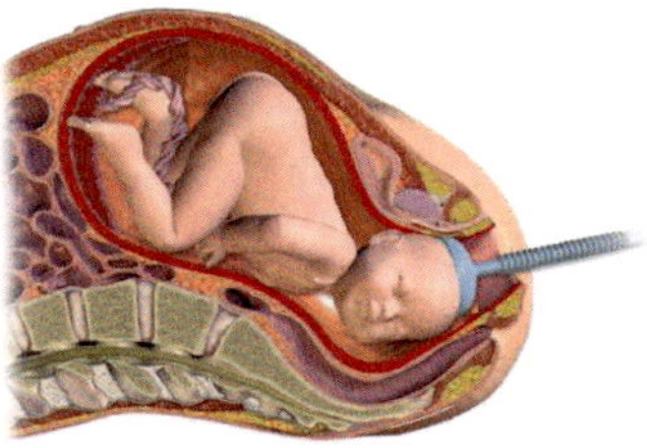

FIGURE 17.1.67 - Vacuum Delivery

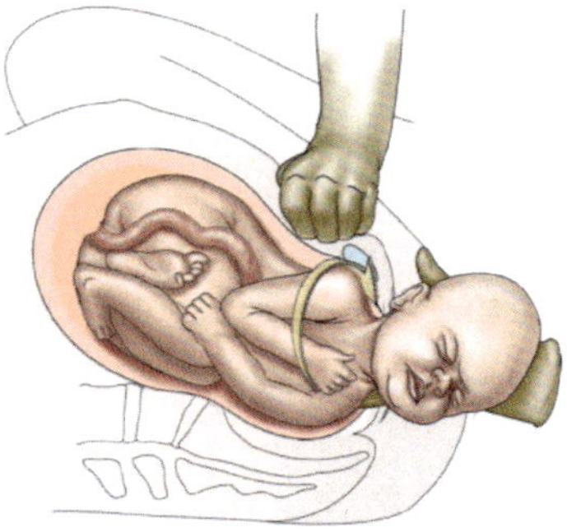

FIGURE 17.1.68 - Shoulder Dystocia

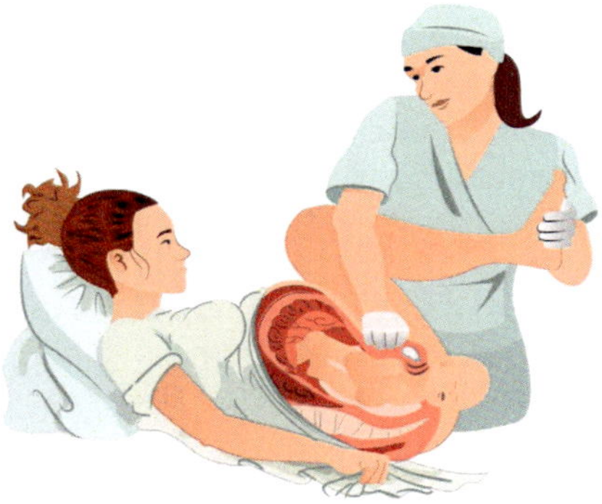

FIGURE 17.1.69 - McRoberts Maneuver

III. Shoulder Dystocia
   A. Lodged anterior shoulder under maternal symphysis pubis after vaginal delivery of fetal head
   B. Most cases are idiopathic
   C. Risk factors
      1. Maternal diabetes and obesity causing fetal macrosomia
      2. Post-term pregnancy
   D. Turtle sign: fetus retracts its head back into vagina
   E. Treatment ("BE CALM")
      1. **B**reath, do not push
      2. **E**levate legs (McRoberts maneuver)
      3. **C**all for help
      4. **A**pply suprapubic pressure
      5. En**L**arge vaginal opening
      6. **M**aneuvers
   F. Rubin maneuver: posterior pressure applied to anterior shoulder to bring baby in oblique position
   G. Woods-Screw maneuver: anterior shoulder pushed towards chest and posterior shoulder pushed towards back
   H. Gaskin maneuver: all fours position with arched back to enlarge pelvic outlet
   I. Zavanelli maneuver: pushing baby's head back and doing C-section
   J. Complications
      1. Brachial plexopathy: usually transient, most commonly Erb's palsy
      2. Clavicle fracture: can be intentional to facilitate delivery of anterior shoulder
      3. Humerus fracture
      4. Death due to hypoxia

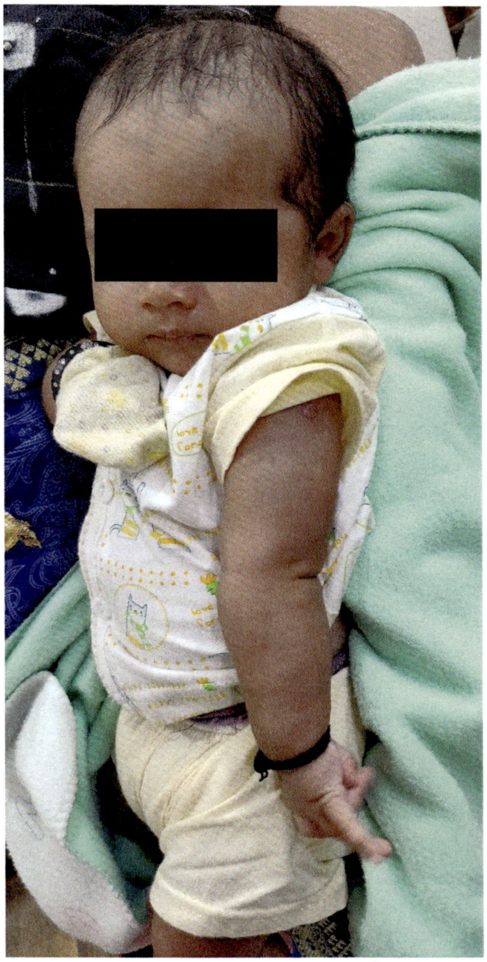

FIGURE 17.1.70 - "Waiter's Tip" Deformity

REVIEW QUESTIONS

1. A 35-year-old G2 P1 woman comes to the physician at 35 weeks of gestation for a routine prenatal visit. Her first baby was delivered via a classical cesarean section. Her vital signs and the physical exam are unremarkable. The patient wants to deliver her current baby vaginally. However, the physician recommends against the vaginal birth. What is the rationale behind the physician's recommendation for this patient?

   - **Since classical cesarean section is performed via vertical uterine incision, and leaves a significant scar on the uterus, trial of labor after classical C-section is associated with the risk for uterine rupture prior classical C-section - risk for uterine rupture in case of vaginal birth.**
   - This patient delivered her first baby via a classical cesarean section, and now she wants to deliver her baby via vaginal birth.
   - This is why the physician recommends against vaginal birth.

2. A 27-year-old G2 P1 woman is brought to the emergency department at 39 weeks of gestation due to severe uterine contractions every three minutes. She has a past medical history of type two diabetes mellitus. Her prepregnancy BMI was 30 kg/m2. Her vital signs include a temperature of 370 C (98.60 F), a blood pressure of 130/80 mmHg, a heart rate of 87 beats/min, and a respiratory rate of 17 breaths/min. The cervix is 6 cm dilated and 50% effaced. Several hours later the fetal head is delivered. However, progression of labor stops due to an inability to deliver the fetal shoulders. Which of the following is the best next step in the management of this patient?

   A. Flex the maternal hips and knees, and apply suprapubic pressure
   B. Apply posterior pressure to the anterior fetal shoulder
   C. Ask the mother to position herself in the all fours position and arch her back
   D. Push the baby's head back into the uterus and do a C-section

   - **The correct answer is option A.**
   - This patient with a past medical history of type two diabetes mellitus and a prepregnancy BMI of 30 kg/m2 presents in labor.
   - Several hours later the fetal head is delivered but then the progression of labor stops due to inability to deliver fetal shoulders.
   - This is a classic description of shoulder dystocia.
   - The best next step in the management of the patient with shoulder dystocia is to perform McRoberts maneuver. In other words, we should flex the maternal hips and knees, and apply suprapubic pressure.
   - Reviewing the treatment for Shoulder Dystocia "Be Calm", the Mc Roberts maneuver is the first maneuver that we apply to the mother in labor.
   - Options B and C are consistent with Rubin and Gaskin maneuvers, respectively. Rubin and Gaskin maneuvers are attempted only if McRoberts maneuver fails.
   - Finally, option D is consistent with the Zavanelli maneuver. Zavanelli maneuver is the last resort for managing shoulder dystocia.

Obstetrics | Section 18: Fetal Growth Restriction, Macrosomia & Amniotic Fluid Disorders

I. Fetal Growth Restriction
   A. Fetal weight < 10th percentile for gestational age
   B. Symmetric
      1. 1st trimester
      2. Chromosomal abnormalities or congenital infections
   C. Asymmetric (head-sparing)
      1. 2nd or 3rd trimester
      2. Uteroplacental insufficiency or maternal malnutrition
   D. Management
      1. Weekly biophysical profiles
      2. Serial umbilical artery Doppler ultrasonography
      3. Serial growth ultrasounds

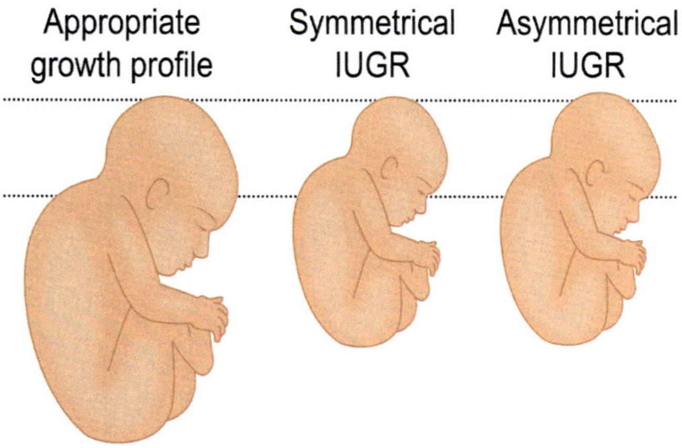

FIGURE 17.1.71 - Symmetric and Asymmetric Fetal Growth Restriction

II. Fetal Macrosomia
   A. Newborn weighs more than 4 kg
   B. Signs
      1. Large fundal height
      2. Polyhydramnios
   C. Risk factors
      1. Maternal diabetes
      2. Pregestational obesity
      3. Excessive gestational weight gain
      4. Prior history of fetal macrosomia
      5. Maternal age > 35
   D. Diagnosis
      1. Prenatal near-term ultrasound
      2. Postnatal weight measurement (> 4 kg)
   E. Prevention
      1. Control of maternal diabetes
      2. Control of gestational weight gain
      3. Regular exercise

III. Amniotic Fluid Disorders
   A. Derived mostly from fetal urine
      1. Renal disorders or placental insufficiency: decreased production
   B. Removed mostly via fetal swallowing
      1. Gastrointestinal or neurological conditions: decreased resorption
   C. Polyhydramnios
      1. Esophageal atresia
      2. Duodenal atresia
      3. Anencephaly
      4. Maternal diabetes
      5. Fetal anemia
      6. Multiple gestations
   D. Oligohydramnios
      1. Maternal hypertension
      2. Bilateral renal agenesis
      3. Posterior urethral valves
   E. Oligohydramnios can cause Potter sequence
      1. Pulmonary hypoplasia
      2. Facial and extremity defects

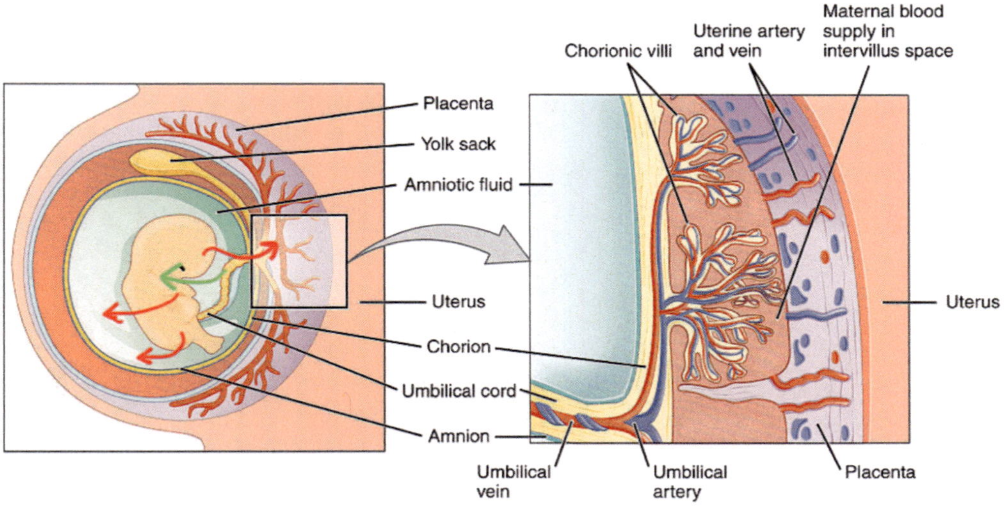

FIGURE 17.1.72 - Normal Amniotic Fluid Circulation

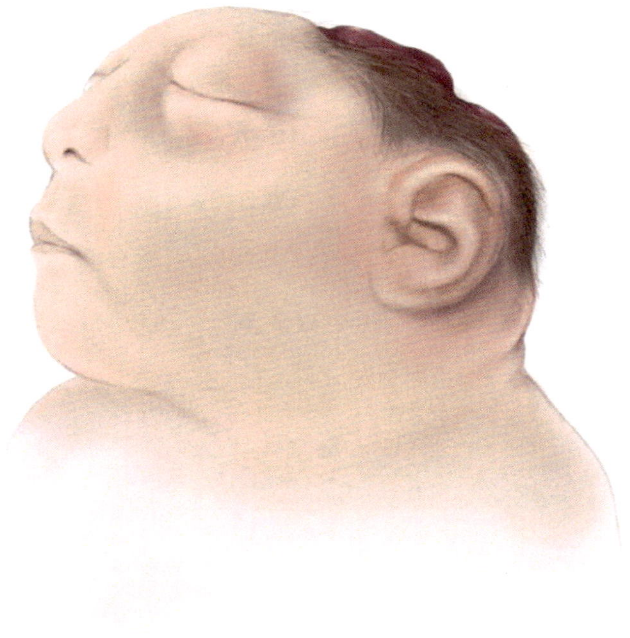

Centers for Disease Control and Prevention, National Center on Birth Defects and Developmental Disabilities, Public domain, via Wikimedia Commons

FIGURE 17.1.35 - Anencephaly

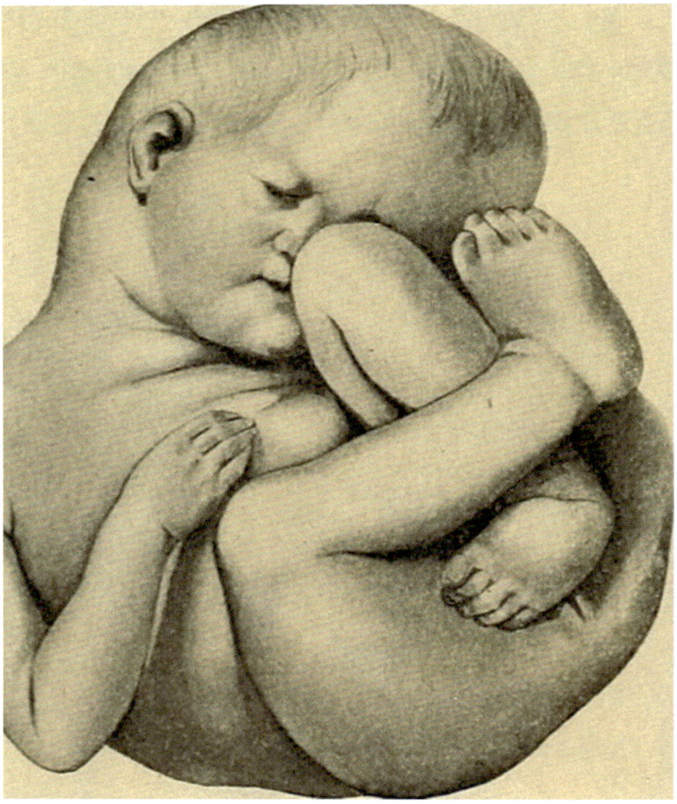

Public Domain

FIGURE 17.1.36 - Potter Sequence

REVIEW QUESTIONS

1. A 32-year-old G3P2 woman comes to her OBGYN at 36 weeks gestation for a routine prenatal visit. She gained 26 lbs (12 kg) during her current pregnancy. Her prepregnancy BMI was 23 kg/m^2. History is significant for gestational diabetes. Ultrasound shows a large baby with an amniotic fluid index of 28 cm. Which aspect of this patient's history contributed the most to fetal macrosomia?

- **The aspect of this patient's history that contributed the most to fetal macrosomia is her gestational diabetes mellitus.**
- This is a 32-year-old woman who has a history of gestational diabetes mellitus.
- She gained 26 lbs (12 kg) during her current pregnancy and prepregnancy her BMI was 23.
- Ultrasound reveals a large baby and polyhydramnios (amniotic fluid index > 24 cm).
- Maternal diabetes causes fetal hyperinsulinemia, which, in turn, results in excessive fat and glycogen deposition in tissues.
- She gained 26 lbs (12 kg), a normal weight gain for her given her normal prepregnancy BMI of 23 kg/m^2, therefore her BMI is unlikely the cause.

Obstetrics | Section 19: Hemolytic Disease of the Newborn

I. Hemolytic Disease of the Newborn: Introduction
   A. Also known as erythroblastosis fetalis

II. Hemolytic Disease of the Newborn: Rh Hemolytic Disease of the Newborn
   A. Rh negative mother and Rh positive fetus
   B. First Rh positive pregnancy is sensitization
   C. Subsequent Rh positive pregnancies at risk for HDN
   D. Prevent by giving RhoGAM to Rh negative patients at 28 weeks and within 72 hours of delivery

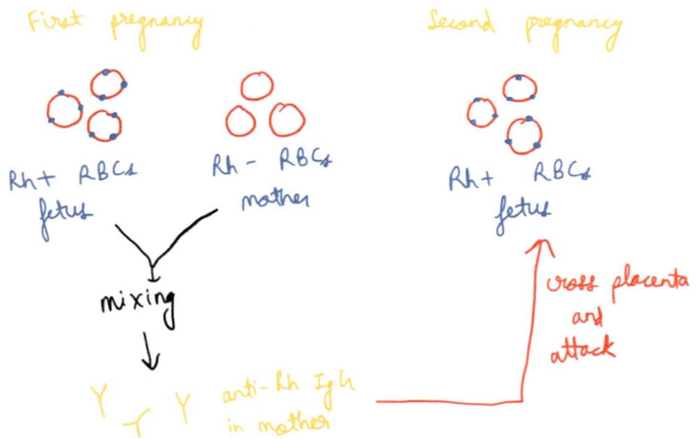

FIGURE 17.1.73 - Pathogenesis of Rh Hemolytic Disease of Newborn

III. Hemolytic Disease of the Newborn: ABO Hemolytic Disease of the Newborn
   A. Type O mother and type A or B fetus
   B. Preexisting maternal anti-A or anti-B IgG antibodies cross placenta and attack fetal RBCs
   C. First pregnancy affected (vs. Rh HDN)
   D. Milder than Rh HDN
   E. ABO incompatibility protects against Rh HDN

IV. Hemolytic Disease of the Newborn: Signs and Symptoms
   A. Hydrops fetalis (Rh HDN)
   B. Jaundice
   C. Kernicterus

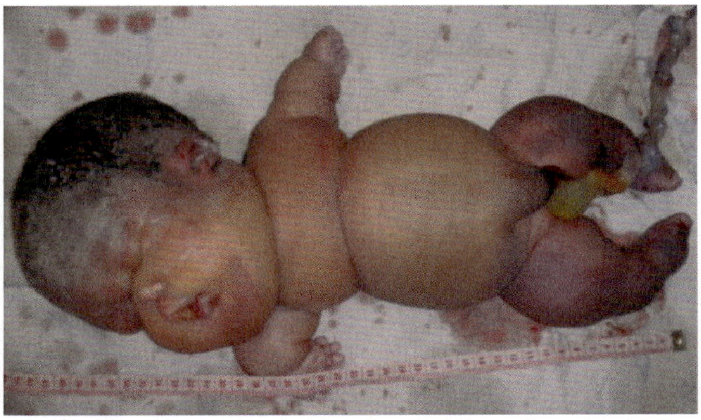

FIGURE 17.1.74 - Hydrops Fetalis

V. Hemolytic Disease of the Newborn: Treatment
   A. Phototherapy
   B. Exchange transfusion

REVIEW QUESTIONS

1. A 23-year-old G P0 woman comes to her primary care physician at 16 weeks gestation because of vaginal bleeding for the past day. She is Rh negative, while her husband is Rh positive. A cervical exam shows 10 cm cervical dilation. An ultrasound exam shows absent fetal cardiac activity. What is the best next step in management?
   - **The next best step in management is to administer anti-RhD immune globulin (RhoGAM) within the next 72 hours to prevent maternal alloimmunization against fetal Rh-positive red blood cells.**
   - This pregnant woman presents with vaginal bleeding, completely open cervical os, and absent fetal cardiac activity consistent with inevitable abortion.
   - She is Rh negative, while her husband is Rh positive.
   - Therefore, the chance of her fetus being Rh-positive is high.
   - RhoGAM should be administered to Rh-negative women if they have a miscarriage or stillbirth of Rh-positive fetus.

Obstetrics | Section 20: Post-Term Pregnancy & Multiple Gestations

I. Post-term Pregnancy
  A. Gestational age ≥ 42 weeks
  B. Risk factors
    1. Prior history of post-term pregnancy
    2. Nulliparity
    3. Obesity
    4. Age ≥ 35
  C. Fetal complications
    1. Macrosomia
    2. Oligohydramnios
    3. Demise
  D. Maternal complications
    1. Severe obstetric laceration
    2. Postpartum hemorrhage
  E. Management
    1. Regularly monitor the fetus via nonstress test
    2. Delivery prior to 43 weeks gestation

II. Multiple Gestations
  A. Dizygotic twins also known as fraternal twins
  B. 2 separate eggs simultaneously fertilized by 2 separate sperm cells
  C. Different genotypes
  D. Always dichorionic diamniotic
  E. Monozygotic twins also known as identical twins
  F. 1 egg fertilized by 1 sperm cell that splits in early pregnancy
  G. Chorionicity and amnionicity determined by time of zygote split
    1. 0 - 4 days: dichorionic diamniotic
    2. 4 - 8 days: monochorionic diamniotic
    3. 8 - 12 days: monochorionic monoamniotic
    4. ≥ 13 days: conjoined twins (shared body and organs)
  H. Twin-twin transfusion syndrome (TTTS)
    1. Abnormal arteriovenous anastomosis between monochorionic twins
    2. Donor twin: hypovolemia, anemia, oligohydramnios
    3. Recipient twin: hypervolemia, polycythemia, polyhydramnios
  I. Management
    1. Serial ultrasound, amnioreduction, laser ablation
  J. Timing of delivery
    1. Dichorionic diamniotic: 38th week of gestation
    2. Monochorionic diamniotic: 36th week of gestation
    3. Monochorionic monoamniotic: 32 - 34 weeks of gestation
  K. Route of delivery
    1. Cephalic/cephalic diamniotic: vaginal delivery of both twins
    2. Non-cephalic/cephalic diamniotic: cesarean delivery of both twins
    3. Non-cephalic/non-cephalic diamniotic: cesarean delivery for both twins
    4. Cephalic/non-cephalic diamniotic: vaginal delivery of twin A and breech extraction of twin B
  L. Timing of triplet delivery
    1. Monoamniotic or diamniotic: 32nd week of gestation
    2. Triamniotic: 35th week of gestation
  M. Route of triplet delivery
    1. Cesarean delivery

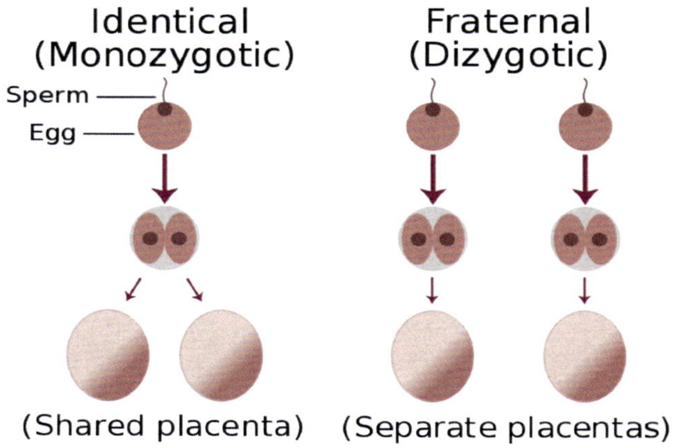

FIGURE 17.1.75 - Dizygotic and Monozygotic Twinning

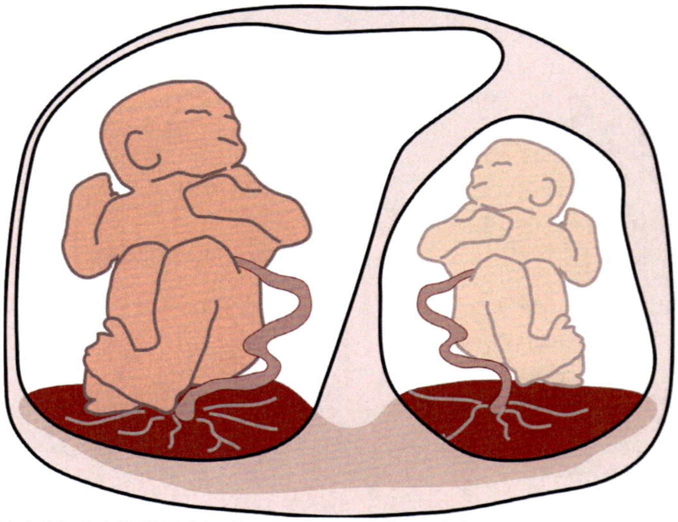

FIGURE 17.1.76 - Twin-Twin Transfusion Syndrome

REVIEW QUESTIONS

1. A 36-year-old G1P0 woman comes to her OBGYN at 42 weeks gestation for a routine prenatal visit. Her pregnancy has been uncomplicated. Ultrasound shows a large baby with increased biparietal diameter and femur length. The physician recommends inducing labor within the next several days. Which complications is this woman most likely to experience during vaginal delivery?

- **Complications this woman is most likely to experience are obstetric lacerations and postpartum hemorrhage.**
- This 36-year-old woman presents at 42 weeks gestation, which is a post-term pregnancy.
- Ultrasound shows a large baby consistent with fetal macrosomia.
- Vaginal delivery of a macrosomic fetus is commonly complicated by severe obstetric lacerations due to cephalopelvic disproportion.
- Another common intrapartum complication of delivery of a macrosomic fetus is a postpartum hemorrhage.

2. A 25-year-old G2P1 woman is admitted to the labor and delivery unit at 38 weeks gestation for planned labor. Her first pregnancy was uncomplicated. She has a history of gestational diabetes mellitus in her current pregnancy. Vital signs include a temperature of 98.6° F (37° C), blood pressure of 115/75 mmHg, heart rate of 95 beats/min, and respiratory rate of 17 breaths/min. Ultrasound shows dichorionic diamniotic non-cephalic/cephalic twins and an amniotic fluid index of 22 cm. Which of the following is the best route of delivery for this patient?

   A. Cesarean delivery of twin A and vaginal delivery of twin B
   B. Vaginal delivery of both twins
   C. Cesarean delivery of both twins
   D. Vaginal delivery for twin A and breech extraction for twin B

- **The correct answer is option C.**
- This patient has a twin pregnancy.
- She has dichorionic diamniotic non-cephalic/cephalic twins.
- This means that twin A is supposed to be delivered first, as it is in any presentation other than cephalic, while twin B should be delivered second, as it is in cephalic presentation.
- Whenever twin A in a diamniotic pregnancy is in non-cephalic presentation, vaginal delivery cannot be performed because there is a high risk of asphyxia. Instead, cesarean delivery of both twins should be performed, even for twin B, who is in cephalic presentation.
- Option A, cesarean delivery of twin A and vaginal delivery of twin B, is incorrect because once the cesarean section is done for the first twin, the second twin can easily be delivered via cesarean section as well.
- Option B, vaginal delivery of both twins, is incorrect because vaginal delivery of non-cephalic twin A is associated with an increased risk of obstetric complications like perinatal asphyxia.
- Option D, vaginal delivery of twin A and breech extraction for twin B, is performed when twin A is in cephalic presentation while twin B is in non-cephalic presentation.

Obstetrics | Section 21: Gestational Hypertension, Preeclampsia and HELLP Syndrome

I. Gestational Hypertension
   A. Blood pressure > 140/90 mm Hg after 20 weeks of gestation
   B. No proteinuria or end-organ damage (vs. preeclampsia)
   C. No pre-existing hypertension (vs. chronic hypertension)
   D. Diagnosis
      1. Documented high blood pressure after 20 weeks of gestation
      2. Proteinuria excluded via urinalysis
      3. End-organ damage excluded via complete blood count, liver function tests, and renal function tests
   E. Treatment
      1. Hydralazine, alpha-methyldopa, labetalol, or nifedipine

II. Preeclampsia Without Severe Features: Pathophysiology
   A. Abnormal cytotrophoblast invasion to the endometrium
   B. No vascular remodeling of the spiral artery
   C. Increased antiangiogenic factors and decreased proangiogenic factors
   D. Maternal vasospasm
   E. Hypertension and end-organ damage

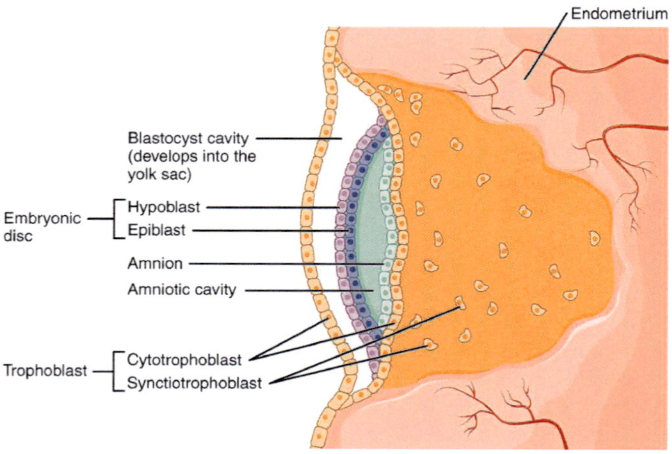

FIGURE 17.1.77 - Embryonic Disc and Trophoblast

III. Preeclampsia Without Severe Features: Risk Factors
   A. Prior preeclampsia
   B. Chronic kidney disease
   C. Chronic hypertension
   D. Diabetes mellitus
   E. Autoimmune disease
   F. Multiple gestation pregnancy

IV. Preeclampsia Without Severe Features: Clinical Manifestations
   A. SBP ≥ 140 mmHg and/or DBP ≥ 90 mmHg at ≥ 20 weeks of gestation
   B. Mild proteinuria (vs. preeclampsia with severe features)
   C. No end-organ damage (vs. preeclampsia with severe features)

V. Preeclampsia Without Severe Features: Management
   A. Antihypertensive medications
   B. Magnesium sulfate for seizure prophylaxis
   C. Delivery at > 37 weeks of gestation
   D. Prevent with low-dose aspirin starting at 12 weeks of gestation

VI. Preeclampsia with Severe Features
   A. Pathophysiology and risk factors: same as for preeclampsia without severe features
   B. Clinical manifestations
      1. SBP ≥ 160 mm Hg and/or DBP ≥ 110 mm Hg at ≥ 20 weeks of gestation
      2. Severe proteinuria, pulmonary and peripheral edema
      3. Visual/cerebral symptoms, high creatinine/LFTs, thrombocytopenia
   C. Management:
      1. Antihypertensive medications
      2. Magnesium sulfate for seizure prophylaxis
      3. Delivery at > 34 weeks of gestation (vs. > 37 weeks gestation)
      4. Prevent with low-dose aspirin starting at 12 weeks of gestation

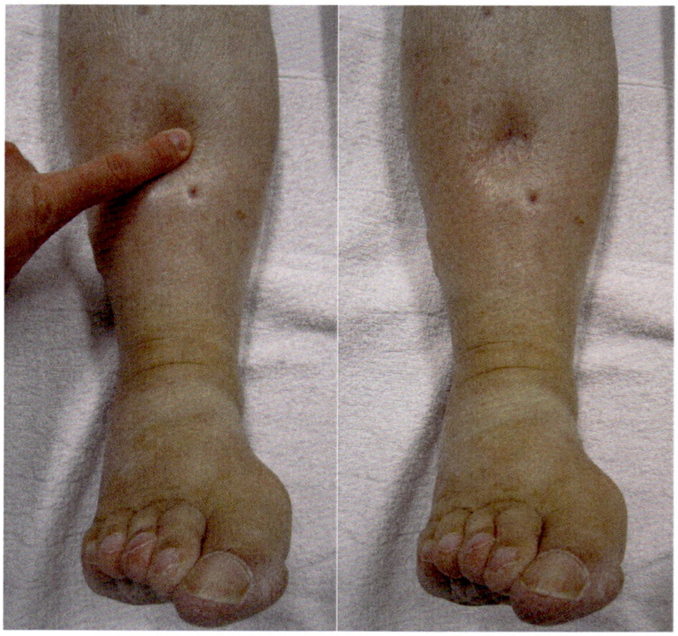

FIGURE 17.1.78 - Pitting Edema

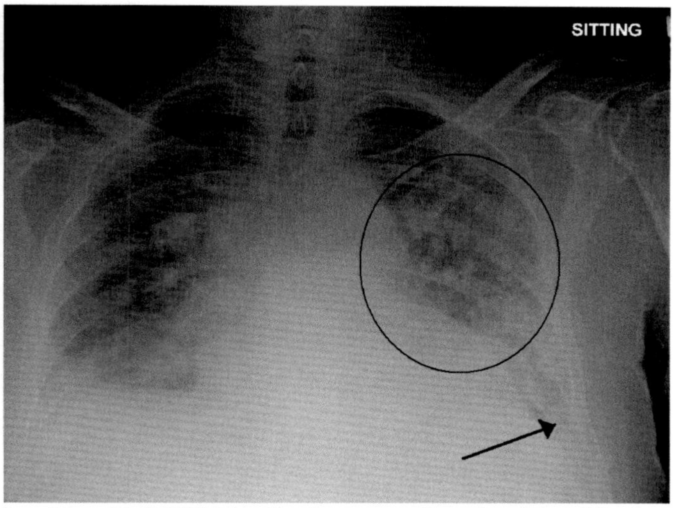

James Heilman, MD, CC BY-SA 3.0 <https://creativecommons.org/licenses/by-sa/3.0>, via Wikimedia Commons

FIGURE 17.1.79 - Chest X-ray: Bilateral Interstitial Infiltrates in Pulmonary Edema

VII. HELLP Syndrome
   A. Subtype of preeclampsia with severe features
   B. Clinical manifestations
      1. <u>H</u>emolysis (microangiopathic hemolytic anemia with high LDH, low haptoglobin, high indirect bilirubin)
      2. <u>E</u>levated <u>L</u>iver enzymes
      3. <u>L</u>ow <u>P</u>latelets (thrombocytopenia)
   C. Treatment
      1. Antihypertensive medications
      2. Magnesium sulfate for seizure prophylaxis
      3. Immediate delivery (obstetric emergency)

REVIEW QUESTIONS

1. A 27-year-old G2P1 woman comes to her OBGYN at 26 weeks gestation due to high blood pressure readings at home. She has never had hypertension before. She has a history of type 1 diabetes mellitus, diagnosed 10 years ago. Physical examination shows a blood pressure of 150/100 mmHg. Urinalysis is significant for 3+ proteinuria. What is the inciting event in the pathophysiology of this patient's condition?
   - **The inciting event in the pathophysiology of this patient's condition is insufficient cytotrophoblast invasion and abnormal spiral artery development.**
   - This pregnant patient, at 26 weeks of gestation, presents with hypertension and proteinuria.
   - She has no previous history of hypertension.
   - This presentation is consistent with the diagnosis of preeclampsia.
   - She has a past medical history of type 1 diabetes mellitus, which further supports the current diagnosis of preeclampsia because diabetes is a well-known risk factor.

2. A 25-year-old G2P2 woman comes to her OBGYN at 14 weeks gestation for a routine prenatal visit. Her two previous pregnancies were complicated by preeclampsia. Vital signs and laboratory findings are unremarkable. Which medication should be initiated in this patient?
   - **The medication that should be initiated is low-dose aspirin.**
   - This pregnant woman comes in at 14 weeks gestation for a routine prenatal visit.
   - She has a history of preeclampsia in both of her prior pregnancies.
   - However, her vital signs and laboratory findings are unremarkable at the current visit.
   - In order to prevent preeclampsia in her current pregnancy, she should be started on low-dose aspirin.

Obstetrics | Section 22: Eclampsia, Acute Fatty Liver of Pregnancy and Chronic Hypertension

I. Eclampsia: Clinical Manifestations
   A. Preeclampsia with severe features and seizures
   B. Generalized tonic-clonic seizures usually lasting less than 1 minute
   C. Postictal state
   D. Hyperreflexia
   E. Visual disturbances (e.g. scotoma)

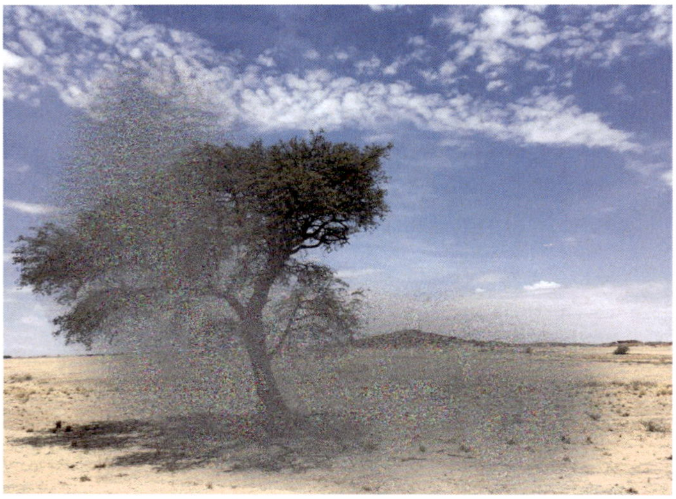

FIGURE 17.1.80 - Visual Field of a Patient with Scotoma

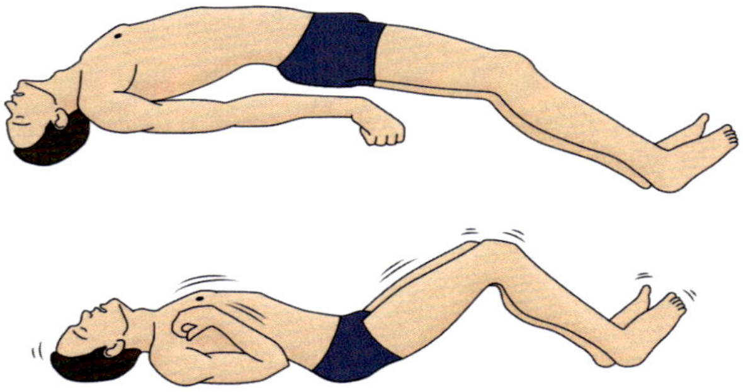

FIGURE 17.1.81 - Tonic-Clonic Seizure

II. Eclampsia: Diagnosis
   A. Preeclampsia and seizures when there is no other neurological condition that could account for seizures
   B. Bilateral frontal and occipital lobe edema on CT scan of the head

III. Eclampsia: Treatment
   A. Antihypertensive medications
   B. Magnesium sulfate for seizure termination
   C. Immediate delivery

IV. Acute Fatty Liver of Pregnancy: Pathophysiology
   A. Fulminant liver failure due to fat deposition

V. Acute Fatty Liver of Pregnancy: Clinical Features
   A. Nausea and vomiting
   B. Right upper quadrant and epigastric pain

VI. Acute Fatty Liver of Pregnancy: Laboratory Findings
   A. High bilirubin
   B. High aminotransferases
   C. Thrombocytopenia
   D. Hypoglycemia
   E. Disseminated intravascular coagulation (DIC)

VII. Acute Fatty Liver of Pregnancy: Treatment
   A. Immediate delivery

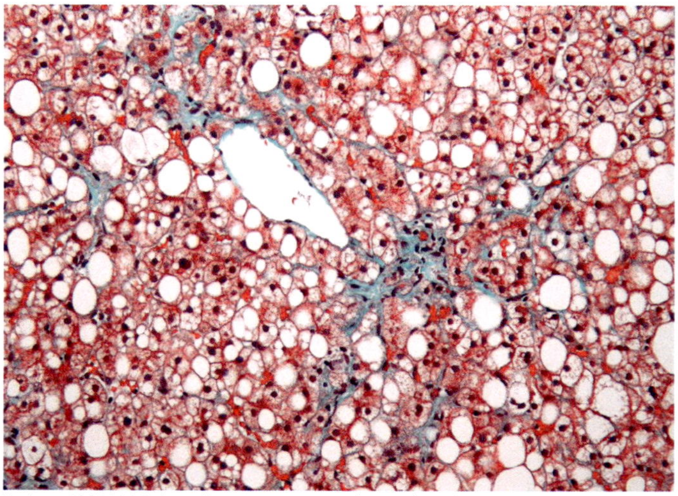

FIGURE 17.1.82 - Liver Biopsy Showing Lipid Droplets

VIII. Chronic Hypertension
   A. SBP ≥ 130 mmHg and/or DBP ≥ 80 mmHg before onset of pregnancy or before 20 weeks of gestation
   B. No proteinuria
   C. No acute end-organ damage
   D. Subacute and chronic end-organ damage might be present

IX. Chronic Hypertension: Treatment
   A. Treatment before pregnancy
      1. ACE inhibitors, ARBs, thiazide diuretics, dihydropyridine calcium channel blockers
   B. Treatment during pregnancy
      1. Hydralazine, alpha-methyldopa, labetalol, nifedipine

X. Chronic Hypertension with Superimposed Preeclampsia
   A. SBP ≥ 130 mmHg and/or DBP ≥ 80 mmHg before onset of pregnancy or before 20 weeks of gestation
   B. After 20 weeks of gestation
      1. Clinical features of preeclampsia
      2. Increase in blood pressure (> 140/90 mmHg)
      3. Proteinuria
      4. Possible end-organ damage

XI. Chronic Hypertension with Superimposed Preeclampsia: Treatment
   A. Treatment before pregnancy
      1. ACE inhibitors, ARBs, thiazide diuretics, dihydropyridine calcium channel blockers
   B. Treatment during pregnancy
      1. Hydralazine, alpha-methyldopa, labetalol, nifedipine

REVIEW QUESTIONS

1. A 31-year-old G1P0 woman comes to her OBGYN at 35 weeks gestation because of nausea and vomiting for the last 2 days. She also complains of right upper quadrant abdominal pain. She has never had similar symptoms before. Her ALT is 3,000 U/L (10 - 40 U/L) and her AST is 2,500 U/L (12 - 38 U/L). Total bilirubin is 15 mg/dL (0.1 - 1.0 mg/dL) and direct bilirubin is 7 mg/dL (0 - 0.3 mg/dL). Blood glucose is 65 mg/dL (70 - 100 mg/dL). What is the best next step in the management?

   - **The best next step in the management of acute fatty liver of pregnancy is immediate delivery.**
   - This woman presents in her third trimester of pregnancy with nausea, vomiting, and right upper quadrant abdominal pain.
   - Laboratory studies are significant for elevated transaminases and mixed hyperbilirubinemia.
   - This presentation is consistent with the diagnosis of acute fatty liver of pregnancy and requires immediate delivery regardless of gestational age.

REVIEW QUESTIONS

2. A 20-year-old G1P0 woman at 38 weeks gestation is brought to the emergency department because of generalized tonic-clonic seizures that started 1 hour ago. She takes no medications other than prenatal vitamins. A previous prenatal visit showed hypertension, and proteinuria. Vital signs include temperature of 98.6° F (37° C), blood pressure of 170/120 mmHg, heart rate of 94 beats/min, and respiratory rate of 18 breaths/min. The patient has a repeated seizure in the emergency department. Which of the following is the next best step in the management of this patient?

   A. IV labetalol
   B. IV magnesium sulfate
   C. IV terbutaline
   D. IV normal saline

   - **The correct answer is option B.**
   - This woman presents with seizures and recently had a prenatal examination showing hypertension and proteinuria concerning for preeclampsia.
   - Given that she has now started to have seizures she has progressed to eclampsia.
   - The first priority in eclampsia is to terminate the seizure and then deliver the baby emergently.
   - The first-line drug used to terminate seizures in pregnant women with eclampsia is IV magnesium sulfate.
   - Option A is incorrect because although IV labetalol will be given urgently to this patient with eclampsia, the first priority is to terminate the seizure. Then we can deal with her hypertension.
   - Option C, IV terbutaline, is incorrect because eclampsia is managed with emergent delivery of the fetus. Terbutaline, on the other hand, is tocolytic and, therefore, it will delay delivery.
   - Option D is incorrect because IV normal saline is not essential in this particular case. It is more important to terminate the seizure first rather than to give her fluids.

Obstetrics | Section 23: Diabetes During Pregnancy

I. Gestational Diabetes Mellitus: Definition
   A. Diabetes mellitus starting after 20 weeks gestation
   B. No history of diabetes before pregnancy

II. Gestational Diabetes Mellitus: Pathophysiology
   A. Human placental lactogen increases insulin resistance
   B. Hyperglycemia
   C. Compensatory hyperinsulinemia by pancreas
   D. GDM if pancreas cannot overcome insulin resistance

III. Gestational Diabetes Mellitus: Risk Factors
   A. Obesity
   B. Family history (1st degree relative)
   C. History of GDM in prior pregnancy

IV. Gestational Diabetes Mellitus: Clinical Features
   A. Mother
      1. Polydipsia
      2. Polyuria and glucosuria
   B. Fetus
      1. Polycythemia
      2. Organomegaly and macrosomia
      3. Neonatal hypoglycemia and birth traumas

V. Fetal Complications: Brachial Plexopathy
   A. Erb palsy or Klumpke palsy
   B. Good prognosis
   C. Erb palsy
      1. Damage of upper trunk (C5 - C6) with "waiter's tip"
   D. Klumpke palsy
      1. Damage of lower trunk (C8 - T1) with "claw hand"

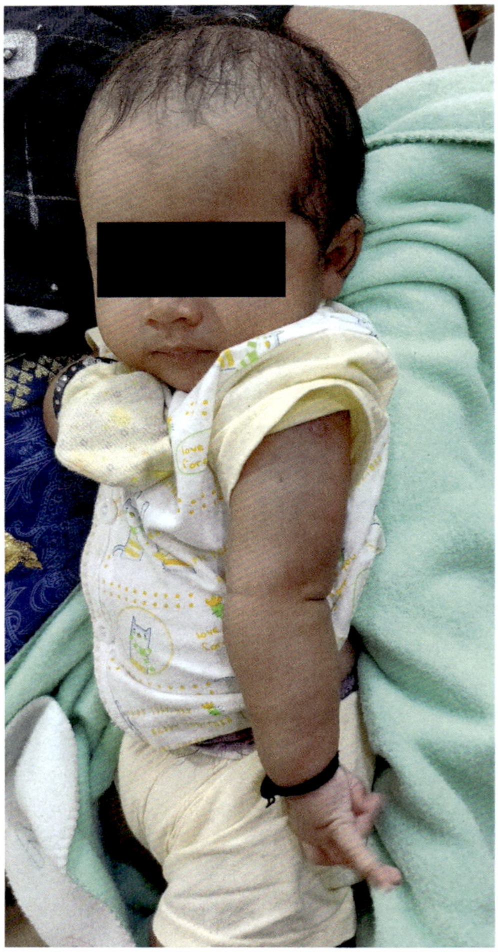

FIGURE 17.1.70 - "Waiter's Tip" Deformity in Erb Palsy

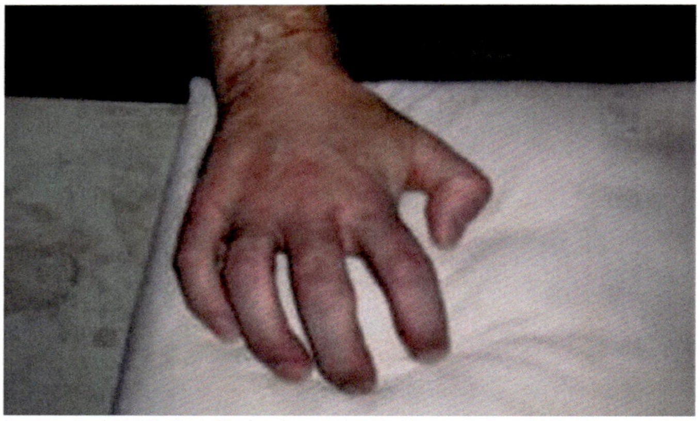

FIGURE 17.1.83 - "Claw Hand" in Klumpke Palsy

VI. Fetal Complications: Shoulder Dystocia
   A. Anterior shoulder lodged under pubic symphysis
   B. Due to fetal macrosomia
   C. Can lead to brachial plexus injury
   D. Special maneuvers necessary for successful management

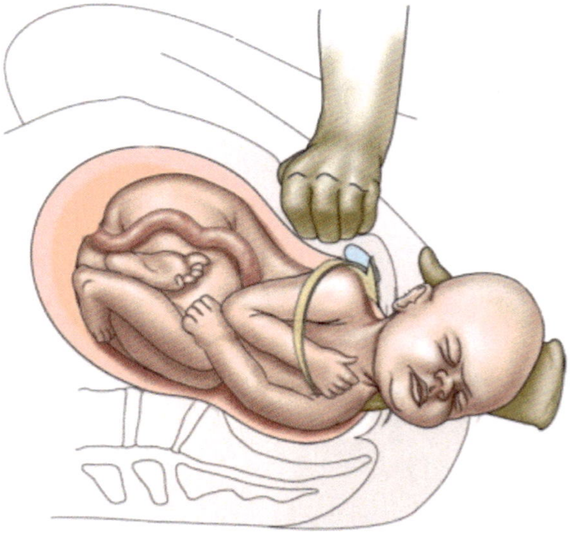

FIGURE 17.1.68 - Shoulder Dystocia

VII. Gestational Diabetes Mellitus: Diagnosis

A. 1-hour glucose challenge test (screening test)
   1. Performed at 24-28 weeks gestation
   2. 50 g of glucose in water ingested
   3. Blood glucose measured 1 hour after ingestion
   4. Blood glucose ≥ 140 mg/dL is positive result
   5. Positive result needs confirmation with 3-hour glucose challenge test

B. 3-hour glucose challenge test (confirmatory test)
   1. 100 g of glucose in water ingested
   2. Blood glucose measured at fasting, 1, 2, and 3 hours after ingestion
   3. Glucose cut-off values:
      a) Fasting: ≥ 95 mg/dL; 1-hour: ≥ 180 mg/dL
      b) 2-hour: ≥ 155 mg/dL; 3-hour: ≥ 140 mg/dL
      c) ≥ 2 criteria met: diagnostic for GDM

VIII. Gestational Diabetes Mellitus: Treatment

A. Mother:
   1. Diet low in carbohydrates
   2. Mild to moderate exercise (upregulates GLUT-4 expression)
   3. If insufficient, add insulin

B. Fetus:
   1. Regular fetal ultrasound
   2. Possible cesarean delivery due to macrosomia

IX. Gestational Diabetes Mellitus: Follow-Up

A. Insulin no longer required after delivery

B. 2-hour glucose challenge test to ensure resolution of GDM
   1. 75 g of glucose ingested
   2. Blood glucose measured 2 hours after ingestion
   3. Glucose < 140 mg/dL confirms resolution of GDM
   4. Glucose 140 - 199 mg/dL is pre-diabetes
   5. Glucose ≥ 200 mg/dL is diabetes

X. Pregestational Diabetes Mellitus: Definition

A. Diabetes mellitus starting before pregnancy or within first 20 weeks of gestation

XI. Pregestational Diabetes Mellitus: Pathophysiology

A. Either type 1 or type 2

B. Type 1
   1. Pancreatic beta-cell destruction

C. Type 2
   1. Insulin resistance

XII. Pregestational Diabetes Mellitus: Risk Factors

A. Family history

B. Obesity (type 2 DM)

C. Other autoimmune disorders (type 1 DM)

XIII. Pregestational Diabetes Mellitus: Clinical Features

A. Mother (polyuria, polydipsia)

B. Fetus
   1. Spontaneous abortion
   2. Transposition of great vessels, transient HOCM
   3. Small left colon syndrome
   4. Caudal regression syndrome
   5. Sirenomelia (mermaid syndrome)

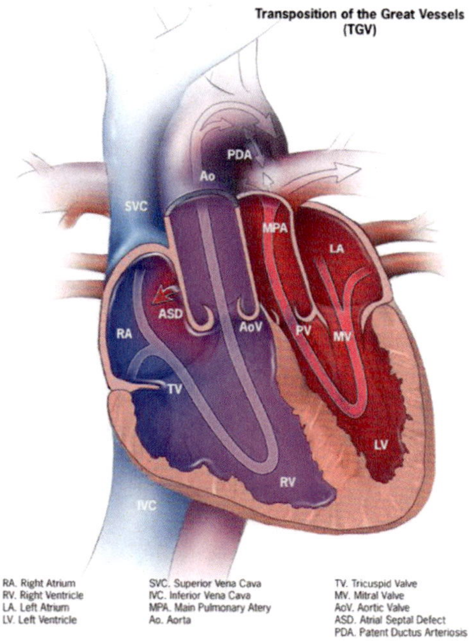

Centers for Disease Control and Prevention, CC0, via Wikimedia Commons

FIGURE 17.1.84 - Transposition of Great Vessels

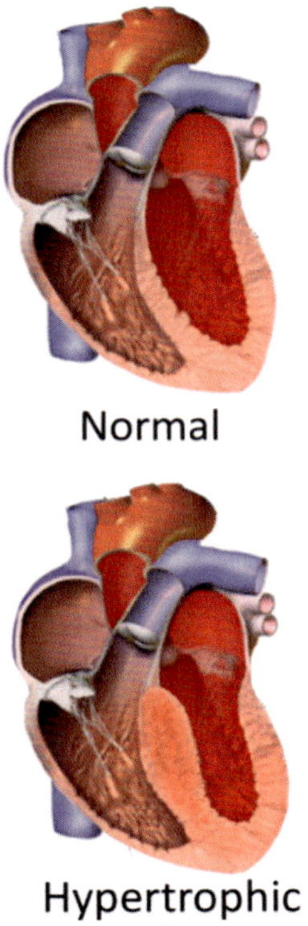

Npatchett at English Wikipedia, CC BY-SA 3.0 <https://creativecommons.org/licenses/by-sa/3.0>, via Wikimedia Commons

FIGURE 17.1.85 - Hypertrophic Obstructive Cardiomyopathy

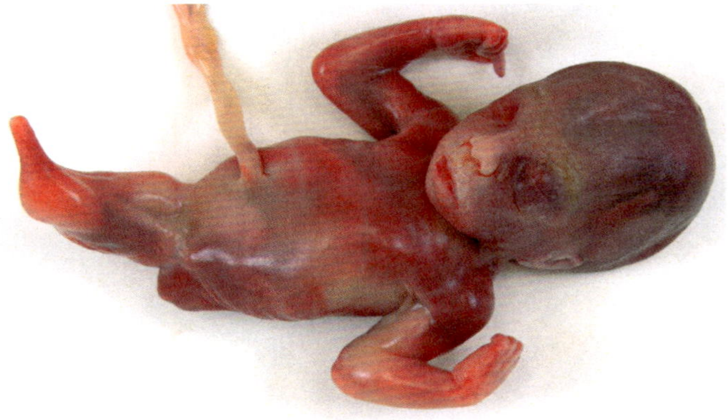

FIGURE 17.1.86 - Sirenomelia (Mermaid Syndrome)

XIV. Pregestational Diabetes Mellitus: Diagnosis
   A. If not diagnosed before conception, measure HbA1c in first trimester
   B. HbA1c ≥ 6.5% is diagnostic for DM
   C. HbA1c shows average glycemic control over past 3 months

XV. Pregestational Diabetes Mellitus: Treatment
   A. Mother
      1. Diet low in carbohydrates
      2. Mild to moderate exercise
      3. Increase insulin dose while pregnant
   B. Fetus
      1. Regular fetal ultrasound
      2. Possible cesarean delivery due to macrosomia

XVI. Pregestational Diabetes Mellitus: Follow-Up
   A. Continue glucose monitoring
   B. Decrease insulin dose after delivery as appropriate

REVIEW QUESTIONS

1. Which hormone plays an essential role in the pathogenesis of gestational diabetes?
   - **The hormone that plays an essential role in the pathogenesis of gestational diabetes is human placental lactogen.**
   - Human placental lactogen is a hormone that induces insulin resistance.

2. A pregnant woman at 26 weeks gestation has a blood glucose level of 120 mg/dL 1 hour after ingesting 50g of glucose dissolved in water. What is the best next step in management?
   - **The next best step in management is to stop screening for gestational diabetes.**
   - A negative 1-hour glucose challenge test is when the measurement is less than 140 mg/dL.
   - Therefore, her expectant management should be continued without the need for a 3-hour glucose challenge test.

REVIEW QUESTIONS

3. A 32-year-old G2P1 woman comes to her OBGYN at 27 weeks gestation for a routine prenatal visit. She has no specific complaints. History includes gestational diabetes mellitus in her previous pregnancy which resolved after delivery. Vital signs include temperature of 96.8° F (36° C), blood pressure of 125/70 mmHg, heart rate of 92 beats/min, and respiratory rate of 16 breaths/min. Physical examination shows a fundal height of 27 cm. A 1-hour glucose challenge test shows a blood glucose level of 150 mg/dL. She also undergoes a 3-hour glucose challenge test that shows a fasting glucose of 110 mg/dL, 1-hour glucose level of 200 mg/dL, 2-hour glucose level of 140 mg/dL, and 3-hour glucose level of 130 mg/dL. Which of the following is the most likely effect of this patient's condition on her child?

   A. Klumpke palsy
   B. Small left colon syndrome
   C. Transposition of great vessels
   D. Sirenomelia

   - **The correct answer is option A.**
   - This pregnant woman presents for a routine prenatal visit at 27 weeks gestation.
   - She has a history of gestational diabetes mellitus in her previous pregnancy which resolved after delivery. Therefore, If she has diabetes now, it cannot be pregestational because her hyperglycemia resolved before her current pregnancy.
   - Gestational diabetes mellitus is diagnosed if ≥ 2 criteria of 3-hour glucose challenge test are met.
   - She meets exactly two criteria, that is, fasting glucose ≥ 95 mg/dL and 1-hour glucose ≥ 180 mg/dL.
   - Gestational diabetes can cause fetal macrosomia with resultant shoulder dystocia. Shoulder dystocia, in turn, can cause brachial plexopathy including Klumpke palsy.
   - Options B, C, and D are incorrect because small left colon syndrome, transposition of great vessels, and sirenomelia occur if a fetus is exposed to maternal hyperglycemia in the first trimester. In other words, these complications happen only in pregestational diabetes mellitus.

Obstetrics | Section 24: Acute Pyelonephritis, *Group B Streptococcus* & Chorioamnionitis

I. Acute Pyelonephritis
   A. Upper urinary tract infection
   B. Risk factors
      1. Diabetes mellitus
      2. Asymptomatic bacteriuria
      3. Age < 20
   C. Pathogens
      1. *E. coli*, *Enterobacter*, *Klebsiella*, Group B *Streptococcus*
   D. Complications
      1. Preterm labor
      2. Low birth weight
   E. Treatment
      1. IV ceftriaxone followed by oral cephalexin if afebrile for 48 hours
      2. Total duration: 5 - 14 days
   F. Preventing recurrence
      1. Low-dose daily prophylaxis
         a) 3rd trimester urine culture
      2. No prophylaxis
         a) Monthly urine culture

II. Group B Streptococcus
   A. Gram positive *Streptococcus*
   B. Colonizes vagina
   C. Most common cause of neonatal
      1. Sepsis
      2. Meningitis
      3. Pneumonia
   D. Can cause chorioamnionitis during pregnancy
   E. Antenatal screening: rectovaginal swab at 35 - 37 weeks
   F. Indications for intrapartum prophylaxis (IV penicillin/ ampicillin)
      1. Prior infant with neonatal GBS infection (no need for swab)
      2. GBS bacteriuria or UTI in current pregnancy (no need for swab)
      3. Unknown GBS status and intrapartum fever, preterm labor, or ROM > 18 hours
      4. GBS positive rectovaginal culture

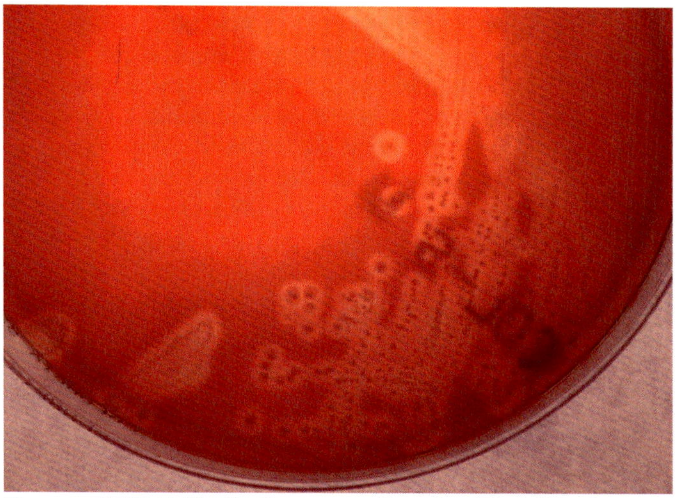

FIGURE 17.1.5 - Blood Agar: Colonies of *Group B Streptococcus*

III. Chorioamnionitis
   A. Risk factors
      1. Prolonged ROM (> 18 hours)
      2. PPROM
      3. Prolonged labor
      4. Internal fetal monitoring device
      5. Repetitive vaginal examination
      6. Presence of genital tract infection
   B. Diagnosis: maternal fever and at least one of the following
      1. Purulent amniotic fluid
      2. Maternal leukocytosis
      3. Fetal tachycardia (> 160 beats/min)
   C. Treatment
      1. Delivery
      2. Broad-spectrum antibiotics (ampicillin and gentamicin)
   D. Maternal complications
      1. Postpartum hemorrhage
      2. Endometritis
   E. Fetal complications
      1. Neonatal sepsis
      2. Pneumonia
      3. Cerebral palsy

REVIEW QUESTIONS

1. A 27-year-old G2P1 woman comes to her OBGYN at 32 weeks gestation for a routine prenatal visit. Her previous pregnancy was complicated by neonatal *Group B Streptococcus* (GBS) pneumonia. The physician tells her that she will need intrapartum penicillin prophylaxis for GBS without the need for a rectovaginal swab. What is the most likely rationale behind administering intrapartum penicillin to this patient without the rectovaginal swab?

- **The rationale behind administering intrapartum penicillin without the rectovaginal swab is previous neonatal GBS infection.**
- This pregnant patient, at 32 weeks gestation, presents for a routine neonatal visit.
- She has a prior history of neonatal *Group B Streptococcus* (GBS) pneumonia in her first child.
- History of previous early-onset neonatal GBS infection is an indication for intrapartum penicillin prophylaxis for GBS in the current pregnancy without the need for a rectovaginal swab
- The swab is not needed because the patient is already at high risk for having GBS vaginal colonization and her fetus is at high risk for acquiring the infection with GBS.

2. A 25-year-old G1P0 woman at 34 weeks gestation is brought to the emergency department by her partner because of rupture of membranes 20 hours ago. She did not have any prenatal care. Her cervix is 80% effaced and 8 cm dilated. Cardiotocography shows a fetal heart rate of 180 beats/min and uterine contractions with an intensity of 300 MVU (Normal: > 200 MVU). Amniotic fluid is purulent. The patient's vital signs include temperature of 102.2° F (39° C), blood pressure of 90/70 mmHg, heart rate of 150 beats/min, and respiratory rate of 18 breaths/min. Basic metabolic panel shows sodium of 138 mEq/L (136 - 145 mEq/L) and potassium of 4 mEq/L (3.5 - 5 mEq/L). Complete blood count is significant for leukocyte count of 20,500 cells/mm^3 (4,500 - 11,000 cells/mm^3). Which of the following is the best next step in management?

   A. IV nifedipine
   B. IV oxytocin
   C. IV ampicillin and gentamicin
   D. IV 0.45% saline

- **The correct answer is option C.**
- This pregnant woman at 34 weeks gestation has prolonged rupture of membranes.
- She has had no prenatal care.
- Vitals are significant for a fever, and her amniotic fluid is purulent, which is concerning for chorioamnionitis.
- Chorioamnionitis is typically a polymicrobial infection; group *B Streptococcus* must be covered, as well as Gram-negative bacteria.
- The next best step in management is broad-spectrum antibiotics, such as IV ampicillin and gentamicin.
- Option A is incorrect because IV nifedipine is a tocolytic agent. Tocolytics are avoided in a patient with suspected chorioamnionitis because these medications will delay the delivery of the fetus.
- Option B, IV oxytocin, is incorrect because this patient has adequate uterine contractions evidenced by a contraction intensity of 300 MVU. Therefore, she does not need augmentation of labor with oxytocin.
- Option D is incorrect because IV 0.45% saline is hypotonic. This patient certainly needs IV fluids because she is hypotensive and tachycardic. However, she needs isotonic, rather than hypotonic, fluids like 0.9% saline or lactated Ringer's solution.

Obstetrics | Section 25: Hepatitis B, Parvovirus & HIV in Pregnancy

I. Hepatitis B
   A. 90% risk of transmission without prophylaxis
   B. < 2% risk of transmission with prophylaxis
   C. Risk factors: high maternal viral load, maternal HBeAg+
   D. Routes of transmission
      1. Transvaginal (most common)
      2. Transplacental
   E. Prevention
      1. HBV vaccine (active immunization)
      2. HBIG (passive immunization)

II. Parvovirus
   A. Infects RBCs and endothelial cells
   B. Mother
      1. Pure RBC aplasia
      2. Rheumatoid arthritis-like arthropathy
   C. Fetus
      1. Hydrops fetalis

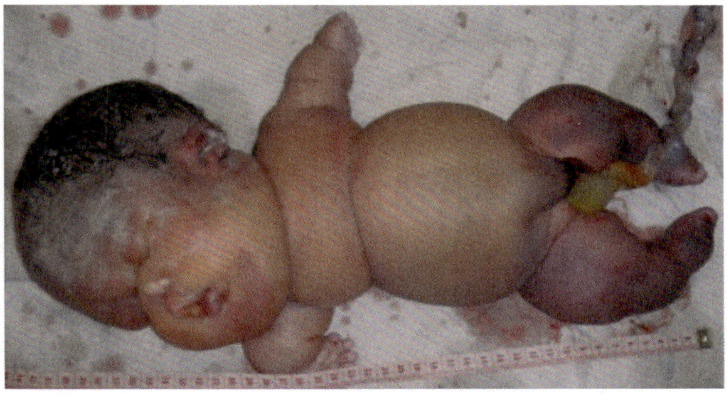

FIGURE 17.1.87 - Hydrops Fetalis

III. HIV
   A. Neonatal HIV
   B. Routes of fetal acquisition: transplacental, transvaginal
   C. Risk factors: high maternal viral load, breastfeeding by infected mother
   D. Signs and symptoms
      1. Chronic diarrhea
      2. Failure to thrive and generalized lymphadenopathy
      3. Pneumocystis infection
   E. Diagnosis
      1. Viral load
      2. Persistence of HIV antibody after 18 months
   F. Treatment
      1. Start antiretroviral therapy as soon as possible
      2. Maternal viral load < 1000 copies/mL at birth: zidovudine in infant
      3. Maternal viral load > 1000 copies/mL at birth: multidrug ART

REVIEW QUESTIONS

1. A newborn baby girl was born 2 hours ago to a G1P1 mother at 37 weeks gestation via vaginal delivery. The pregnancy and delivery were uncomplicated. The mother has a history of chronic hepatitis B. Vital signs and physical examination of the neonate are unremarkable. What is the next best step in the management of this newborn?
   - **The best next step in the management of this newborn is to administer the HBV vaccine and HBIG.**
   - This neonate was born to a mother with chronic hepatitis B.
   - Newborns of mothers with chronic hepatitis B (HBV) receive hepatitis B vaccine, just like all newborns, regardless of the maternal HBV status.
   - Additionally, this child should receive hepatitis B immune globulin (HBIG) to reduce the risk of perinatal HBV transmission.

REVIEW QUESTIONS

2. A 3-hour-old baby boy, born at 38 weeks gestation to a G3P2 mother via vaginal delivery. Apgar scores were 8 and 9 at 1 and 5 minutes, respectively. The pregnancy and delivery were uncomplicated. The mother has a history of HIV infection treated with antiretroviral therapy, and her intrapartum HIV viral load was 200 copies/mm^3. Neonatal vital signs include a temperature of 96.8° F (36° C), blood pressure of 60/40 mmHg, heart rate of 150 beats/min, and respiratory rate of 52 breaths/min. Physical examination is unremarkable. Which of the following is the best initial step in the management of this patient?

   A. Measure HIV viral load
   B. Measure anti-HIV IgG antibody
   C. Start antiretroviral therapy
   D. Isolate the patient from the mother

- **The correct answer is option A.**
- This neonate is born to a mother with HIV infection.
- Maternal intrapartum HIV viral load was <1000 copies/$mm^{3,}$ which explains why she delivered the boy via vaginal delivery.
- Even in cases of low maternal intrapartum HIV viral load, there is still a chance of perinatal HIV transmission. Therefore, the neonatal HIV status must be checked. This is done via neonatal HIV viral load measurement.
- Option B is incorrect because this baby boy will likely have a positive anti-HIV IgG antibody from transplacental antibody transfer. However, the presence of the antibody at birth does not necessarily mean that the neonate is also infected. It is only the persistence of anti-HIV antibodies beyond 18 months of age that confirms HIV infection in infants.
- Option C is incorrect because the newborn must first be diagnosed with HIV before starting antiretroviral therapy.
- Option D is incorrect because there is no need to isolate the patient from the mother physically. HIV is not transmitted via aerosols or respiratory droplets, although it can be transmitted via breastfeeding.

Obstetrics | Section 26: TORCHES Infections

I. Overview
   A. T = Toxoplasmosis
   B. O = Other (Zika and Varicella zoster virus)
   C. R = Rubella
   D. C = Cytomegalovirus
   E. He = Herpes simplex virus
   F. S = Syphilis

II. Toxoplasmosis
   A. Congenital toxoplasmosis
   B. Routes of maternal acquisition: undercooked pork, cat feces
   C. Neonatal manifestations: triad
      1. Diffuse intracranial calcifications
      2. Hydrocephalus
      3. Chorioretinitis
   D. Treatment: pyrimethamine and sulfadiazine

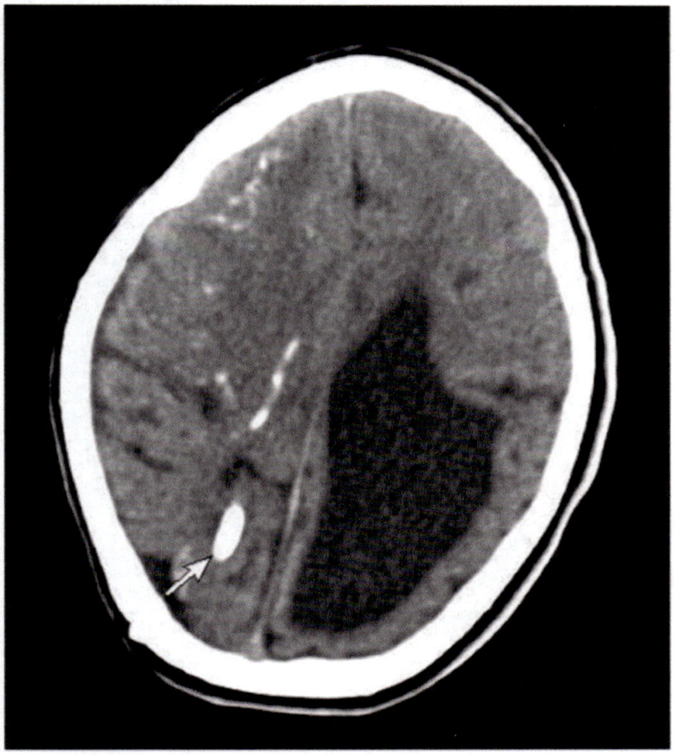

FIGURE 17.1.88 - CT Scan of Head: Intracranial Calcifications and Hydrocephalus in Congenital Toxoplasmosis

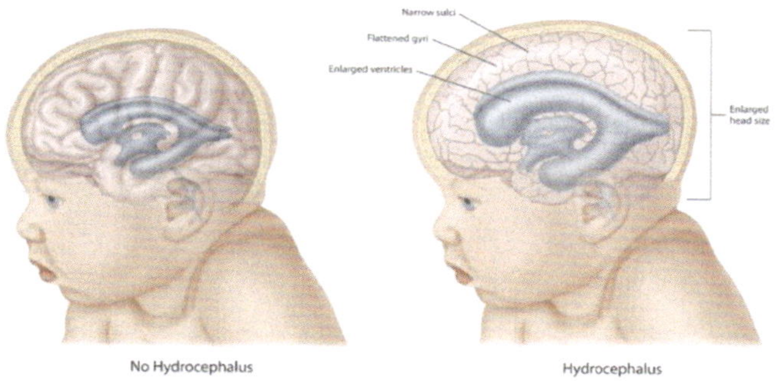

FIGURE 17.1.89 - Hydrocephalus

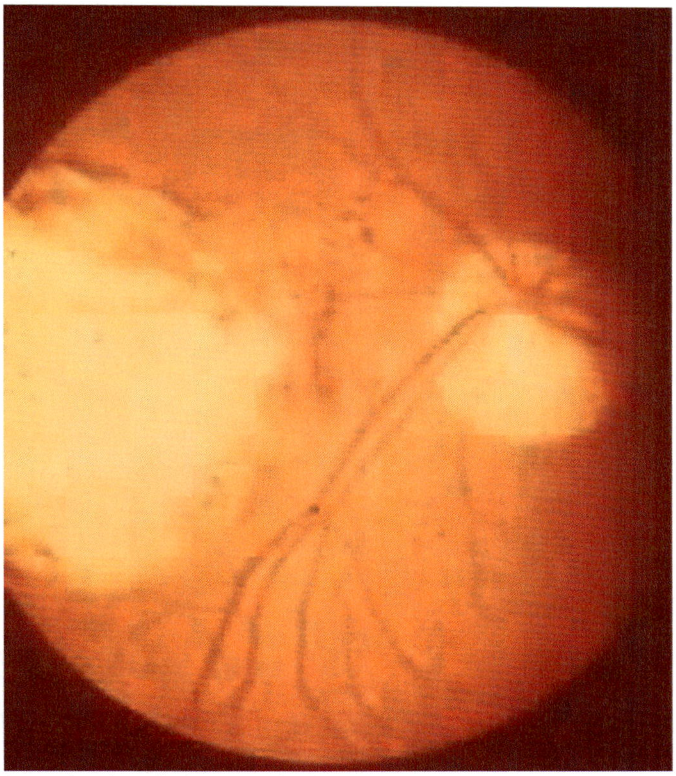

FIGURE 17.1.90 - Fundoscopy: Chorioretinitis

III. Zika Virus
   A. Congenital Zika syndrome
   B. Flavivirus mostly transmitted by *Aedes* mosquito bite
   C. Sexual and vertical transmission can occur
   D. Neonatal findings
      1. Subcortical calcifications
      2. Ventriculomegaly
      3. Microcephaly, spasticity, and ocular abnormalities
   E. Diagnosis
      1. RT-PCR
      2. Serology
   F. Treatment: supportive

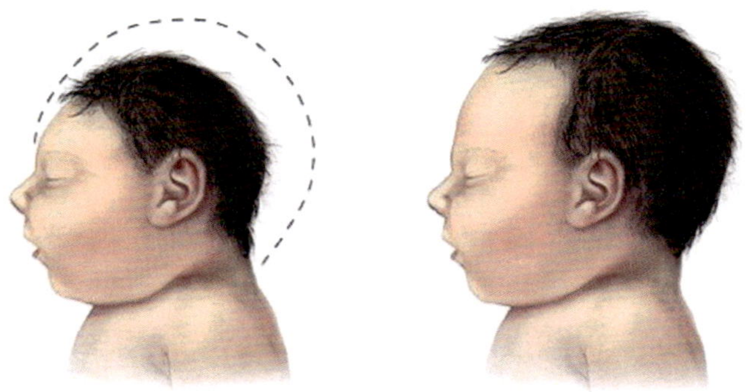

Centers for Disease Control and Prevention, Public domain, via Wikimedia Commons

FIGURE 17.1.91 - Microcephaly

IV. Varicella Zoster Virus
   A. Varicella zoster virus (HHV-3)
   B. Acquired by pregnant woman via air droplets
   C. Fetal manifestations
      1. Skin vesicles
      2. Skin scarring
      3. Limb hypoplasia
      4. Hydrocephalus and seizures
   D. Prevention
      1. Avoidance of infected individuals
      2. VZV vaccine contraindicated during pregnancy
      3. VZV vaccination after delivery if not previously vaccinated
   E. Post-exposure prophylaxis: varicella zoster immune globulin (VZIG)

V. Rubella
   A. Rubella (togavirus)
   B. Transmission: air droplets
   C. Maternal manifestations
      1. Fever, rash, arthralgia, lymphadenopathy
   D. Fetal manifestations: triad
      1. Congenital cataracts
      2. PDA and sensorineural hearing loss

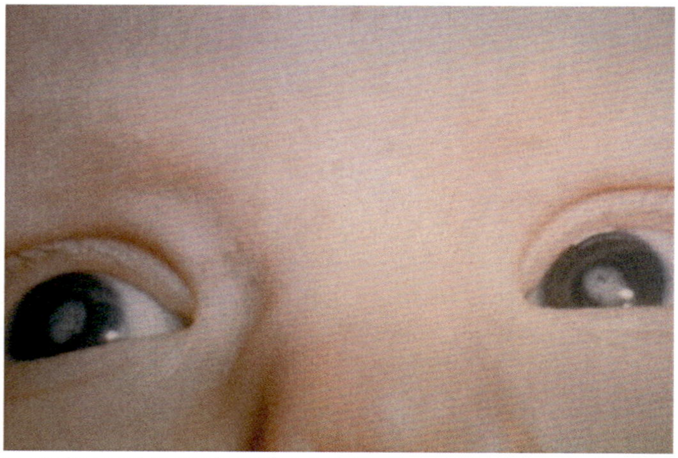

See page for author, Public domain, via Wikimedia Commons

FIGURE 17.1.92 - Bilateral Cataracts

VI. Cytomegalovirus
   A. Cytomegalovirus (HHV-5)
   B. Routes of maternal acquisition: sexual contact, saliva, urine, transplant, blood transfusion
   C. Maternal manifestations
      1. Mononucleosis-like symptoms
   D. Fetal manifestations
      1. Periventricular calcifications, seizure, “blueberry muffin” rash

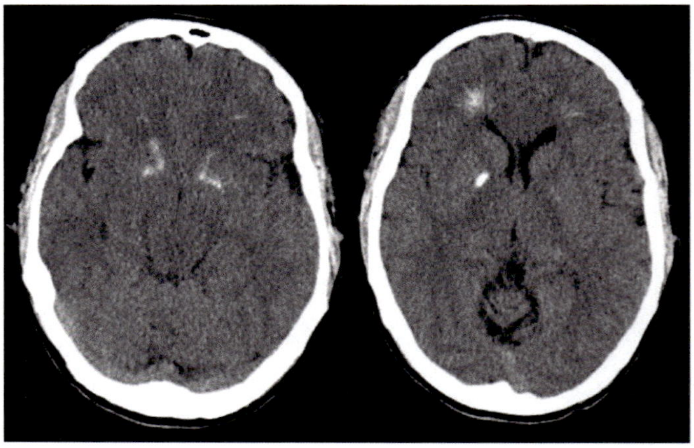

Adriano R Tonelli1, Kalyan Kosuri1, Sainan Wei2, and Davoren Chick1 [Modified]

FIGURE 17.1.93 - CT Scan of Head: Periventricular Calcification in Congenital CMV

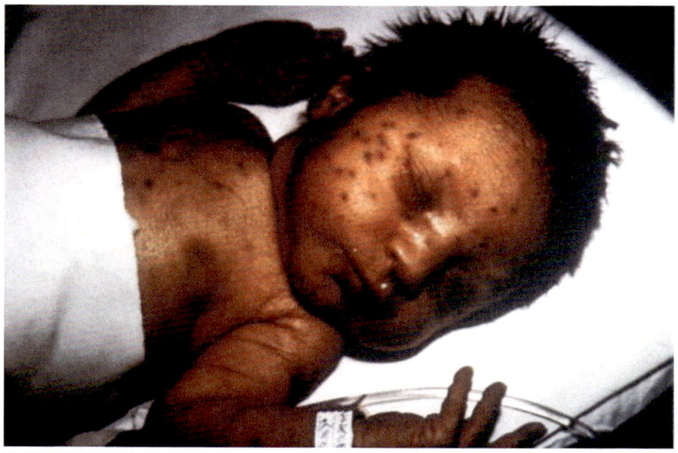

CDC [Public domain]

FIGURE 17.1.94 - “Blueberry Muffin” Rash

VII. Herpes Simplex Virus
   A. Herpes simplex virus (HSV-1 or HSV-2)
   B. Acquired via vaginal secretions
   C. Diffuse vesicles on neonatal skin
   D. Dissemination possible
   E. Disseminated neonatal herpes involves CNS
   F. Meningoencephalitis
   G. Prevention
      1. History of previous genital herpes: acyclovir suppression therapy from 36 weeks
      2. No genital vesicles or prodromal symptoms (burning, itching): vaginal delivery
      3. Genital vesicles or prodromal symptoms: cesarean delivery

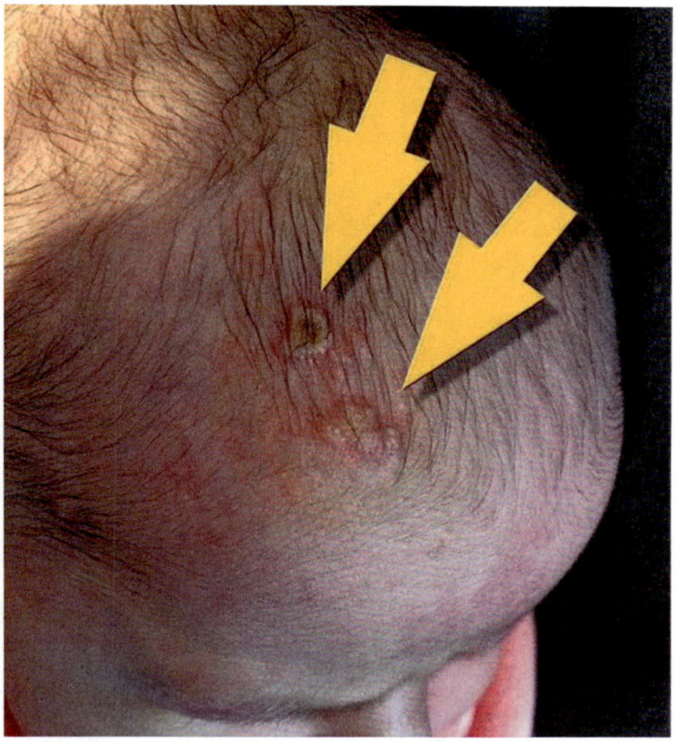

FIGURE 17.1.95 - Vesicular Rash in Herpes Simplex Virus Infection

VIII. Syphilis

A. Congenital syphilis
B. Route of maternal acquisition: unprotected sexual intercourse
C. Route of fetal acquisition: transplacental transmission
D. Neonatal findings
    1. Snuffles (nasal discharge), rhagades (angular cheilitis)
    2. Saddle nose, Hutchinson's teeth, mulberry molars
    3. Short maxilla, bowed legs, sensorineural deafness
E. Prevention: condoms
F. Treatment
    1. Intramuscular benzathine penicillin G
G. Treatment in penicillin-allergic patients
    1. Desensitize and give intramuscular benzathine penicillin G

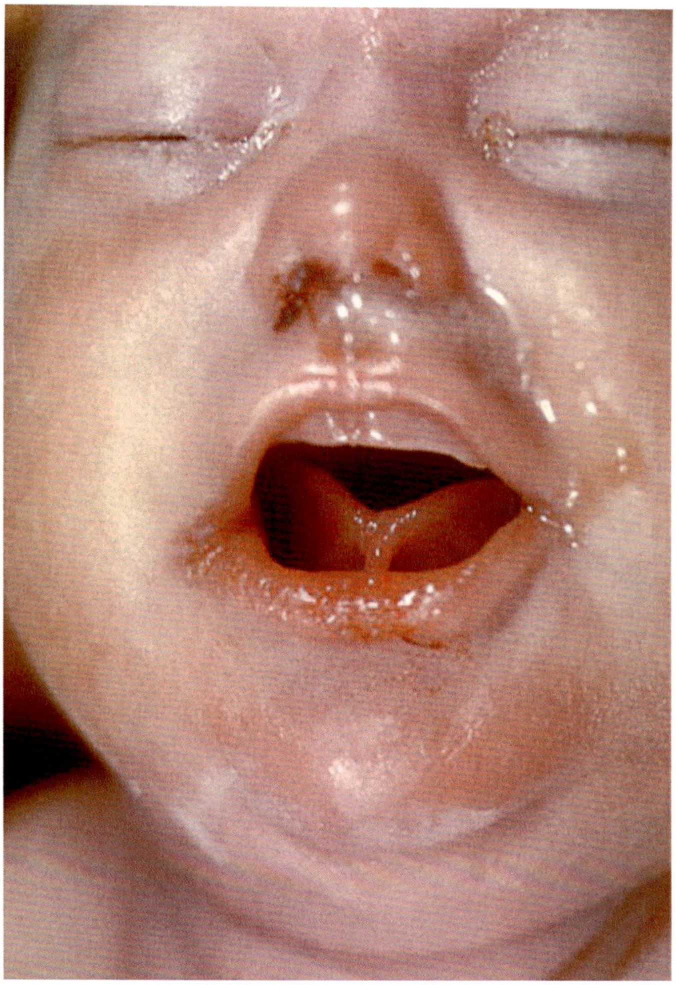

FIGURE 17.1.96 - Snuffles and Rhagades in Congenital Syphilis

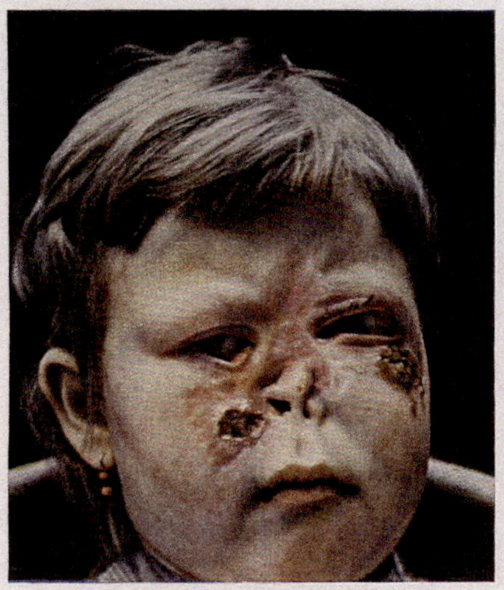

CONGENITAL SYPHILIS.

Destruction of nasal bones with major portion of skin of nose and its vicinity. The skin is replaced by cicatricial tissue. Ectropion of the lower lids owing to contraction of scar. The scars themselves are affected by recent ulceration.

FIGURE 17.1.97 - Saddle Nose Deformity in Congenital Syphilis

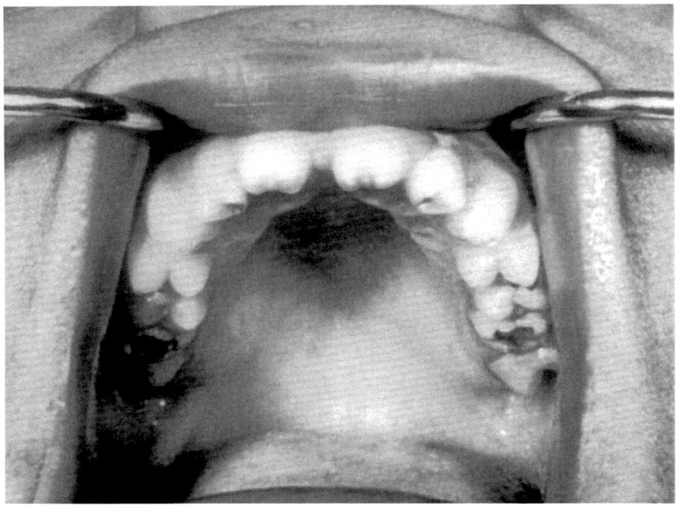

CDC/Susan Lindsley, Public domain, via Wikimedia Commons

FIGURE 17.1.98 - Hutchinson Teeth and Mulberry Molars in Congenital Syphilis

REVIEW QUESTIONS

1. A 2-day-old girl is brought to the emergency department by her parents because of rhythmic bilateral upper and lower extremity movements for the past few minutes. An electroencephalogram shows a generalized seizure. She was born at 39 weeks gestation to a G2P2 woman. She had a fever and hepatosplenomegaly in the second trimester. Physical examination of the neonate shows a head circumference at the 97th percentile. Fundoscopic exam shows bilateral retinal exudates and edema. An MRI of the brain reveals diffuse parenchymal calcifications. What is the best treatment option for this neonate?

- **The best treatment option for this neonate is pyrimethamine and sulfadiazine.**
- This neonate is evaluated and found to be having a generalized seizure.
- She has a head circumference at the 97th percentile, consistent with macrocephaly concerning for hydrocephalus.
- She also has bilateral retinal exudates and edema consistent with chorioretinitis.
- Her brain MRI shows diffuse parenchymal calcifications.
- The triad of hydrocephalus, chorioretinitis, and diffuse intracranial calcifications is consistent with congenital toxoplasmosis.
- Treatment for congenital toxoplasmosis is pyrimethamine and sulfadiazine.

Obstetrics | Section 27: Medical Complications of Pregnancy

I. Hyperemesis Gravidarum
   A. Severe form of morning sickness
   B. Weight loss and ketosis
   C. Can last until term in severe cases
   D. Unclear etiology
      1. May be related to elevated β-hCG or thyroid hormones
      2. Increased risk in molar pregnancies

II. Hyperemesis Gravidarum: Diagnosis
   A. Persistent vomiting
   B. Weight loss of > 5% pre-pregnancy weight
   C. Ketonuria

III. Hyperemesis Gravidarum: Treatment
   A. Maintain adequate nutrition; frequent and small meals
   B. May require feeding tube or parenteral nutrition
   C. If dehydrated, rehydrate with IV fluids and replete electrolytes
   D. May also need thiamine supplementation to prevent Wernicke's
   E. Antiemetics: first-line promethazine
   F. B_6 and doxylamine

IV. Thyroid Disease in Pregnancy
   A. Physiologic changes in pregnancy
      1. Increased thyroxine-binding globulin and sex hormone-binding globulin
      2. Decreased amount free active hormone
      3. Increased metabolic demands in pregnancy

V. Thyroid Disease in Pregnancy: Hypothyroid
   A. Most commonly due to Hashimoto's disease or previous ablation
   B. Increase levothyroxine dose by 25 - 30%
      1. Adjust every four weeks until TSH stable
      2. Monitor TSH once per trimester when stable
   C. Fetal complications: IUGR, congenital thyroid deficiency, stillbirth

VI. Thyroid Disease in Pregnancy: Hyperthyroid
   A. Most commonly due to Graves disease
   B. Check TSH-receptor stimulating antibodies at first prenatal visit
      1. Can lead to fetal goiter if elevated; monitor with ultrasound
   C. Management:
      1. 1st trimester: propylthiouracil
      2. 2nd and 3rd trimester: methimazole
      3. Follow symptoms and TSH; serial non-stress tests
   D. Symptoms of hyperthyroidism can be treated with beta-blockers
   E. Thyroid storm
      1. May be precipitated by infection, surgeries, labor, delivery
      2. Fever > 103° F, severe tachycardia, changes in mental status
      3. High risk for maternal heart failure

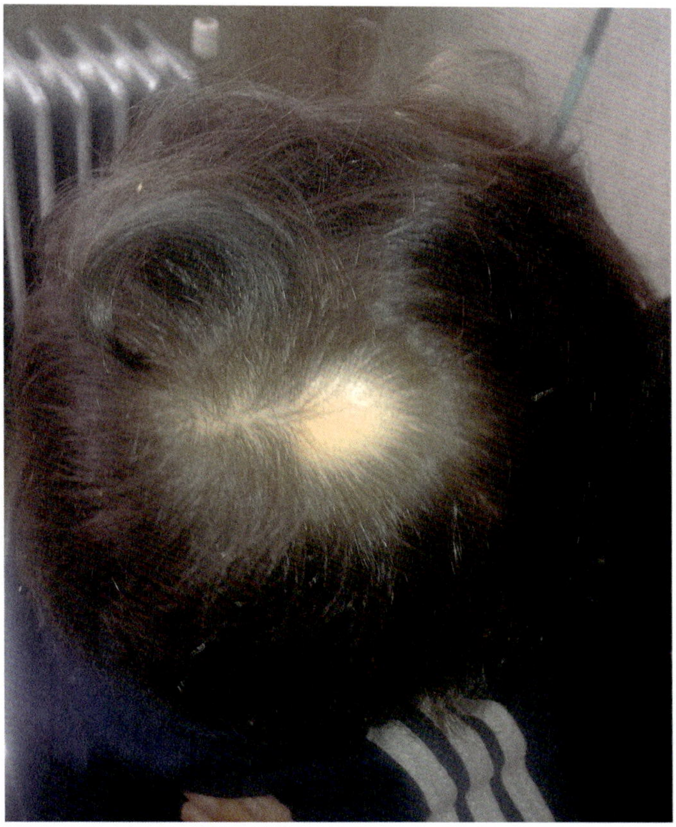

FIGURE 17.1.99 - Aplasia Cutis

VII. Thyroid Disease in Pregnancy: Postpartum Thyroiditis
   A. Subacute autoimmune inflammation → inflammation and lymphocytic infiltration
   B. Destruction of follicular cells → release of thyroid hormone
   C. May present as hypothyroidism, hyperthyroidism, or hyperthyroidism followed by hypothyroidism
   D. Most women will be euthyroid at one year postpartum

VIII. Neonatal Lupus
   A. Complications of lupus such as hypertension and renal disease can affect pregnancy
   B. Increased risk of preeclampsia, IUGR, preterm delivery, and miscarriages in first and second trimesters
   C. Continue aspirin and corticosteroids
   D. Discontinue cyclophosphamide and methotrexate

E. Maternal antigen-antibody complexes can cross the placenta and cause lupus symptoms in the neonate

F. Dermatologic manifestations
   1. Erythematous annular lesions
   2. Primarily on scalp and periorbital area
   3. Rash can persist even after maternal antibodies levels decrease

G. Congenital heart block
   1. anti-Ro and anti-La antibodies are tissue-specific to the cardiac conduction system → destruction of AV node → heart block
   2. Screen for Ro or La antibodies at first visit
   3. Most commonly presents during 2nd trimester
   4. Can be irreversible; may require pacemaker insertion

IX. Peripartum Cardiomyopathy

A. Heart failure secondary to dilated cardiomyopathy

B. Can occur immediately before, during, or after birth

C. May be associated with baseline cardiomyopathy or postinfectious cardiomyopathy

D. Diagnosis
   1. Echocardiogram: dilated heart with ejection fraction of 20 - 40%

E. Management
   1. > 34 weeks should be delivered
   2. If earlier, give betamethasone for lung maturity
   3. Follow typical heart failure management: diuretics, digoxin, vasodilators, supplemental oxygen
   4. Avoid ACE inhibitors, ARBs, and mineralocorticoid antagonists

F. Most patients will return to baseline

REVIEW QUESTIONS

1. A 27-year-old G1P0 woman at 15 weeks gestation is brought to the emergency department by her husband because of worsened confusion for the past 3 hours. She has been forgetting her husband's name for the last 2 weeks. She reports severe nausea and vomiting in her first pregnancy. Her pre-pregnancy weight was 154 lbs, while her current weight is 143 lbs. Physical examination shows an irregular, ataxic gait, slow extraocular movements, and horizontal nystagmus. Supplementation with what substance could have prevented these neurological findings?
   - **Supplementation of thiamine could have prevented this patient's current neurological findings.**
   - This patient presents with a recent onset of confusion. Additionally, she reports severe nausea and vomiting in her first pregnancy.
   - She has ataxia and ophthalmoplegia manifested as slow extraocular movements as well as nystagmus.
   - She has lost more than 5% of her prepregnancy weight in the current pregnancy.
   - This presentation is most consistent with Wernicke encephalopathy caused by hyperemesis gravidarum.
   - Thiamine supplementation should be initiated in pregnant women with hyperemesis gravidarum to prevent the development of Wernicke encephalopathy.

REVIEW QUESTIONS

2. A 23-year-old woman comes to her primary care physician to discuss pregnancy planning. She has no specific complaints. Her past medical history is significant for Hashimoto thyroiditis, treated with levothyroxine. Vital signs include a temperature of 96.8° F (36° C), blood pressure of 125/80 mmHg, heart rate of 82 beats/min, and respiratory rate of 16 breaths/min. What modification should be made to her levothyroxine dose during pregnancy?

- **After this patient gets pregnant, her medication regimen should be modified by Increasing the levothyroxine dose by 25-30%.**
- This patient presents for a preconception visit.
- She has a past medical history of Hashimoto thyroiditis treated with levothyroxine.
- Higher estrogen levels during pregnancy stimulate the hepatic synthesis of thyroxine-binding globulin, causing free thyroxine levels to decrease.

3. A 24-year-old G1P0 woman is admitted to the labor and delivery unit at 39 weeks gestation after spontaneous rupture of membranes. Her pregnancy has been uncomplicated. She has a past medical history of systemic lupus erythematosus treated with hydroxychloroquine. Her cervix is dilated to 4 cm and effaced by 60%. Several hours after admission, she delivers a baby boy. The newborn's physical examination shows a diffuse rash, most prominent in the periorbital regions. His AST is 1,000 U/L (12 - 38 U/L), and his ALT is 1,500 U/L (10 - 40 U/L). An electrocardiogram shows severe bradycardia with complete atrioventricular dissociation. What is the most likely pathophysiology of this newborn's presentation?

- **The most likely pathophysiology of this newborn's presentation is the transplacental passage of maternal anti-Ro antibodies that damage multiple fetal tissues, causing neonatal lupus.**
- This patient has a past medical history of systemic lupus erythematosus.
- She delivers a baby boy with diffuse rash, severe transaminitis marked by increased levels of AST and ALT, and ECG findings consistent with third-degree AV block.
- All of these clues point to the diagnosis of neonatal lupus.
- Neonatal lupus is caused by transplacental passage of maternal anti-Ro antibodies that damage multiple fetal tissues, including the cardiac conduction system.
- Transplacental passage of maternal anti-Ro antibodies → neonatal lupus.

Obstetrics | Section 28: Substance Use and Teratogenic Medications in Pregnancy

I. Substance Use in Pregnancy: Alcohol
   A. No safe amount of alcohol in pregnancy
   B. Most detrimental effects seen in patients who drink 2 - 5 drinks daily
   C. Fetal alcohol syndrome
   D. Growth retardation, CNS effects such as intellectual disability
   E. Abnormal facies
   F. Aggressive counseling for mother, monitor for nutritional deficiencies

Craniofacial features associated with fetal alcohol syndrome

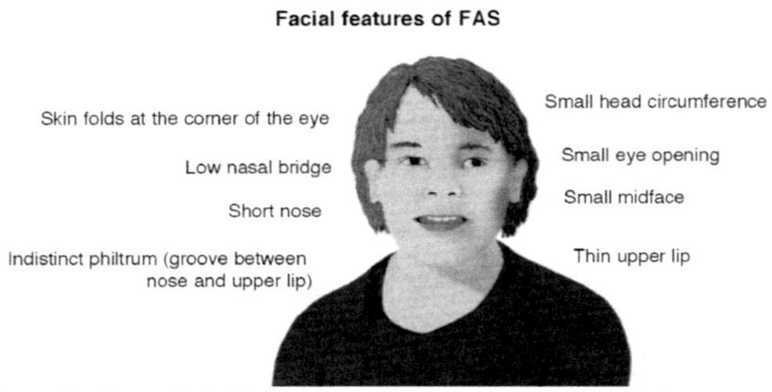

FIGURE 17.1.100 - Facial Features of Fetal Alcohol Syndrome

II. Substance Use in Pregnancy: Tobacco
   A. Increased risks with increased amounts of smoking
   B. Risk for spontaneous abortions, preterm birth, placental abruptions
   C. Infants exposed to tobacco in utero and after birth are at increased risk for sudden infant death syndrome
   D. Patients should be encouraged to at least decrease the amount of smoking

III. Substance Use in Pregnancy: Cocaine
   A. Increased risk for IUGR, preterm labor, placental abruption
   B. Due to vasoconstrictive effects
   C. Social services should be involved in the patient's care
   D. Mother should be encouraged to detox

IV. Substance Use in Pregnancy: Opiates
   A. Most commonly used in pregnancy: oxycodone, heroin, methadone
   B. Not directly teratogenic
   C. Withdrawal can lead to miscarriage, preterm delivery, fetal death
   D. Mothers should be encouraged to start a methadone program rather than quit
   E. Infant will require weaning off of opiates at birth

V. Teratogenic Medications: Warfarin
   A. Easily crosses placenta
   B. Exposure 6 - 9 weeks: nasal and midface hypoplasia
   C. Later in pregnancy: hydrocephalus

VI. Teratogenic Medications: ACE Inhibitors
   A. Limb contractures
   B. Growth restriction

VII. Teratogenic Medications: Isotretinoin
   A. Fetal loss
   B. Craniofacial defects
   C. Thymic defects
   D. Cardiac defects
   E. CNS defects

VIII. Teratogenic Medications: Lithium
   A. Ebstein anomaly

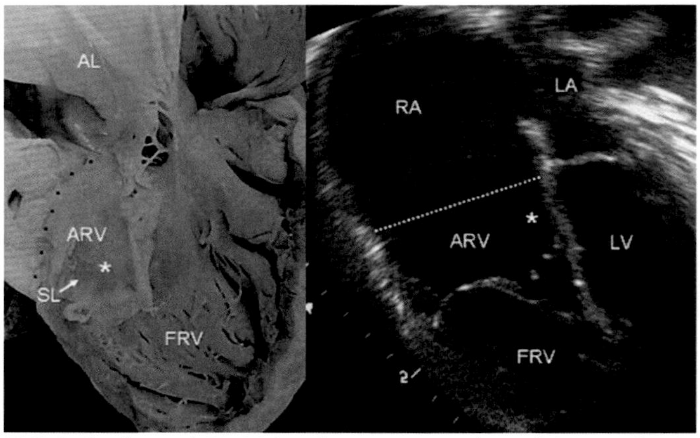

FIGURE 17.1.101 - Ebstein's Anomaly

IX. Teratogenic Medications: Antiepileptics
   A. Carbamazepine: neural tube defects
   B. Valproic acid: neural tube defects
   C. Phenytoin
      1. Folate antagonist
      2. Abnormal facies, cleft lip/palate, microcephaly, growth deficiency, neural tube defects

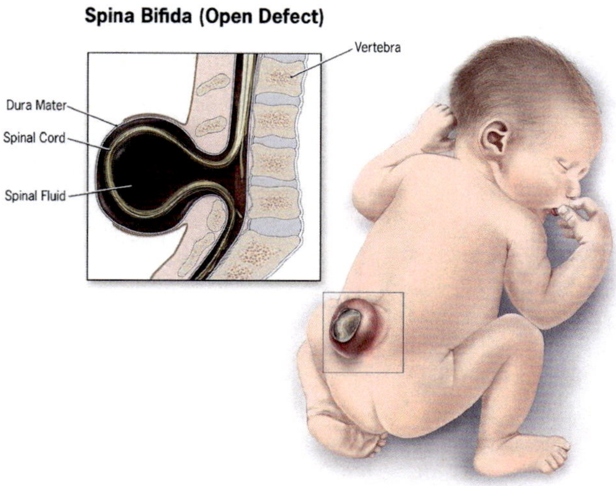

Centers for Disease Control and Prevention, Public domain, via Wikimedia Commons

FIGURE 17.1.102 - Spina Bifida

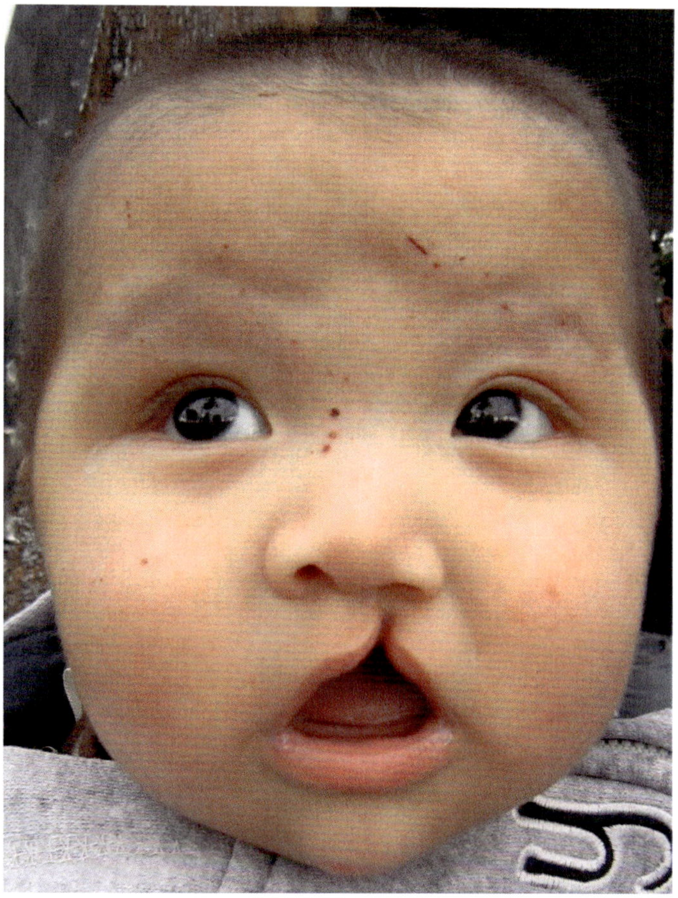

James Heilman, MD, CC BY-SA 3.0 <https://creativecommons.org/licenses/by-sa/3.0>, via Wikimedia Commons

FIGURE 17.1.103 - Cleft Lip

Substance/Medication	Effect on the Fetus
Alcohol	- Fetal alcohol syndrome: intellectual disability, characteristic facial features
Tobacco	- Spontaneous abortion, preterm birth, placental abruption
Cocaine	- IUGR, preterm labor, placental abruption
Opiates	- Withdrawal can lead to spontaneous abortion
Warfarin	- Nasal and midface hypoplasia, hydrocephalus
ACE inhibitors	- Limb contractures, IUGR
Methimazole	- Aplasia cutis, omphalocele, tracheoesophageal fistulas, choanal atresia
Isotretinoin	- Fetal loss, congenital malformations
Lithium	- Ebstein's anomaly
Carbamazepine and valproic acid	- Neural tube defects
Phenytoin	- Abnormal facies, cleft lip/palate, microcephaly, growth deficiency, neural tube defects

TABLE 17.1.3- Effects of Certain Substances and Medications on the Fetus

REVIEW QUESTIONS

1. A 15-day-old boy is brought to his primary care physician by his parents for a routine check-up. He was born at 38 weeks gestation via vaginal delivery. The patient is exclusively breastfed, and he has already regained his birth weight. His mother smokes 1 pack of cigarettes per day. His vital signs and physical examination are unremarkable. What is this neonate at risk for due to his exposure to cigarette smoke?

   - **This neonate is at risk for sudden infant death syndrome due to his exposure to cigarette smoke.**
   - This neonate was born at term via vaginal delivery.
   - He is exclusively breastfed and has regained his birth weight.
   - Although the patient's overall condition is satisfactory, his exposure to cigarette smoke can predispose him to sudden infant death syndrome or SIDS, which is an unexpected death of the baby before 1 year of age.

2. A 6-year-old boy is brought to his primary care physician by his parents because of problems at school for the past year. Teachers report that he has a hard time listening and gets distracted easily, requiring lots of redirection. He also blurts out the answers to questions without considering his classmates. He was born at 39 weeks gestation and had an uncomplicated pregnancy. Vital signs are within normal limits. Physical examination shows a smooth philtrum, a thin upper lip, a short nasal bridge, and small palpebral fissures. In utero exposure to which of the following substances is the most likely cause of this patient's current condition?

   A. Alcohol
   B. Cocaine
   C. Tobacco
   D. Heroin

   - **The correct answer is option A.**
   - This 6-year-old boy exhibits signs of ADHD at school with frequency distraction, outbursts, and requiring lots of redirection.
   - Physical examination shows smooth philtrum, thin upper lip, short nasal bridge, and small palpebral fissures; A classic description of fetal alcohol syndrome.
   - Therefore, in utero, exposure to alcohol is the most likely cause of this patient's current condition.
   - Option B, cocaine, and option C, tobacco, are incorrect because in utero, exposure to either of them is most likely associated with preterm birth, intrauterine growth restriction, or spontaneous abortion.
   - Option D, heroin, is incorrect because maternal heroin abuse during pregnancy is associated with neonatal abstinence syndrome, which is characterized by neonatal irritability, diarrhea, sneezing, tachypnea, tremors, and possible seizures.

Obstetrics | Section 29: Postpartum Hemorrhage Overview, Uterine Rupture, Inversion and Lacerations

I. Postpartum Hemorrhage: Overview
   A. > 1000 mL of blood loss after a vaginal delivery or C-section
   B. Risk factors
      1. Prolonged labor course
      2. Instrument-assisted delivery (e.g. forceps)
      3. Large baby (e.g. > 4000 g)
      4. Hypertensive disorder of pregnancy
      5. Induction of labor
   C. Findings associated with blood loss
      1. Hypotension
      2. Tachycardia
      3. Decreased hemoglobin and hematocrit
      4. Hypothermia
      5. Acidosis

<u>Causes of Postpartum Hemorrhage</u>

The **4 Ts**

- **T**rauma (uterine inversion, uterine rupture, genital tract lacerations and hematomas)
- **T**one (uterine atony)
- **T**issue (placenta accreta spectrum, retained products of conception)
- **T**hrombin (coagulopathy)

FIGURE 17.1.104 - Causes of Postpartum Hemorrhage

II. Uterine Inversion: Risk Factors
   A. Uncontrolled traction on the umbilical cord
   B. Excessive fundal pressure
   C. Macrosomia
   D. Placenta accreta
   E. Fundal placenta
   F. Abnormal labor course

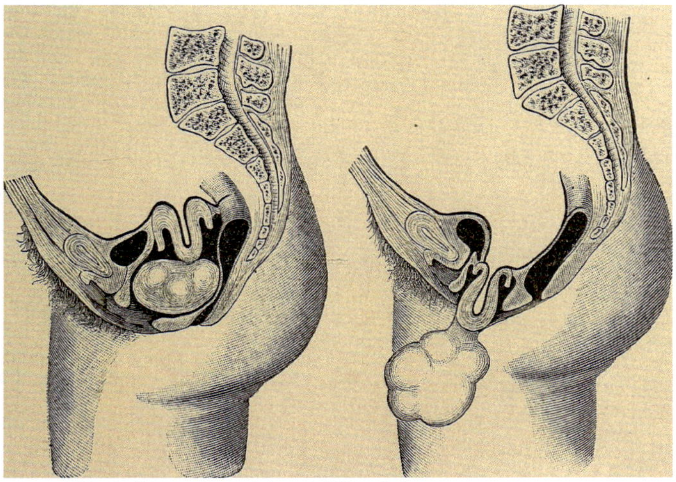

FIGURE 17.1.105 - Uterine Inversion Diagram

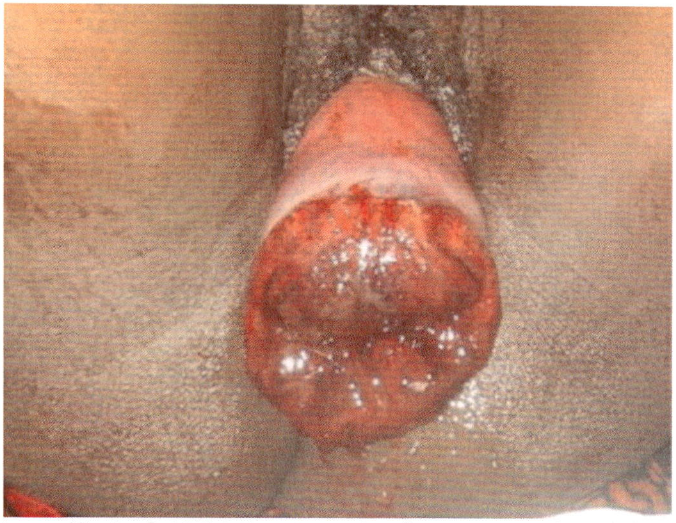

FIGURE 17.1.106 - Uterine Inversion

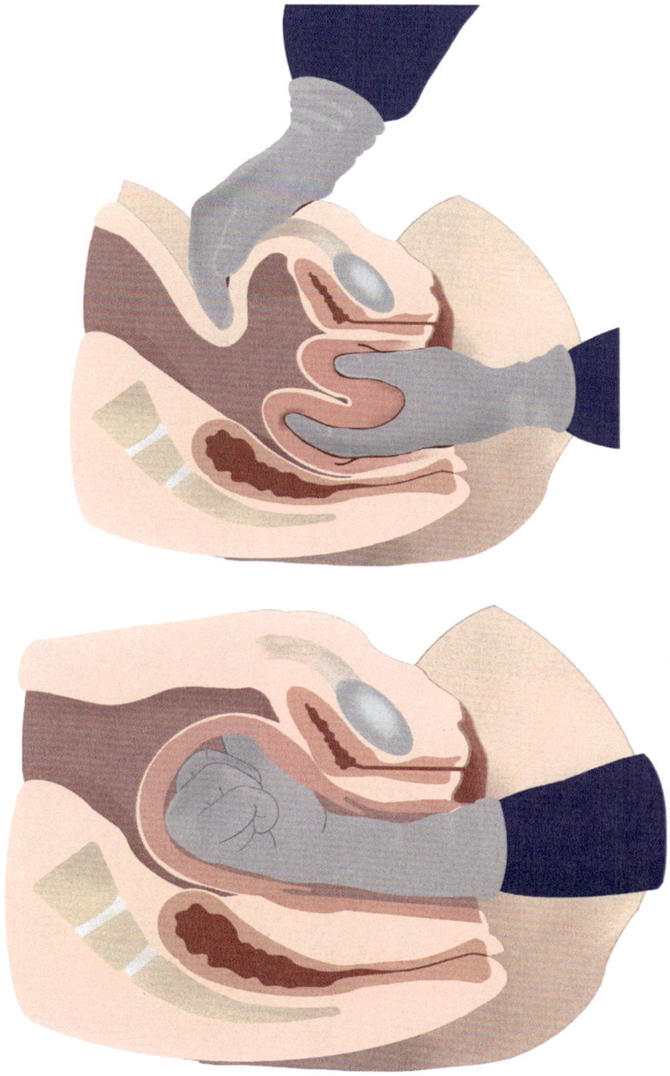

FIGURE 17.1.107 - Manual Replacement of Inverted Uterus

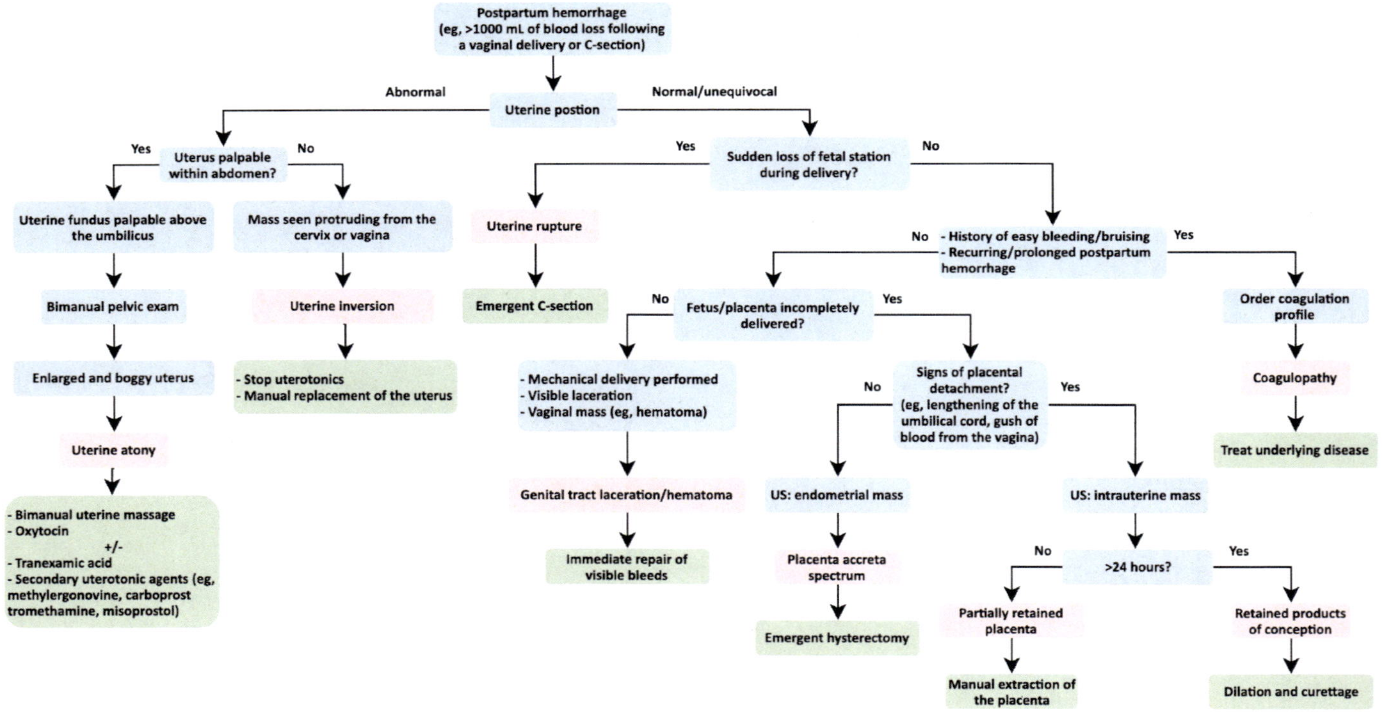

FIGURE 17.1.108 - Evaluation and Management of Postpartum Hemorrhage

III. Uterine Inversion: Clinical Presentation
   A. Severe abdominal pain
   B. Profuse bleeding with clots
   C. Hypotension

IV. Uterine Inversion: Diagnosis
   A. Clinical diagnosis made at the bedside
   B. Radiographic imaging is unnecessary

V. Uterine Rupture
   A. Uterus opens up during the labor process
   B. The number one risk factor is a history of a prior C-section
   C. Patients can have a "popping" sensation accompanied by abdominal pain, back pain, vaginal bleeding, and unstable vital signs
   D. Irregular protuberance is felt in the abdomen
   E. Treatment is an emergent C-section
   F. May lead to significant postpartum hemorrhage

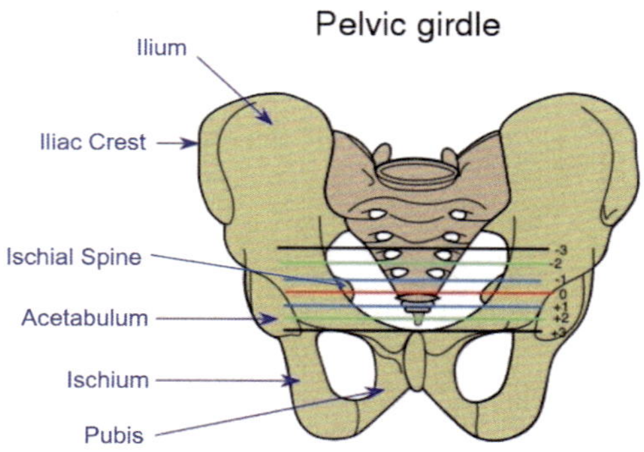

FIGURE 17.1.50 - Fetal Stations

VI. Genital Tract Lacerations and Hematomas: Definition
   A. Post-delivery lacerations are breaks in the epithelium that can occur at the perineum, labia, periurethral area, deeper vagina, and cervix
   B. Hematomas occur when a blood vessel ruptures underneath the epithelium and blood pools

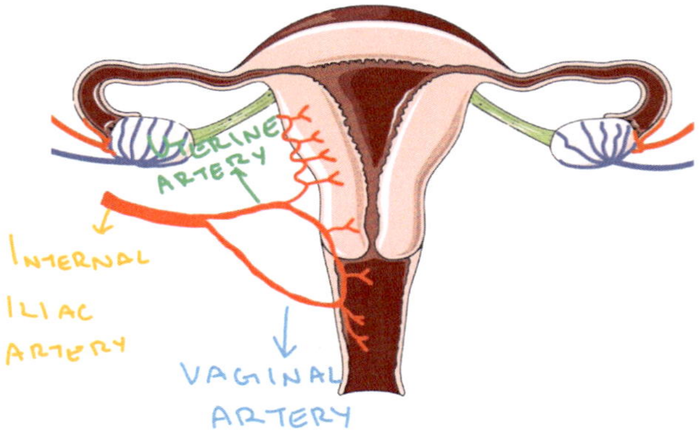

FIGURE 17.1.109 - Major Blood Supply of Uterine, Cervix, and Vagina

VII. Genital Tract Lacerations and Hematomas: Risk Factors
   A. Operative vaginal delivery, particularly forceps
   B. Cervical lacerations
      1. Rapidly dilating cervix
      2. Strong expulsive efforts during labor
   C. Hematoma
      1. Large baby
      2. Nulliparity

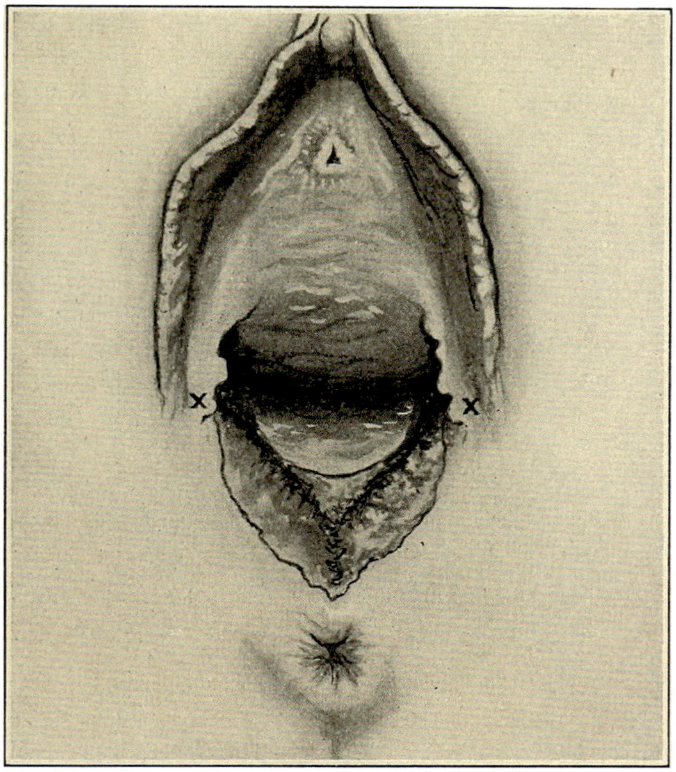

Internet Archive Book Images, No restrictions, via Wikimedia Commons

FIGURE 17.1.110 - Vaginal Laceration

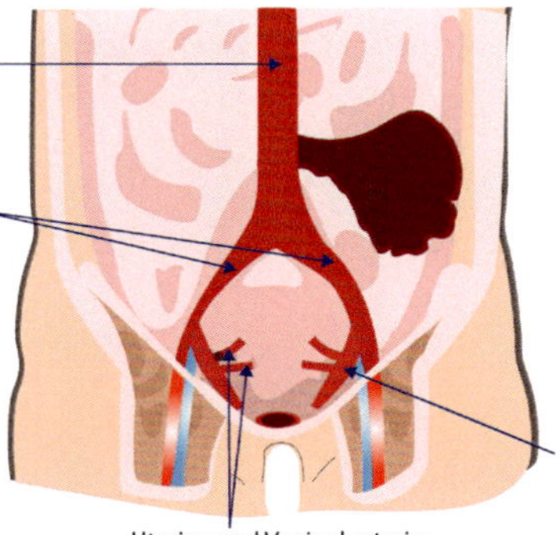

FIGURE 17.1.111 - Retroperitoneal Hematoma

REVIEW QUESTIONS

1. Why should uterotonic medications such as oxytocin be stopped in a patient who has experienced uterine inversion?
    - **Uterotonic medications should be stopped in a patient who has experienced uterine inversion in order to relax the uterus to facilitate manual replacement.**
    - The most important thing to do for patients with uterine inversion is to correct the inverted uterus as soon as possible manually.
    - To help facilitate this, the uterus needs to be relaxed. Stopping the uterotonic medications helps with this. In some instances, uterine relaxants such as terbutaline and nitroglycerin may need to be added.
    - However, relaxing the uterus too much could lead to uterine atony and further bleeding.
2. In a patient who suffers uterine rupture, what happens to the fetal station?
    - **In a patient who suffers uterine rupture, the fetal station becomes more negative.**
    - Fetal station is a system used to describe the position of the baby's head relative to the ischial spine of the mother.
    - 0 station is when the top of the head is level with the ischial spine.
    - Negative values are given when the baby's head is superior to this landmark, while positive values are given when the baby's head is inferior to this landmark.
    - In the case of uterine rupture, the opening up of the uterus provides an alternative pathway for the baby, and the fetal parts will often move through it.
    - Therefore, the baby moves up in the pelvis, and the value of the fetal station becomes more negative. This will often be referred to as loss of fetal station.

REVIEW QUESTIONS

3. A 34-year-old woman presents to the emergency department because of severe lower back and rectal pain. She recently gave birth 2 weeks ago. During labor, forceps were used to assist with vaginal delivery. Physical examination of the vagina and cervix shows no evidence of bleeding. Hemoglobin and hematocrit are 6.3 g/dL (12 - 16 g/dL) and 19.1% (36 - 46%), respectively. What is the most likely diagnosis?

   - **The most likely diagnosis is a retroperitoneal hematoma.**
   - This woman presents with severe lower back and rectal pain shortly after forceps-assisted vaginal delivery.
   - Her hemoglobin and hematocrit are low, which strongly suggests bleeding.
   - The first source is to assess for vaginal bleeding.
   - However, the physical examination of the vagina and cervix shows no evidence of bleeding.
   - Given that she is experiencing pain in the lower back and rectum, the most likely diagnosis is a retroperitoneal hematoma.

4. A patient presents to her primary care provider for routine follow-up. One week ago, she gave birth to a baby boy. Delivery was complicated by postpartum hemorrhage. Vitals include BP 87/52 mmHg and pulse 106/min. She notes that she is not producing much milk to breastfeed and has started to use formula. What is the most likely diagnosis?

   - **The most likely diagnosis is Sheehan syndrome.**
   - The question stem presents a classic description of Sheehan syndrome, which is a complication of postpartum hemorrhage. Sheehan syndrome is the result of ischemia to the pituitary gland.
   - During pregnancy, the pituitary gland becomes enlarged, and its function can be significantly reduced without adequate blood flow.
   - Patients with this pathology will show symptoms specific to the deficient pituitary hormones.
   - Low ACTH can lead to anorexia and hypotension. Low levels of prolactin result in difficulty with milk production. Low FSH and LH manifests as amenorrhea, hot flashes, and atrophy of the vagina. Decreased growth hormone means less lean body mass. Low TSH can lead to fatigue and bradycardia.
   - Treatment is to replace the deficient hormones. However, bringing back the ability to lactate is not feasible.

Obstetrics | Section 30: Uterine Atony, Placenta Accreta, Retained Products of Conception & Coagulopathy

I. Causes of Postpartum Hemorrhage: The 4 Ts
   - **A.** **T**rauma (uterine inversion, uterine rupture, genital tract lacerations and hematomas)
   - **B.** **T**one (uterine atony)
   - **C.** **T**issue (placenta accreta spectrum, retained products of conception)
   - **D.** **T**hrombin (coagulopathy)

II. Uterine Atony: Definition
   - A. Inadequate contraction of the muscle layer of the uterus after delivery

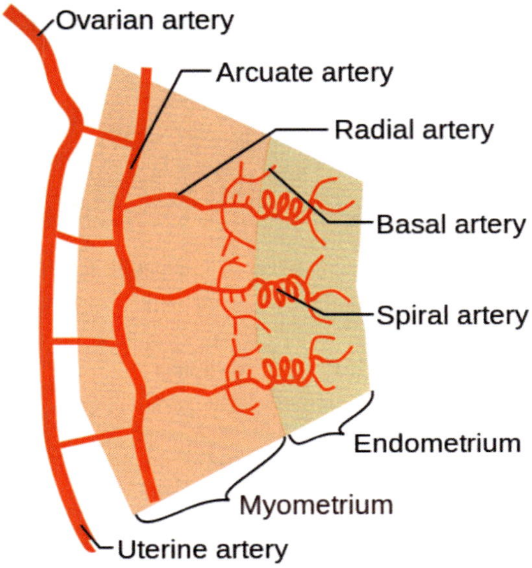

Mikael Häggström, Public domain, via Wikimedia Commons

FIGURE 17.1.112 - Blood Supply to the Uterus

III. Uterine Atony: Pathophysiology
   - A. Vessels throughout the placental bed rely on compression from the contracted uterus to stop bleeding
   - B. Without proper constriction of the vessels, the patient bleeds

IV. Uterine Atony: Risk Factors
   - A. Tired uterine muscle (e.g. prolonged, induced, or precipitous delivery)
   - B. Enlarged uterus (e.g. multiple gestations, macrosomia, polyhydramnios)
   - C. Intraamniotic infection
   - D. Magnesium sulfate

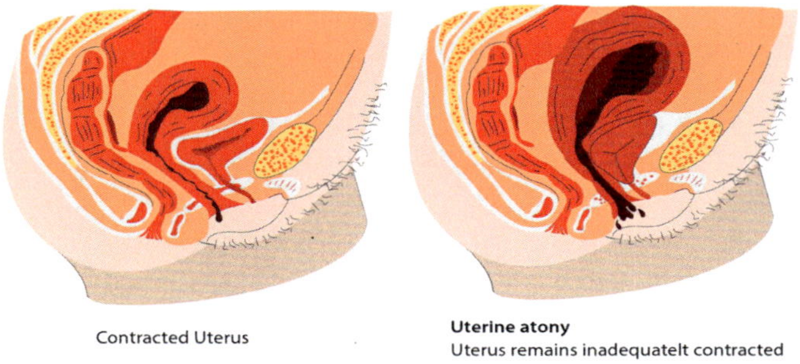

FIGURE 17.1.113 - Normal Uterus (Left) vs. Uterine Atony (Right)

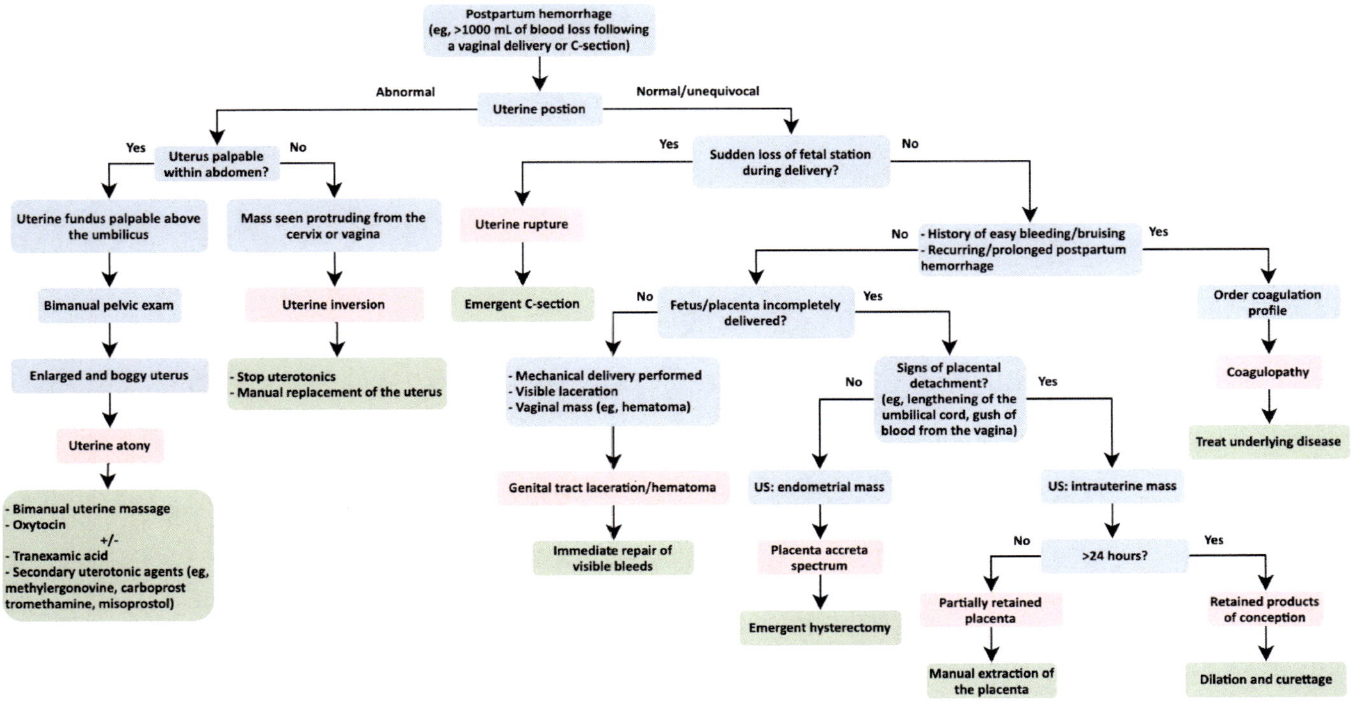

FIGURE 17.1.114 - Evaluating a Patient with Postpartum Hemorrhage

V. Placenta Accreta Spectrum: Definition
   A. Abnormal placentation where the placenta villi are attached to the myometrium instead of the decidua of the uterus

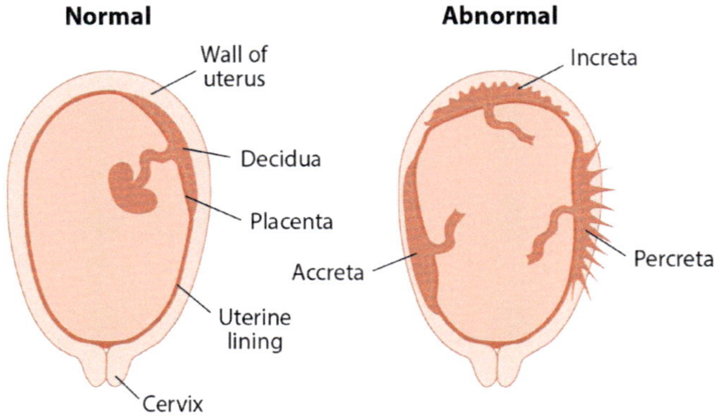

FIGURE 17.1.115 - Normally Attached Placenta (Left) vs. Placenta Accreta Spectrum (Right)

VI. Placenta Accreta Spectrum: Risk Factors
   A. Placenta previa following a prior delivery by C-section
   B. Areas of scarring within the uterus caused by dilation and curettage, myomectomy, or C-section

VII. Retained Products of Conception: Definition
   A. Tissue from the baby or placenta stays inside the uterus after pregnancy
   B. This retained tissue can lead to significant bleeding

VIII. Retained Products of Conception: Risk Factors
   A. Succenturiate placenta
   B. Manual extraction
   C. Prior uterine surgery
   D. Intraamniotic infection

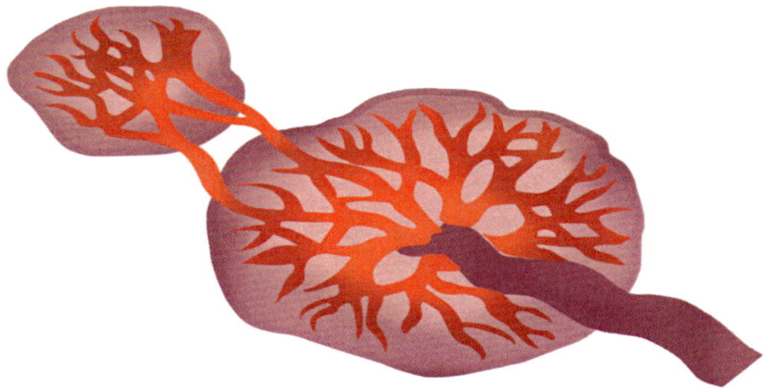

FIGURE 17.1.116 - Succenturiate Placenta

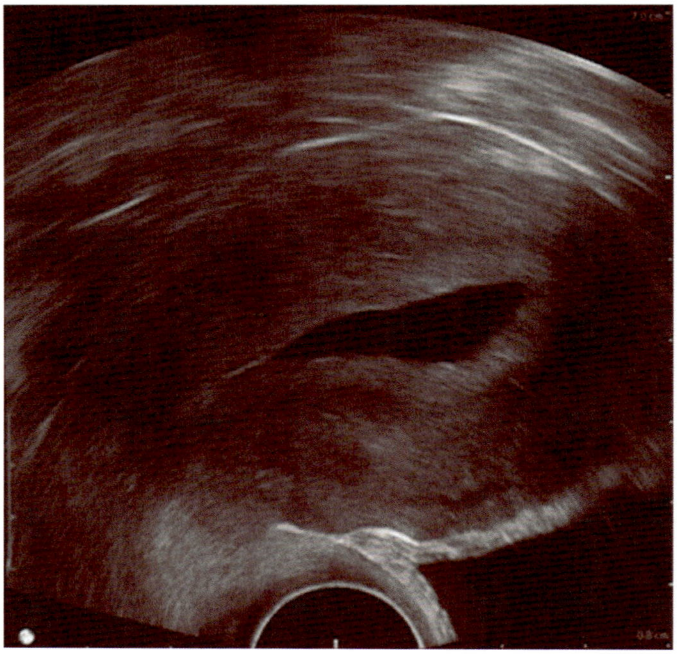

FIGURE 17.1.117 - Pelvic Ultrasound: Normal, Non-Pregnant Uterus

IX. Postpartum Hemorrhage: Treatment
   A. "Last resort" management
      1. Intrauterine balloon tamponade
      2. Bilateral O'Leary sutures to clamp off the uterine arteries
      3. B-Lynch suture to compress the uterus
      4. Hypogastric artery ligation
      5. Hysterectomy

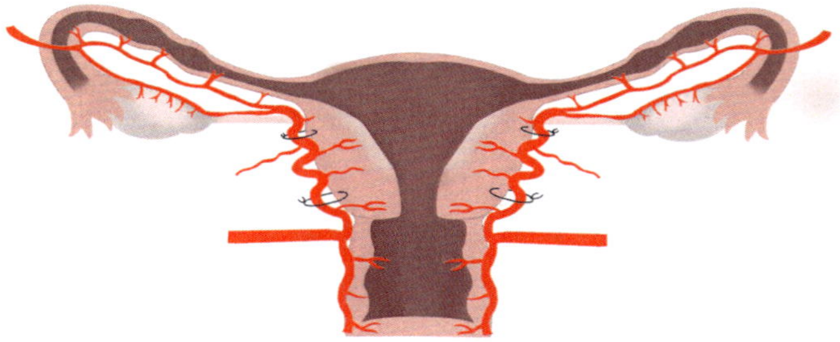

FIGURE 17.1.118 - O'Leary Suture

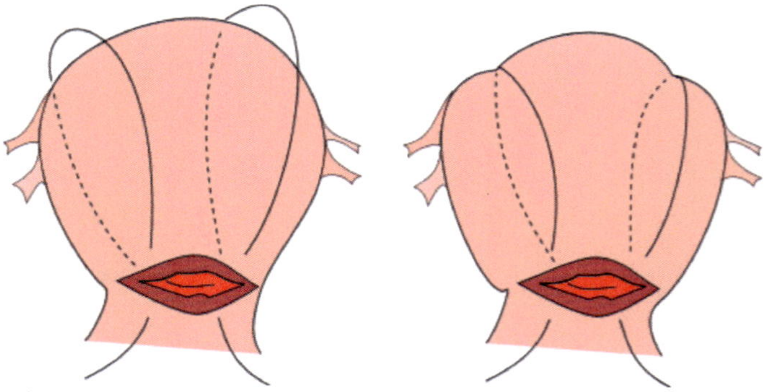

FIGURE 17.1.119 - B-lynch Suture Technique

REVIEW QUESTIONS

1. Why does the administration of magnesium sulfate increase the risk of uterine atony?
   - **The administration of magnesium sulfate increases the risk of uterine atony because of its secondary effect on uterine relaxation. Uterine atony and subsequent postpartum hemorrhage can result.**
   - Magnesium sulfate is commonly used during pregnancy, particularly as a way of preventing seizures in patients with pre-eclampsia. In addition to its anti-seizure effects, this drug has tocolytic properties, meaning that it decreases the contractility of the uterus.
   - In practice, this drug is rarely used for this purpose because it is not effective in decreasing preterm delivery, and prolonged use may lead to defective fetal bone mineralization.

2. Methylergonovine is contraindicated in the treatment of postpartum hemorrhage in patients with what condition?
   - **Methylergonovine is contraindicated in patients with hypertension as it increases the risk of stroke.**
   - Methylergonovine is a drug that is used to contract down the uterus in instances of postpartum hemorrhage, particularly when uterine atony is the cause.
   - In addition to being a uterotonic medication, this drug acts as a vasoconstrictor.

3. Carboprost tromethamine in the treatment of postpartum hemorrhage is contraindicated in patients with what condition?
   - **Given the mechanism of action, carboprost tromethamine can also result in bronchospasm and is thus contraindicated in patients with asthma/reactive airway disease.**
   - Like methylergonovine, carboprost tromethamine is a drug used to clamp down the uterus and decrease bleeding.
   - It works as a prostaglandin F2⍰ analog.

4. Should the placenta be delivered before a hysterectomy in a patient with placenta accreta?
   - **No, the placenta should not be delivered before a hysterectomy in a patient with placenta accreta.**
   - In these patients, the placenta is so tightly attached to the uterine wall that attempts to remove it are likely to cause additional bleeding.
   - Instead, a hysterectomy with the placenta in situ is performed.

5. Two days after a vaginal delivery that required manual extraction of the placenta, a woman presents to the clinic for moderate lower abdominal tenderness. Her vitals show she is febrile to 100.6° F (38.1° C). What is the most likely diagnosis?
   - **The most likely diagnosis is postpartum endometritis.**
   - This is an infection of the endometrium that is more common in patients requiring manual removal of the placenta.
   - Two of three criteria need to be met to make this diagnosis. The criteria are fever, lower abdominal or uterine tenderness without another known cause, and purulent uterine drainage.

REVIEW QUESTIONS

6. A 28-year-old G1P2 woman is assessed at the bedside for moderate vaginal bleeding that has continued for 20 minutes post-delivery. She vaginally delivered twins, weighing 3 kg (6 lb 10 oz) and 2.7 kg (5 lb 15 oz), after being in labor for 18 hours. She has a 5-year history of hypertension that has been well-controlled throughout her pregnancy with nifedipine. She currently feels lightheaded and weak. Vitals show a temperature of 98.0 ° F (36.7° C), respiratory rate of 15 breaths/min, heart rate of 92 beats/min, and blood pressure of 104/71 mmHg. The uterine fundus is palpable above the umbilicus. Vaginal examination shows no evidence of lacerations. A bimanual uterine massage is performed. What is the best next step in the management of this patient's bleeding?

   A. Tranexamic acid
   B. Carboprost tromethamine
   C. High-dose oxytocin
   D. Intrauterine balloon tamponade

- **The correct answer is option C.**
- This patient is experiencing postpartum hemorrhage, and the uterine fundus is palpable above the umbilicus.
- There is no evidence of vaginal lacerations.
- All of this together indicates uterine atony.
- The first step for a patient with uterine atony is to perform a bimanual uterine massage, which is already being done.
- Next, oxytocin should be given.
- Option A is incorrect because tranexamic acid isn't given until after oxytocin has been started.
- Option B is incorrect because carboprost tromethamine is more of a second-line agent for treating postpartum hemorrhage after other interventions have been undergone. If a secondary uterotonic agent were needed, this would be a great option since methylergonovine is contraindicated in this patient, given her history of hypertension.
- Option D is incorrect because the usage of intrauterine balloon tamponade is more of a "last resort" treatment option after traditional medical management has failed.

GYNECOLOGY

Gynecology | Section 1: Polyps and Fibroids

I. Uterine Polyps: Definition
  A. Benign growth of focal endometrial tissue
  B. Common in women 40 - 50s

II. Uterine Polyps: Etiology
  A. Idiopathic
  B. Hormonal (estrogen levels)

III. Uterine Polyps: Risk Factors
  A. Obesity
  B. Hypertension
  C. Tamoxifen
  D. Hormone replacement therapy (HRT)

IV. Uterine Polyps: Clinical Features
  A. Asymptomatic
  B. Menstrual disturbances: irregular, heavy menstruation; spotting, postmenopausal bleeding
  C. Decreased fertility and increased miscarriages: failure of implantation

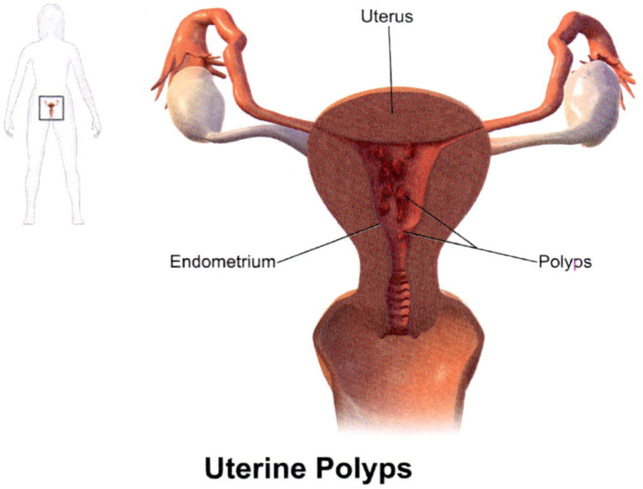

FIGURE 17.2.1 - Uterine Polyps

V. Uterine Polyps: Diagnosis
  A. Transvaginal ultrasound
  B. Hysteroscopy
  C. Endometrial biopsy

VI. Uterine Polyps: Management
  A. Observation and follow-up: asymptomatic patients
  B. Surgical excision: symptomatic patients
  C. Hysterectomy: patients with evidence of malignant cells on biopsy

VII. Fibroids: Definition
  A. Benign neoplasm of smooth muscle cells of the uterus
  B. Also called "leiomyomas"
  C. Most common tumor of the female genital tract

VIII. Fibroids: Pathophysiology
  A. Hormone-sensitive tumors that have upregulated hormone receptors such as estrogen and progesterone receptors
  B. Overproduction of extracellular matrix

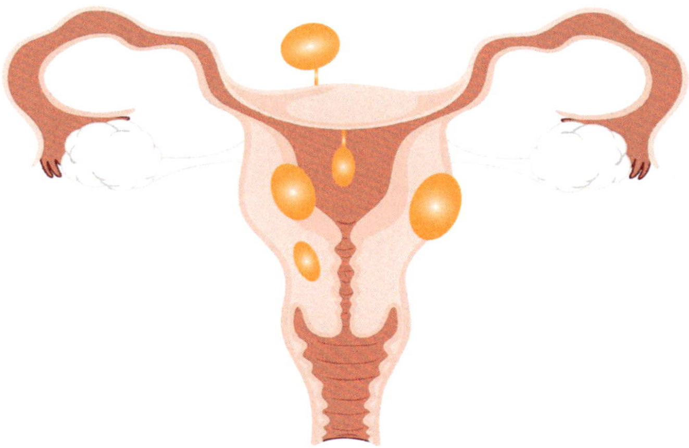

FIGURE 17.2.2 - Uterine Fibroids

IX. Fibroids: Risk Factors
  A. African American women
  B. Factors associated with ↑ estrogen exposure
    1. Nulliparity, early menarche, women in reproductive age (25 - 45 years), obesity
  C. Family history

X. Fibroids: Clinical Features
  A. Could be asymptomatic
  B. Nonspecific symptoms (e.g. back, pelvic pain)
  C. Menstrual disturbances: heavy, painful menstruation; abnormal uterine bleeding
  D. Infertility: especially with submucosal leiomyomas
  E. Mass effect depending on the location
    1. Urinary symptoms: stress incontinence, hydronephrosis and urinary retention due to ureteral obstruction
    2. Bowel symptoms: constipation
  F. Iron deficiency anemia due to menorrhagia
  G. Complications during pregnancy: premature birth, extrauterine pregnancy, fetal growth restriction

XI. Fibroids: Diagnosis

A. Physical exam: enlarged, firm, and irregular uterus

B. Ultrasound: best initial test

   1. Findings include hypoechoic, concentric, heterogenous mass; may contain calcifications

C. Hysteroscopy

D. MRI

E. Biopsy

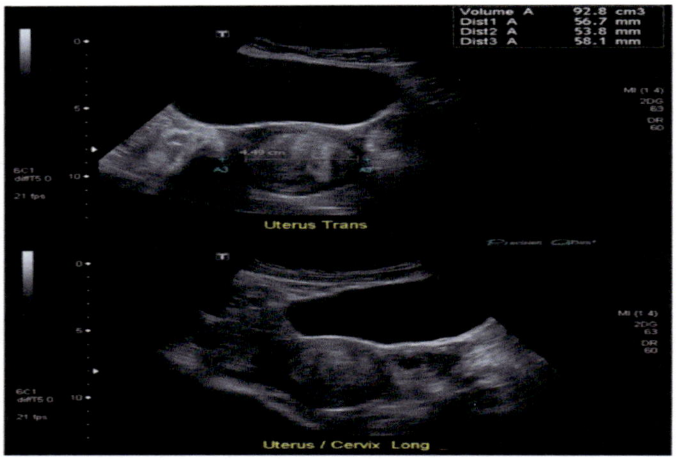

FIGURE 17.2.3 - Transvaginal Ultrasound: Uterine Leiomyoma

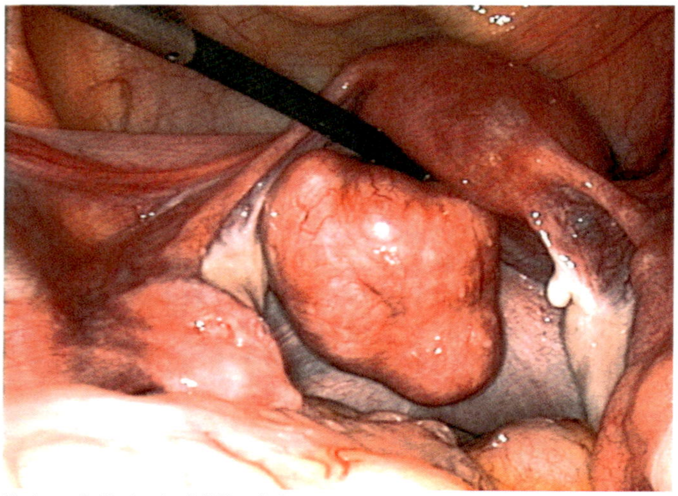

FIGURE 17.2.4 - Subserosal Uterine Leiomyoma

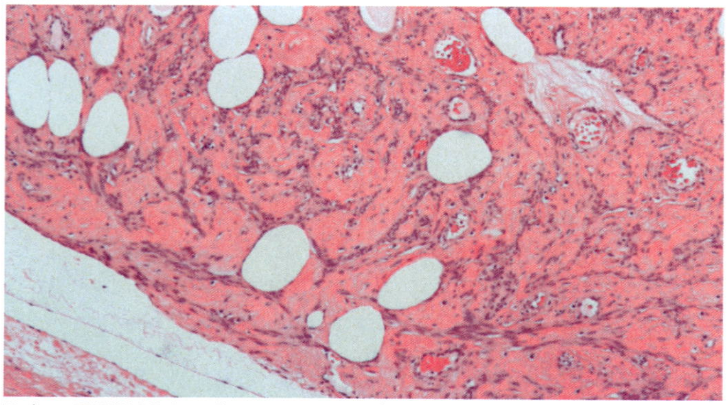

FIGURE 17.2.5 - Light Microscopy: Uterine Leiomyoma

XII. Fibroids: Management

A. Depends on whether the patient is symptomatic or not

B. The goal is to relieve the symptoms

C. Asymptomatic

   1. Observation
   2. Follow-up every 6 - 12 months to monitor growth

D. Symptomatic

   1. Pharmacological treatment
   2. Uterine artery embolization
   3. Surgical treatment

E. Pharmacological treatment

   1. Hormonal: combined OCPs (1st line), IUD, GnRH agonists (e.g. leuprolide)
   2. Androgen agonist (e.g. danazol); many side effects
   3. Antifibrinolytics (e.g. tranexamic acid)
   4. NSAIDs for pain management

F. Uterine artery embolization

   1. Shrinking the fibroid by decreasing its blood supply through injecting polyvinyl alcohol into the supplying arteries
   2. Not used in women who wish to conceive
   3. Not a definitive treatment

G. Surgical treatment

   1. Myomectomy: for women who wish to conceive
   2. Hysterectomy: in case of malignancy, for recurrent disease, or for women who do not wish to conceive

	Uterine Polyps	Fibroids
Definition	- Growth of focal endometrial tissue	- Benign neoplasm of smooth muscle cells of the uterus
Key features	- Abnormal vaginal bleeding (irregular, heavy, and postmenopausal bleeding)	- Heavy menstruation - Infertility - Urinary, bowel symptoms - Enlarged, irregular, firm uterus

TABLE 17.2.1 - Uterine Polyps and Fibroids

REVIEW QUESTIONS

1. A 29-year-old nulliparous African American woman comes to her primary care physician because of pelvic pain and heavy menstruation for the past 6 months. Her periods are regular and usually last for 8 days. She and her husband have also been trying to conceive for the past year but have not been successful. A pelvic exam shows an irregularly enlarged uterus. What is the best next step in management?

    - **The best next step in the diagnosis is a pelvic ultrasound.**
    - This patient presents with pelvic pain and heavy menstruation for the past 6 months.
    - She has an irregularly enlarged uterus.
    - This is most consistent with uterine fibroids.
    - The best initial test to confirm the diagnosis is a pelvic ultrasound. Uterine fibroids appear as concentric, hypoechoic and heterogeneous masses on ultrasound.
    - Her infertility may be directly related to the fibroids.

Gynecology | Section 2: Adenomyosis and Endometriosis

I. Adenomyosis: Definition
   A. A benign condition where endometrial tissue grows into the myometrium
   B. Mostly found in multiparous women > 40 years

II. Adenomyosis: Pathophysiology
   A. Exact cause is unknown
   B. Usually coexists with endometriosis and leiomyomas
   C. Endometrial tissue in myometrium → tissue grows with every cycle → enlarged, boggy uterus

III. Adenomyosis: Clinical Features
   A. Can be asymptomatic
   B. New-onset dysmenorrhea (painful menstruation)
   C. Menorrhagia (heavy menstruation)
   D. Abnormal uterine bleeding
   E. Chronic pelvic pain

IV. Adenomyosis: Diagnosis
   A. Diagnosis is mainly clinical with supportive imaging findings
   B. Pelvic physical exam: symmetrically enlarged, boggy, mobile, soft, and tender uterus
   C. Imaging: US or MRI
   D. Biopsy: confirms the diagnosis

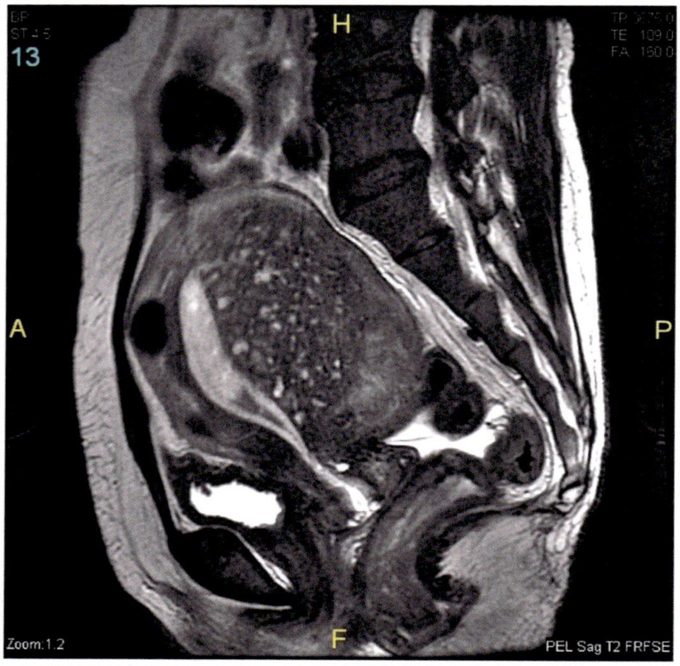

FIGURE 17.2.6 - Pelvic MRI: Adenomyosis

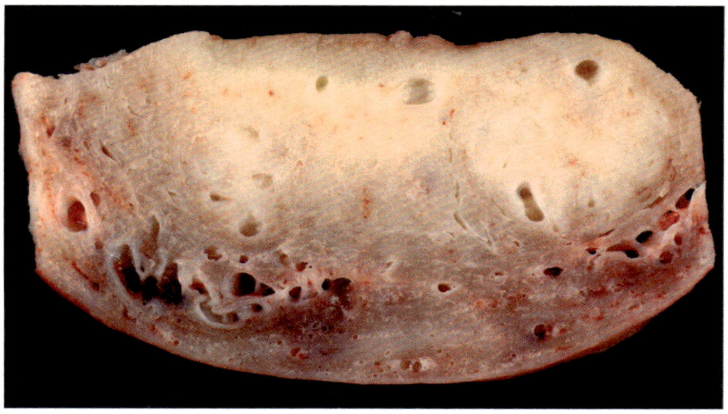

FIGURE 17.2.7 - Adenomyosis

V. Adenomyosis: Management
   A. Pharmacological treatment
      1. NSAIDs, combined OCPs, IUDs, GnRH agonists, progestins (e.g. levonorgestrel)
   B. Interventional treatment
      1. Endometrial ablation, uterine artery embolization
   C. Surgical treatment is definitive
      1. Hysterectomy

VI. Endometriosis: Definition
   A. A condition where endometrial tissue is present outside of the uterus

VII. Endometriosis: Pathophysiology
   A. Not clearly understood; retrograde menstruation theory
   B. This extrauterine endometrial tissue reacts to the hormones and undergoes similar changes to normal uterine tissue during the menstrual cycle

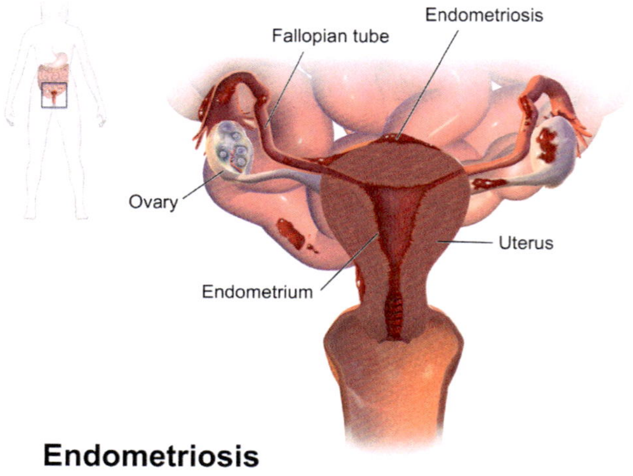

FIGURE 17.2.8 - Endometriosis

VIII. Endometriosis: Clinical Features

A. Can be asymptomatic
B. Cyclical and chronic pelvic pain; worsens before menses
C. Dysmenorrhea: painful but not heavy menstrual bleeding
D. Dyspareunia, infertility
E. Dyschezia: painful defecation; rectal pain

IX. Endometriosis: Diagnosis

A. History
B. Pelvic physical exam
    1. Non-enlarged, non-tender, immobile uterus
    2. Cervical motion tenderness; rectovaginal tenderness
    3. Adnexal mass (chocolate cyst)
C. Transvaginal US: best initial test
    1. Normal sized uterus
    2. Ovarian endometrial cyst
    3. Nodules on bladder, rectovaginal septum, cul-de-sac
D. Laparoscopy: confirmatory test
    1. Blue-black lesions
    2. Gunpowder appearance

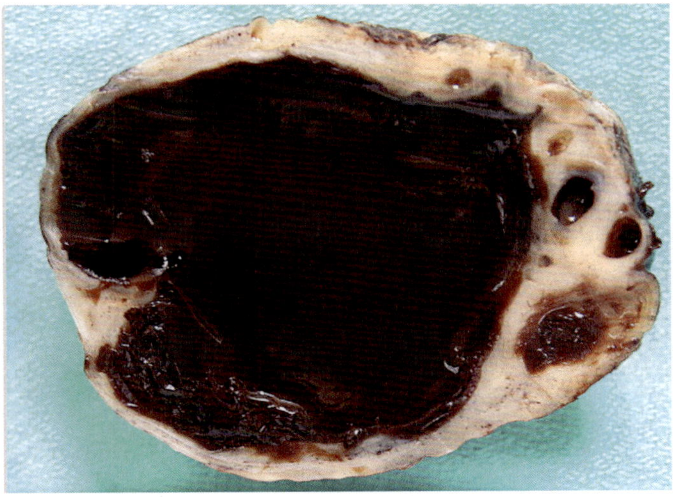

Image courtesy of: Dr. Bulent Celasun, Ankara, Turkey. Used with permission.

FIGURE 17.2.9 - Chocolate Cyst

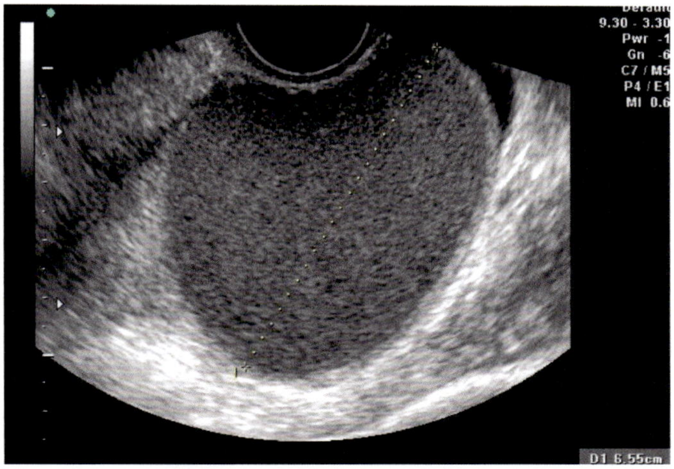

"Figure 1. : "Ultrasound imaging of the ovarian cystic lesion." in: Endometriosis in a postmenopausal woman without previous hormonal therapy: a case report:" by Manuel Garcia Manero, Pedro Royo, Begona Olartecoechea & Juan Luis Alcazar, Journal of Medical Case Reports, licensed under CC BY-SA 4.0. Modifications: Text deleted.

FIGURE 17.2.10 - Transvaginal Ultrasound: Ovarian Endometrial Cyst

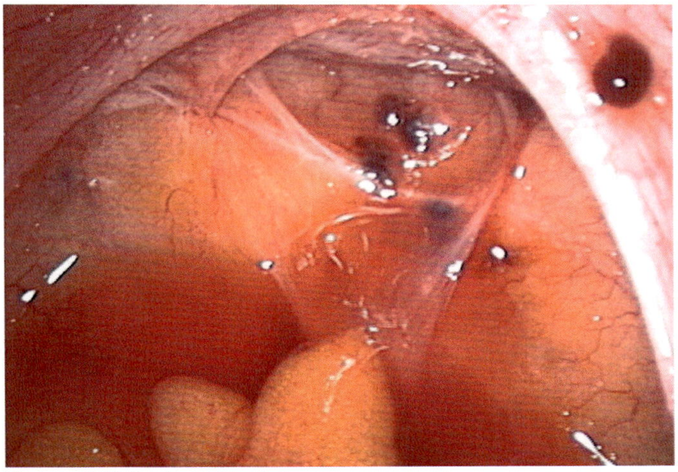

Hic et nunc, Public domain, via Wikimedia Commons

FIGURE 17.2.11 - Laparoscopy: Lesions of Endometriosis in Douglas Space and on Sacrouterine Ligament

X. Endometriosis: Management

A. Medical therapy: NSAIDs, OCPs, GnRH agonists, aromatase inhibitors
B. Surgical resection
    1. Laparoscopy (first line): excision and ablation of endometrial tissue
    2. Hysterectomy (second line) +/- oophorectomy
C. Consider factors such as:
    1. Desire to conceive
    2. Contraindications to medical therapy

	Adenomyosis	Endometriosis
Definition	- Endometrial tissue grows into the myometrium	- Endometrial tissue outside of the uterus
Key features	- Heavy, painful menstruation - Enlarged, globular, tender uterus	- Pain prior to menses - Heavy but not painful menstruation - Dyspareunia, dyschezia - Normal-sized, non-tender, immobile uterus

TABLE 17.2.2 - Adenomyosis and Endometriosis

REVIEW QUESTIONS

1. A 35-year-old woman comes to her primary care physician because of very painful menstruation for the past several months. She says the pain is so severe that she has to miss work during those days. Pelvic ultrasound shows a symmetrically enlarged, globular uterus. What is the likely underlying mechanism of this patient's condition?

   - **The likely underlying mechanism of this patient's condition is endometrial tissue growth into the myometrium.**
   - This middle-aged patient has very painful menstruation.
   - There is a symmetrically enlarged, globular uterus on ultrasound.
   - This is most consistent with adenomyosis, a condition where endometrial tissue grows into the myometrium.

2. A 31-year-old woman comes to her primary care physician because of cyclical pelvic pain that worsens before the onset of her period. Her menses occur at a regular 28-day interval and have moderate to light flow. Over-the-counter analgesics have not helped. She also complains of painful sexual intercourse and occasionally has pain during defecation. Physical examination shows the uterus is normal-sized, non-tender, and no adnexal masses are palpated. What is the next step in managing this patient's symptoms?

   - **The next step in managing the symptoms of this patient is prescribing combined oral contraceptives.**
   - This patient is presenting with cyclical pelvic pain that worsens before the onset of her period, painful sexual intercourse, and pain during defecation.
   - Physical examination shows a normal-sized and non-tender uterus.
   - These signs and symptoms are most likely consistent with endometriosis.
   - She has tried over-the-counter analgesics, but they have not helped.
   - This makes the best next step in management combined oral contraceptives, which will help decrease the severity of pain and the size of endometriotic lesions.

3. A 32-year-old woman comes to her primary care physician because of pelvic pain that starts a couple of days before her menses and gets better after she starts menstruating. Over-the-counter painkillers have not relieved her symptoms. She also complains of pain during sexual intercourse. Menses occur at a regular 30-day interval and last for 5 days. She is currently sexually active and uses combined oral contraceptives. Physical exam shows clear vaginal discharge and rectovaginal tenderness. The remaining portion of the workup, including a transvaginal ultrasound, is normal. What is the best next step in management?

   A. Laser ablation
   B. Hysteroscopy
   C. CT scan of the pelvis
   D. Laparoscopy

   - **The correct answer is option D.**
   - This patient is presenting with characteristic pain of endometriosis, where her pain starts a couple of days before her menses and gets better after she starts menstruating. She also has pain during sexual intercourse.
   - Physical examination shows rectovaginal tenderness.
   - These features are suggestive of endometriosis.
   - Since painkillers have not helped, using combined oral contraceptives has not resolved her symptoms, and the ultrasound was inconclusive; the next best step in management is laparoscopy to confirm the diagnosis of endometriosis.
   - Laparoscopy will also allow laser ablation or excision of the endometriotic lesions once the diagnosis has been confirmed.
   - Option A is incorrect because, before the initiation of any invasive treatments, such as laser ablation, the diagnosis of endometriosis should be first confirmed, given the normal ultrasound findings.
   - Option B is incorrect because hysteroscopy is used in the diagnosis of uterine fibroids and not endometriosis. Patients with fibroids do not usually present with rectovaginal tenderness.
   - Option C is incorrect because a CT scan of the pelvis is not recommended for diagnosing endometriosis due to non-specific findings.

Gynecology | Section 3: Bacterial Vaginosis, Candida Vulvovaginitis, and Trichomonas Vaginali

I. Bacterial Vaginosis
  A. Causative agent: *Gardnerella vaginalis*, anaerobic bacteria
  B. Related to sexual activity but not sexually transmitted
  C. Increases the risk for preterm delivery in pregnant women
  D. Risk factors
    1. Vaginal douching, woman having sex with woman
  E. Signs and symptoms
    1. Painless thin gray vaginal discharge with fishy smell
  F. Diagnosis (≥ 3 out of 4 Amsel criteria)
    1. Vaginal pH ≥ 4.5
    2. Thin gray-white discharge
    3. Positive whiff test
    4. Clue cells on wet mount (*Gardnerella vaginalis* surrounding vaginal epithelial cells)
  G. Treatment: metronidazole or clindamycin

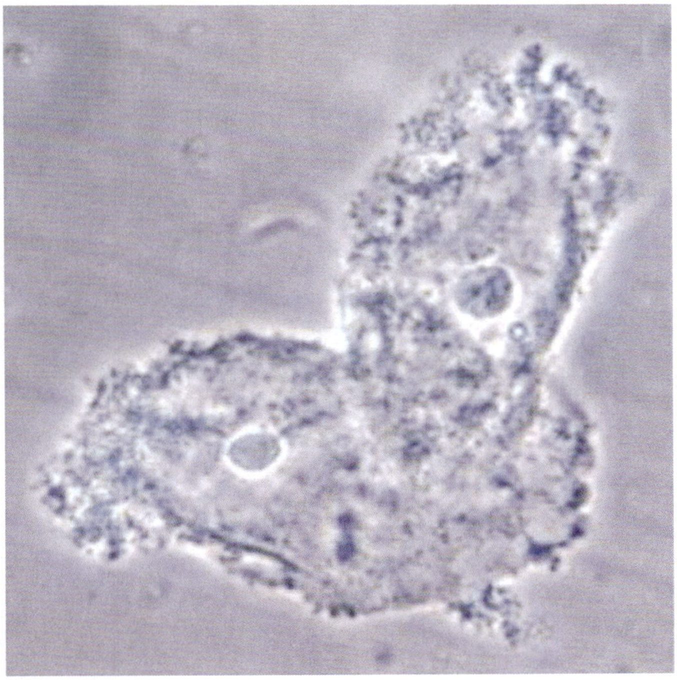

CDC/ M. Rein, Public domain, via Wikimedia Commons

FIGURE 17.2.12 - Microscopic Image Showing a Clue Cell

II. *Candida* vulvovaginitis
  A. Causative agent: *Candida albicans*
  B. Risk factors
    1. Diabetes mellitus
    2. Recent antibiotic use
  C. Signs and symptoms
    1. Thick "cottage cheese" discharge
    2. Painful (vs. bacterial vaginosis which is painless)

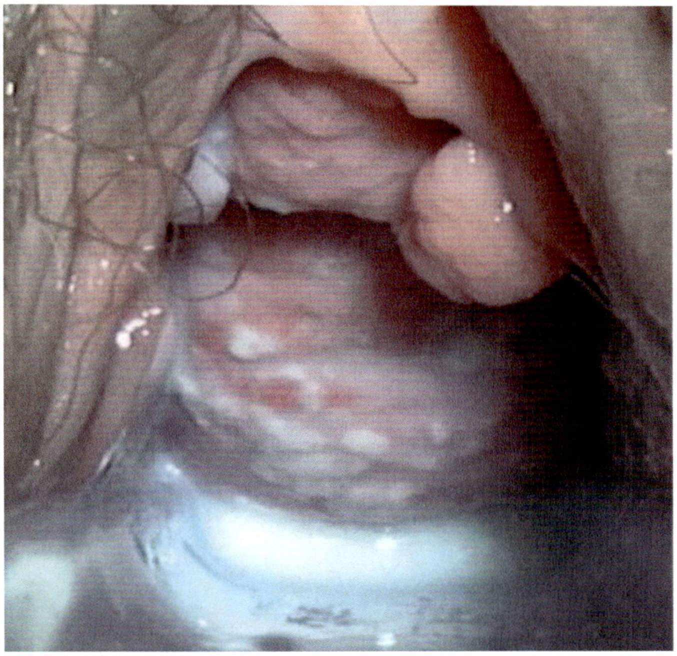

Mikael Häggström, CC0, via Wikimedia Commons

FIGURE 17.2.13 - Image Showing Thick "Cottage Cheese" Discharge In Candida Vulvovaginitis

III. *Candida* Vulvovaginitis
  A. Diagnosis
    1. Vaginal pH 3.8-4.5
    2. Thick "cottage cheese" discharge
    3. Yeast cells and pseudohyphae on microscopy
  B. Treatment: "-azoles" (e.g. oral or topical fluconazole)

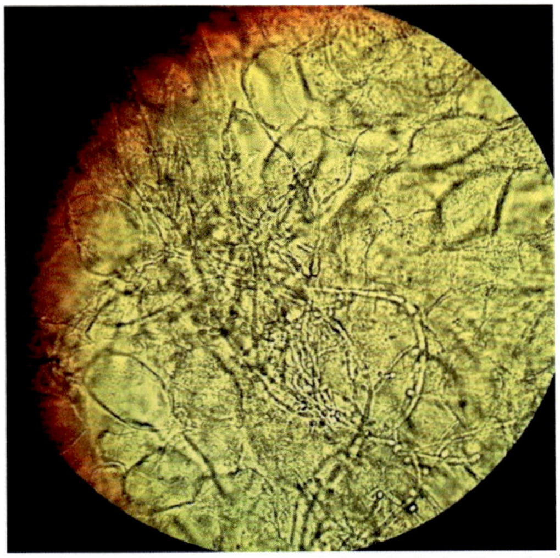

Mikael Häggström.When using this image in external works, it may be cited as:Häggström, Mikael (2014). "Medical gallery of Mikael Häggström 2014". WikiJournal of Medicine 1 (2). DOI:10.15347/wjm/2014.008. ISSN 2002-4436. Public Domain.orBy Mikael Häggström, used with permission., CC0, via Wikimedia Commons

FIGURE 17.2.14 - Photomicrograph Showing Yeast Cells and Pseudohyphae of *Candida albicans*

IV. Trichomonas vaginalis

A. Sexually transmitted protozoal infection
B. Risk factors
   1. Multiple sexual partners
   2. Unprotected sexual intercourse
C. Signs and symptoms
   1. Yellow-green, frothy, foul-smelling discharge
   2. Painful (vs bacterial vaginosis which is painless)
D. Diagnosis
   1. Vaginal pH ≥ 4.5
   2. Yellow-green, frothy, foul-smelling discharge
   3. "Strawberry cervix" (inflamed cervix with punctate hemorrhages)
   4. Motile pear-shaped trichomonads on wet mount
   5. Nucleic acid amplification test (NAAT) - preferred
E. Treatment: metronidazole for the patient and the partner(s)

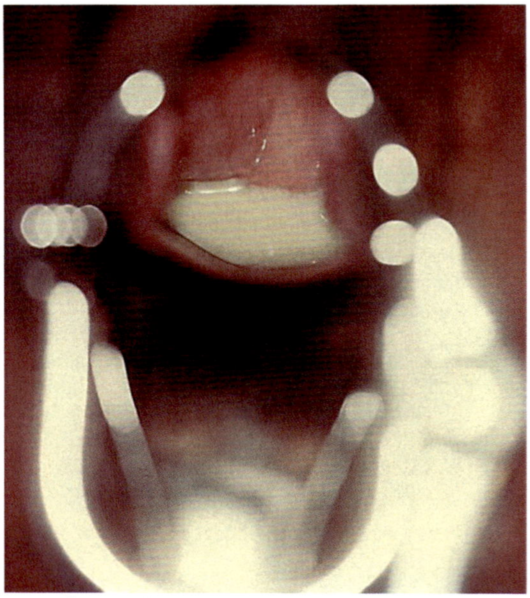

FIGURE 17.2.15 - A Colposcopy Image Showing Thick White-Yellowish Discharge

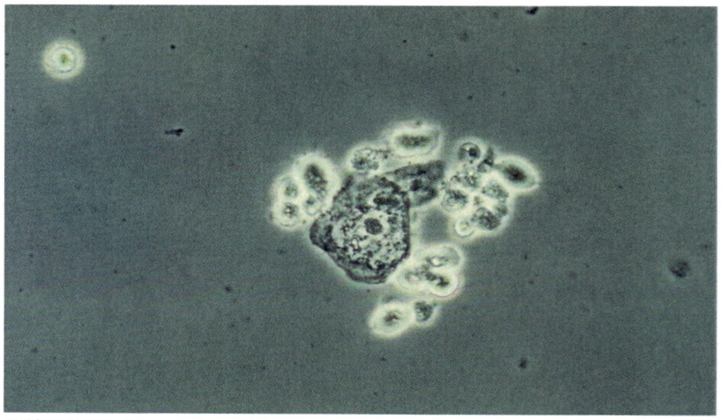

FIGURE 17.2.16 - A Photomicrograph Showing Motile Pear-Shaped Trichomonads

Condition	Etiology	Key Features
Bacterial vaginosis	- *Gardnerella vaginalis* and anaerobic bacteria	- Thin, gray or off-white discharge with fishy odor - Positive whiff test - Clue cells on microscopy - Vaginal pH > 4.5 - Treatment: metronidazole or clindamycin
Trichomoniasis	- *Trichomonas vaginalis*	- Yellow-greenish foul-smelling discharge - "Strawberry cervix" - Pear-shaped motile trichomonads on microscopy - Vaginal pH > 4.5 - Treatment: metronidazole
Candida vulvovaginitis	- *Candida Albicans*	- Thick white "cottage-cheese" discharge - Vaginal inflammation - Yeasts cells and pseudohyphae on microscopy - Normal vaginal pH (3.8 - 4.5) - Treatment: fluconazole

TABLE 17.2.3 - Bacterial Vaginosis, Candida Vulvovaginitis, and Trichomonas Vaginalis

REVIEW QUESTIONS

1. A 23-year-old woman comes to her primary care physician because of vaginal itching and discharge for the past 2 weeks. She has just become sexually active with her boyfriend. She states they use condoms for protection. Vital signs are unremarkable. Physical examination shows a thin off-white discharge with an exacerbating odor upon adding 10% potassium hydroxide solution. What will likely be found on microscopic analysis of this patient's discharge?

    - **Microscopic analysis of the vaginal discharge from the patient with bacterial vaginosis shows clue cells, which are vaginal epithelial cells with peripheral stippling.**
    - This sexually active patient has thin off-white vaginal discharge with exacerbating odor upon adding 10% potassium hydroxide.
    - This presentation is classic for bacterial vaginosis.

2. A 34-year-old woman comes to her primary care physician because of severe vaginal pain and discharge for the past week. She is sexually active with 4 male partners, and she takes oral contraceptive pills. Vital signs are significant for a temperature of 100.4° F (38° C). Physical examination shows yellow-green vaginal discharge. The wet mount shows motile pear-shaped microorganisms. What is the preferred antimicrobial agent for this patient's condition?

    - **The preferred antimicrobial agent for trichomoniasis is metronidazole.**
    - This patient presents with fever and yellow-green vaginal discharge.
    - She has multiple sexual partners, but she does not use barrier contraception.
    - Additionally, the wet mount shows motile pear-shaped microorganisms.
    - All of these findings are consistent with the diagnosis of trichomonas vaginalis infection.

3. A 29-year-old woman comes to her primary care physician because of vaginal itching and discharge for the past 5 days. She had a history of gonococcal cervicitis 3 years ago and atypical pneumonia treated with azithromycin 2 weeks ago. Vital signs are unremarkable. Physical examination shows thick white vaginal discharge. Microscopy shows yeast cells and pseudohyphae. What predisposed this patient to her current condition?

    - **Recent antibiotic use most likely predisposed this patient to her current condition.**
    - This patient has thick white vaginal discharge accompanied by microscopic findings of yeast cells and pseudohyphae.
    - This presentation is classic for candida vulvovaginitis.
    - She was treated with azithromycin 2 weeks ago, which likely disrupted her normal vaginal flora allowing for candida overgrowth.

Gynecology | Section 4: Bartholin Gland Abscess

I. Bartholin Gland Abscess
    A. Bartholin glands (greater vestibular glands) are located at 4 and 8 o'clock positions of the vaginal orifice
    B. Complication of Bartholin gland cyst
    C. Infection of mucus accumulated in Bartholin gland
    D. Causative agents
        1. Polymicrobial
        2. *E.coli* and *Neisseria gonorrhea*
    E. Signs and symptoms
        1. Difficulty sitting and walking
        2. Painful sexual intercourse
        3. Enlarged erythematous mass at the vaginal orifice
        4. Fever
    F. Treatment
        1. Incision and drainage
        2. Antibiotics for: recurrent cases, pregnant, immunocompromised patients, and those with systemic infection (fever, chills)
        3. Word catheter for first or second recurrence
        4. Marsupialization as a last resort for continual drainage

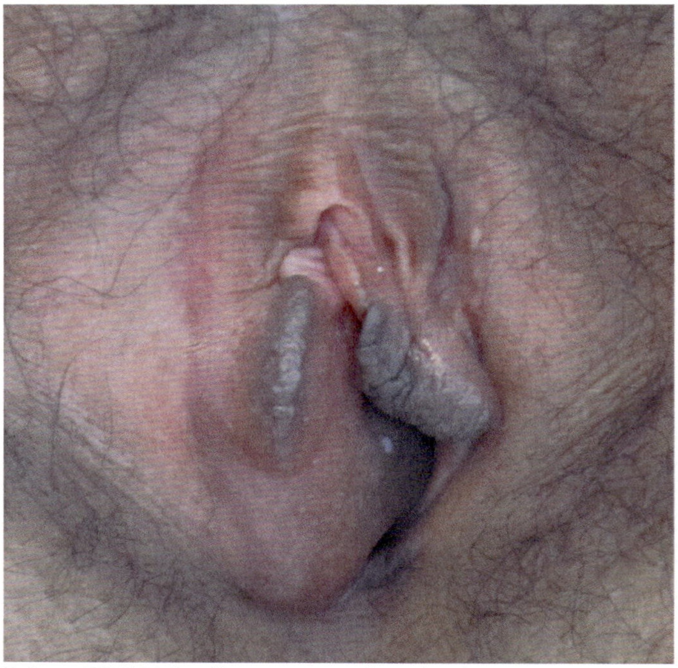

FIGURE 17.2.18 - Bartholin Gland Abscess

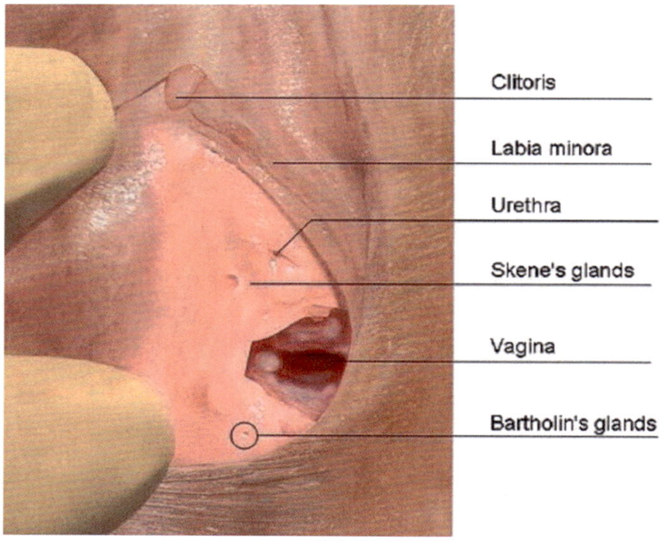

FIGURE 17.2.17 - Normal Anatomy of Bartholin Glands

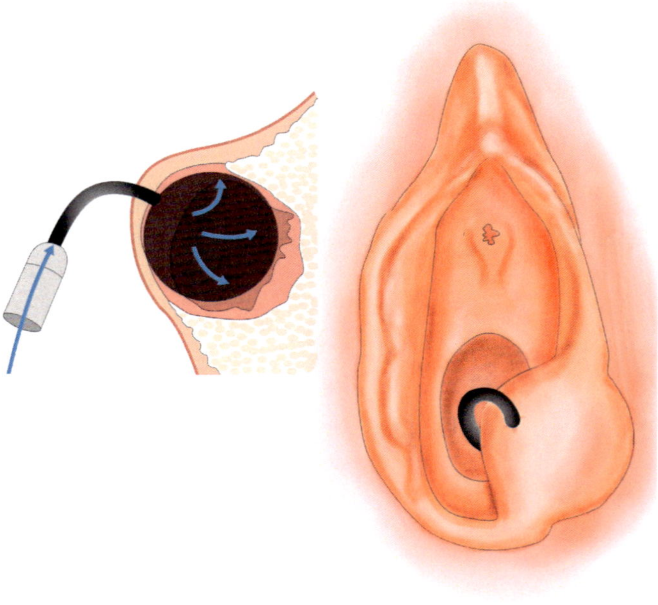

FIGURE 17.2.19 - Word Catheter Placement in Bartholin Gland

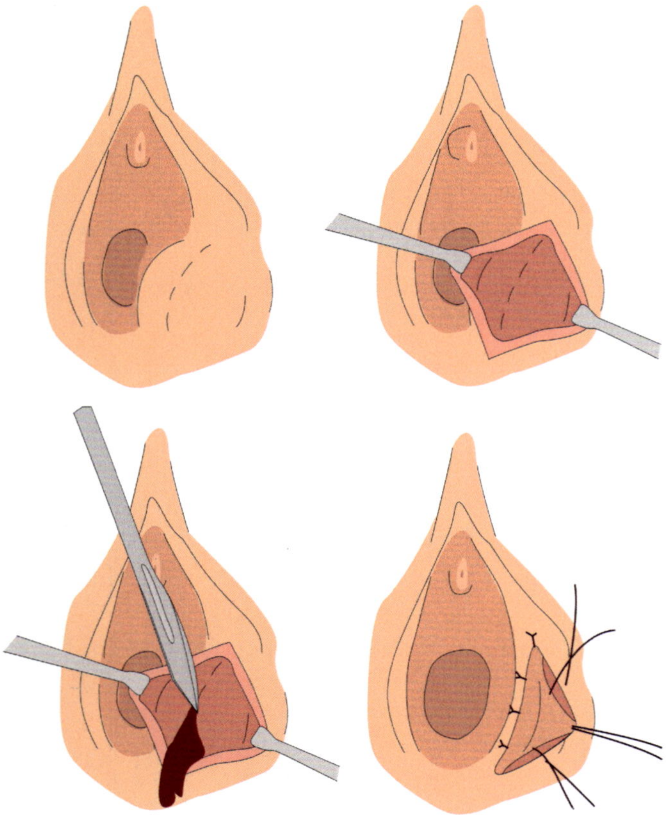

FIGURE 17.2.20 - Marsupialization of the Bartholin Gland

REVIEW QUESTIONS

1. A 27-year-old woman comes to her primary care physician because of severe vulvar pain for the last 4 days. She has trouble walking and sitting due to her pain. She also experiences pain during sexual intercourse, which has put a strain on her relationship with her boyfriend. She has never had a similar problem before. Vital signs include a temperature of 96.8° F (36° C), blood pressure of 125/70 mmHg, heart rate of 92 beats/min, and respiratory rate of 16 breaths/min. Physical examination shows an enlarged erythematous tender mass at the 4 o'clock position of the vulva. Palpation of the mass elicits exquisite pain. Which of the following is the next best step in the management?

   A. Antibiotics
   B. Word catheter placement
   C. Incision and drainage
   D. Marsupialization

- **The correct answer is option C.**
- This patient presents with severe vulvar pain, trouble walking and sitting, and dyspareunia.
- Physical examination shows an enlarged erythematous tender mass at the 4 o'clock position of the vulva.
- This description is most consistent with Bartholin gland abscess.
- Since this is her first occurrence, the best next step in the management is incision and drainage.
- Option A is incorrect because antibiotics are usually reserved for recurrent cases, pregnant and immunocompromised patients, and for those with systemic signs of infection like fever and chills. This patient is afebrile.
- Option B is incorrect because Word catheter is placed after the second or third recurrence of Bartholin gland abscess. This patient has never had a similar problem before.
- Option D is incorrect because marsupialization is the last resort for treating Bartholin gland abscess after using Word catheter.

Gynecology | Section 5: Endometritis and Pelvic Inflammatory Disease

I. Endometritis: Definition
   A. Inflammation of uterine endometrium
   B. Acute and chronic

II. Endometritis: Pathophysiology
   A. Retained material in uterus is nidus for bacteria
   B. Most commonly due to *Chlamydia trachomatis* or *Neisseria gonorrhoeae*
   C. Mycobacterium tuberculosis (rare)

III. Endometritis: Risk Factors
   A. Retained products of conception after delivery (postpartum endometritis)
   B. Spontaneous abortion
   C. Iatrogenic pregnancy termination
   D. Intrauterine device

IV. Endometritis: Clinical Features
   A. Fever (acute endometritis)
   B. Abnormal uterine bleeding
   C. Pelvic pain
   D. Uterine tenderness
   E. Asymptomatic (chronic endometritis)

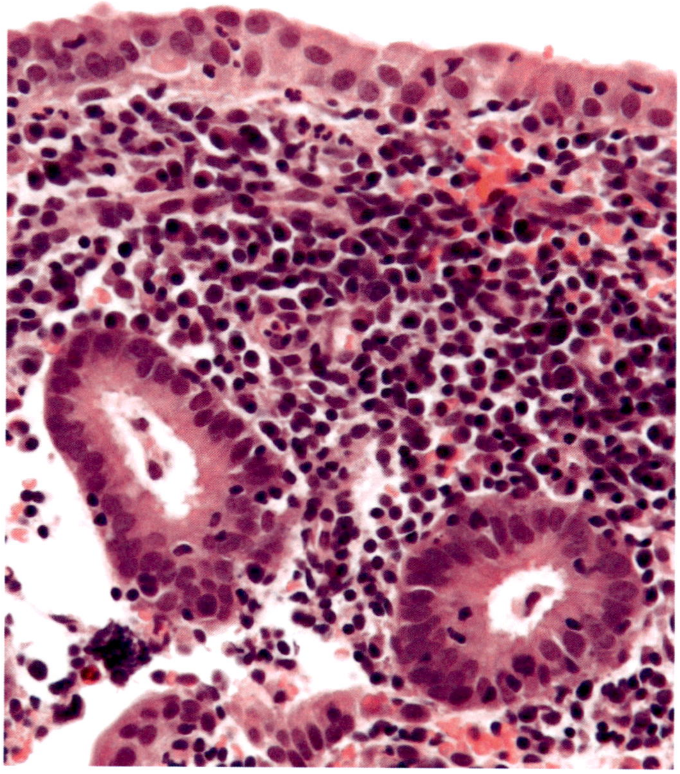

FIGURE 17.2.21 - Histological Appearance of Chronic Endometritis

V. Endometritis: Diagnosis
   A. Most clinical
   B. CBC and urine culture
   C. Endometrial biopsy with culture and acid-fast stain
   D. Histological finding: plasma cells (chronic endometritis)
   E. Menstrual blood culture (better than biopsy for TB endometritis)
   F. Latter two tests not routinely performed

VI. Endometritis: Treatment
   A. Acute endometritis
      1. Clindamycin and gentamicin +/- ampicillin (GBS colonization)
   B. Chronic endometritis
      1. Doxycycline

VII. Pelvic Inflammatory Disease: Definition
   A. Inflammation of upper reproductive tract
   B. Cervicitis: inflammation of cervix
   C. Endometritis: inflammation of endometrium
   D. Salpingitis: inflammation of fallopian tubes
   E. Oophoritis: inflammation of ovaries
   F. Tubo-ovarian abscess: inflamed mass involving tube and ovary
   G. Perihepatitis: inflammation of perihepatic (Glisson's) capsule

VIII. Pelvic Inflammatory Disease: Pathophysiology
   A. Usually polymicrobial infection
   B. Main pathogens: *Chlamydia trachomatis* (more common) or *Neisseria gonorrhoeae*

IX. Pelvic Inflammatory Disease: Risk Factors
   A. Multiple sexual partners
   B. Inconsistent use of barrier contraception
   C. Prior history of PID
   D. Age 15 - 25
   E. Partner with sexually transmitted infection

X. Pelvic Inflammatory Disease: Clinical Features
   A. Fever > 38.3° C (100.94° F)
   B. Cervical motion tenderness
   C. Pelvic pain
   D. Mucopurulent cervical discharge
   E. Fitz-Hugh-Curtis syndrome
      1. Right upper quadrant pain
      2. "Violin string" adhesions of peritoneum to liver

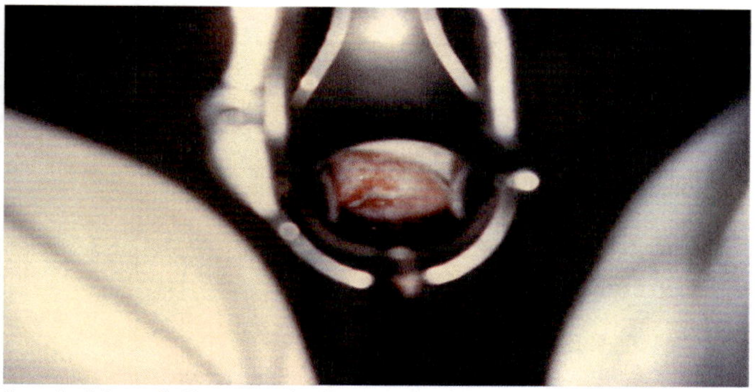

FIGURE 17.2.22 - Colposcopy: Mucopurulent Cervical Discharge Consistent With Pelvic Inflammatory Disease

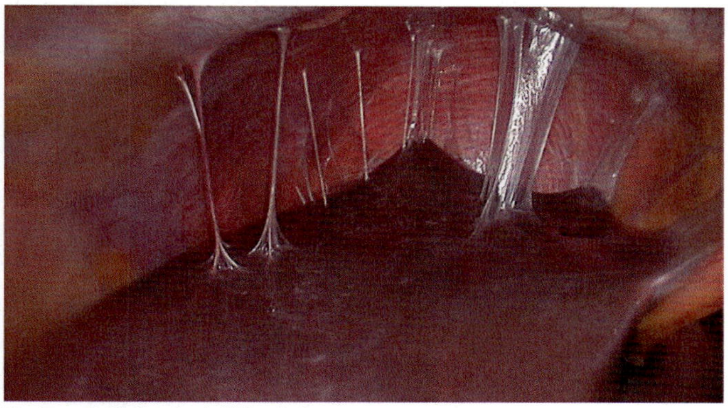

FIGURE 17.2.23 - "Violin String" Adhesions

XI. Pelvic Inflammatory Disease: Diagnosis
   A. Clinical symptoms
   B. Cervical nucleic acid amplification test (NAAT) for chlamydia and gonorrhea

XII. Pelvic Inflammatory Disease: Treatment
   A. Outpatient
      1. Ceftriaxone and doxycycline
   B. Inpatient
      1. IV cefoxitin and doxycycline
      2. Alternative: IV gentamicin and clindamycin
   C. Indications for hospitalization:
      1. Failed outpatient treatment
      2. Pregnancy
      3. Inability to tolerate oral medications
      4. Noncompliant with outpatient therapy
      5. Severe presentation (e.g. vomiting, high fever)
      6. Complications (e.g. tubo-ovarian abscess, perihepatitis)

REVIEW QUESTIONS

1. A 32-year-old woman comes to her primary care physician because of lower abdominal pain for the last 5 days. The pain is dull and constant. She underwent a spontaneous abortion 7 days ago. Vital signs are significant for a temperature of 101.3° F (38.5° C). Lower abdominal palpation shows uterine tenderness. Purulent cervical discharge is noticed on colposcopy. What is the best choice of antimicrobial therapy for this patient?

   - **The best choice of antimicrobial therapy for this patient is clindamycin and gentamicin.**
   - This patient presents with lower abdominal pain, fever, and uterine tenderness starting after spontaneous abortion.
   - Additionally, there is purulent cervical discharge on colposcopy.
   - This combination of findings is most consistent with acute endometritis.

2. A 24-year-old woman comes to her primary care physician because of pelvic pain for the last week. She has recently noticed malodorous vaginal discharge. She had 6 sexual partners over the last 2 months, and she takes oral contraceptive pills. She has a temperature of 104° F (40° C). Colposcopy shows an erythematous cervix with mucopurulent discharge. A cervical nucleic acid amplification test is performed. What is the most likely pathogen responsible for this patient's condition?

   - **The most likely pathogen responsible for this patient's condition is chlamydia.**
   - This patient presents with pelvic pain, fever, and mucopurulent discharge.
   - She has multiple sexual partners, and she does not use barrier contraception.
   - All of these clues are consistent with the pelvic inflammatory disease (PID).
   - Although PID is usually a polymicrobial infection, chlamydia is the most common pathogen responsible for the initial inflammation

Gynecology | Section 6: Tubo-Ovarian Abscess and Toxic Shock Syndrome

I. Tubo-Ovarian Abscess: Definition
  A. Inflammatory mass involving fallopian tube, ovary, and, sometimes, bladder or bowel

II. Tubo-Ovarian Abscess: Pathophysiology
  A. Complication of pelvic inflammatory disease
  B. Usually polymicrobial infection
  C. Commonly isolated pathogens: *E. coli*, *Bacteroides fragilis*, *Prevotella*, *Peptostreptococcus*, other anaerobes

III. Tubo-Ovarian Abscess: Risk Factors
  A. Multiple sexual partners
  B. Inconsistent use of barrier contraception
  C. Prior history of PID
  D. Age 15 - 25
  E. Partner with sexually transmitted infection

IV. Tubo-Ovarian Abscess: Clinical Features
  A. Fever > 38.3° C (100.94° F)
  B. Pelvic pain
  C. Mucopurulent cervical discharge
  D. Adnexal mass on pelvic exam

V. Tubo-Ovarian Abscess: Diagnosis
  A. Clinical symptoms
  B. Pelvic exam showing adnexal mass
  C. Typical ultrasound findings: complex mass with cystic and, sometimes, solid components

VI. Tubo-Ovarian Abscess: Treatment
  A. Hemodynamically stable, no rupture, abscess < 7 cm, response to antibiotic therapy, premenopausal
    1. Only antibiotics
  B. No response to antibiotics and no clinical deterioration
    1. Antibiotics and abscess drainage
  C. No response to antibiotics and clinical deterioration
    1. Antibiotics and open surgery

VII. Toxic Shock Syndrome: Definition
  A. Systemic inflammatory condition from *Staphylococcus aureus* or *Streptococcus pyogenes*

VIII. Toxic Shock Syndrome: Pathophysiology
  A. TSST-1 from *S. aureus*; erythrogenic exotoxin A from *S. pyogenes*
  B. Cross-link beta region of TCR on T-helper 1 cell to MHC II on macrophage
  C. Excessive release of IL-2, IFN-gamma, IL-1, and TNF-alpha
  D. Cytokine storm causes shock

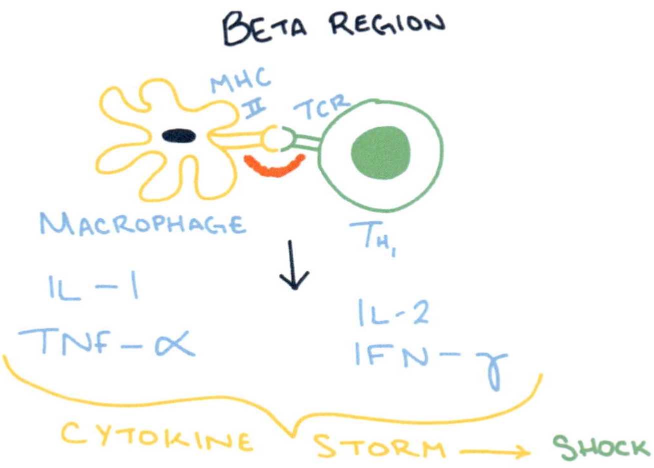

FIGURE 17.2.24 - Pathogenesis of Toxic Shock Syndrome

IX. Toxic Shock Syndrome: Risk Factors
  A. Toxic shock syndrome by *S. aureus*
    1. Prolonged use of vaginal tampon
    2. Nasal or wound packing
  B. Toxic shock-like syndrome by *S. pyogenes*
    1. Painful skin infection (erysipelas, cellulitis)

X. Toxic Shock Syndrome: Clinical Features
  A. Fever
  B. Vomiting and diarrhea
  C. Desquamating rash
  D. End-organ failure
    1. Acute kidney injury, altered consciousness
    2. Acute liver failure
    3. Muscle damage

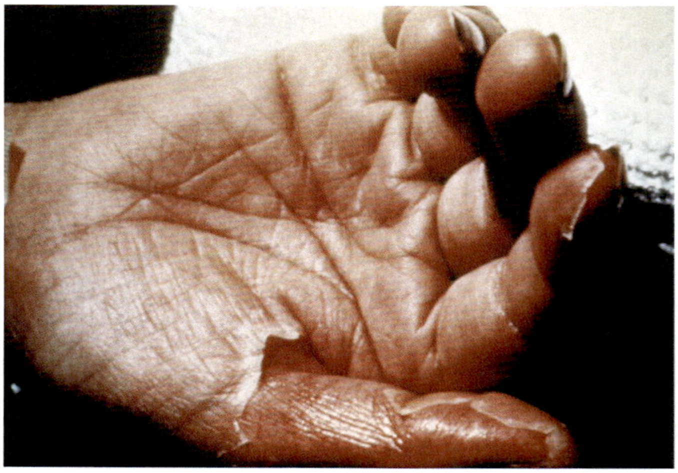

FIGURE 17.2.25 - Desquamating Rash in Toxic Shock Syndrome

XI. Toxic Shock Syndrome: Diagnosis
   A. Clinical symptoms
   B. Known risk factors
   C. Laboratory findings indicating end-organ failure:
      1. Increased AST, ALT, total bilirubin
      2. Increased CK
      3. Increased BUN and creatinine

XII. Toxic Shock Syndrome: Treatment
   A. Removal of packing from the wounds or tampons from vagina
   B. Wound debridement
   C. IV fluids and vasopressors if needed
   D. IV antibiotics
      1. Nafcillin/oxacillin and clindamycin for MSSA
      2. Vancomycin and clindamycin for MRSA
   E. IVIG rarely used in patients unresponsive to fluids and antibiotics

REVIEW QUESTIONS ?

1. A 45-year-old woman comes to her primary care physician because of left lower abdominal pain. She initially had generalized pelvic pain, which lateralized to the left side 3 days ago. She is sexually active with her male partner, and they do not use any contraception. Vital signs are significant for a temperature of 105.8° F (40° C). Her white blood cell count is 25,000/mm^3. Pelvic ultrasound shows a left ovarian mass with cystic and solid components. What is the best next step of management for this patient's ovarian mass?

- **The best management for the ovarian mass is broad-spectrum antibiotics with or without abscess drainage.**
- This patient has left lower abdominal pain.
- She is sexually active with her male partner, and they do not use any contraception.
- She has high fever and severe leukocytosis.
- This presentation is most consistent with pelvic inflammatory disease (PID).
- Her pelvic ultrasound shows a left ovarian mass with cystic and solid components. This mass, in the context of PID, is most likely a tubo-ovarian abscess.
- Tubo-ovarian abscess is treated with broad-spectrum antibiotics with or without abscess drainage.

2. A 34-year-old woman is brought to her primary care physician by her husband because of a rash and diarrhea that started 8 hours ago. She vomited several times on the way to the hospital. She has a history of heavy menstrual bleeding. She saturates pads and tampons frequently. Her last menstrual period started 2 days ago. Vital signs include a temperature of 104° F (40° C), blood pressure of 60/40 mmHg, heart rate of 150 beats/min, and respiratory rate of 25 breaths/min. Laboratory studies shows white blood cell count of 30,000/mm^3 (4,500 - 11,000/mm^3). AST of 4,000 U/L (12 - 38 U/L), ALT of 3,000 U/L (10 - 40 U/L), and total bilirubin of 6 mg/dL (0.1 - 1.0 mg/dL). As well as BUN of 90 mg/dL (7 - 18 mg/dL) and creatinine of 4 mg/dL (0.6 - 1.2 mg/dL). Which of the following is the best next step in management?

   A. Intravenous normal saline
   B. Wound debridement
   C. Intravenous vancomycin and clindamycin
   D. Intravenous immune globulin

- **The correct answer is option A.**
- This patient presents with acute-onset rash and diarrhea.
- She has a history of heavy menstrual bleeding, which started 2 days ago.
- She has high fever, severe hypotension, and tachycardia.
- Her white blood cell count is elevated.
- Her alanine aminotransferase (ALT) and aspartate aminotransferase (AST) are extremely elevated, likely due to ischemic hepatitis.
- Additionally, her BUN to creatinine ratio is more than 20, indicating prerenal acute kidney injury likely due to shock.
- All of these findings are consistent with toxic shock syndrome.
- The very first measure is providing intravenous normal saline to increase the patient's blood pressure.
- Whenever a patient has a life-threatening condition, the ABCDEs must be considered first: A for airway, B for breathing, C for circulation, D for neurological defect, and E for exposure. This patient first needs circulatory support.
- Option B is incorrect because wound debridement would be performed after giving intravenous normal saline and antibiotics.
- Option C is incorrect because intravenous vancomycin and clindamycin would be given after administering intravenous fluids.
- Option D is incorrect because intravenous immune globulin is rarely used in patients unresponsive to initial therapy of fluids and antibiotics.

Gynecology | Section 7: Pelvic Organ Prolapse

I. Pelvic Organ Prolapse: Definition
   A. Abnormal herniation of pelvic organs such as the bladder, uterus, or rectum through the vagina

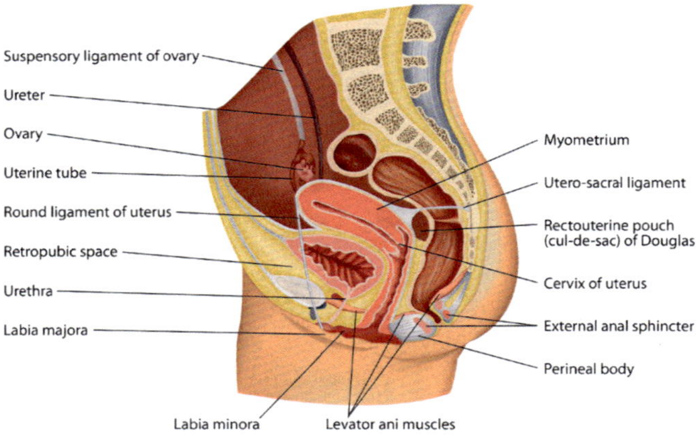

FIGURE 17.2.26 - Female Pelvis and Pelvic Organs

II. Pelvic Organ Prolapse: Pathophysiology
   A. Weak pelvic support and increased intra-abdominal pressure → herniation of organs into the vaginal vault
   B. Could be partial or complete (protrusion beyond the vaginal opening)
   C. Types
      1. Anterior: herniation of bladder (cystocele)
      2. Posterior: herniation of rectum (rectocele) or intestines (enterocele)
      3. Apical: herniation of the uterus or vaginal apex
      4. Uterine procidentia: herniation of all vaginal walls

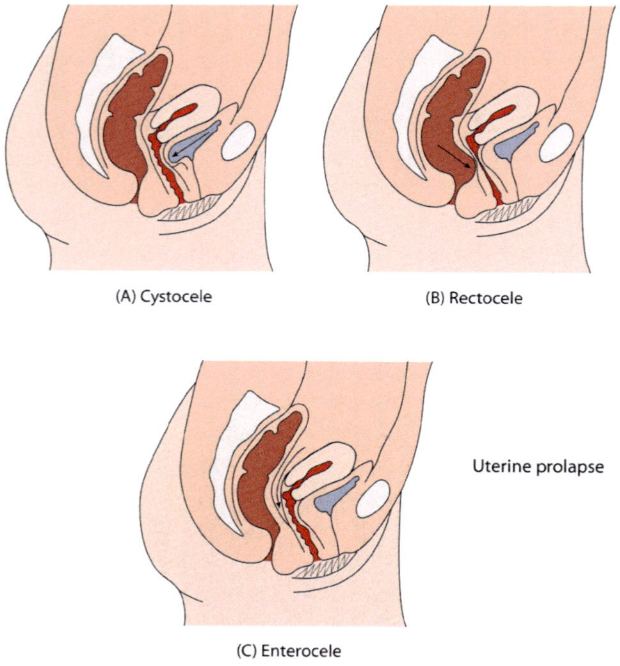

FIGURE 17.2.27 - Cystocele, Rectocele, and Enterocele

III. Pelvic Organ Prolapse: Risk Factors
   A. Multiparity
   B. Vaginal birth
   C. Advanced age
   D. Pelvic surgery (e.g. hysterectomy)
   E. Connective tissue disorders
   F. Conditions increasing intra abdominal pressure (e.g. obesity, constipation, chronic cough)

IV. Pelvic Organ Prolapse: Clinical Features
      1. Sensation of pelvic pressure or fullness
      2. Protrusion from the vagina; "something falling out of the vagina"
      3. Urinary dysfunction
      4. Stress urinary incontinence: urine leakage with coughing or sneezing
      5. Urinary retention (obstructive uropathy): sensation of incomplete bladder emptying
   A. Defecation dysfunction
      1. Constipation
      2. Fecal incontinence
   B. Dyspareunia
   C. Urinary tract infections

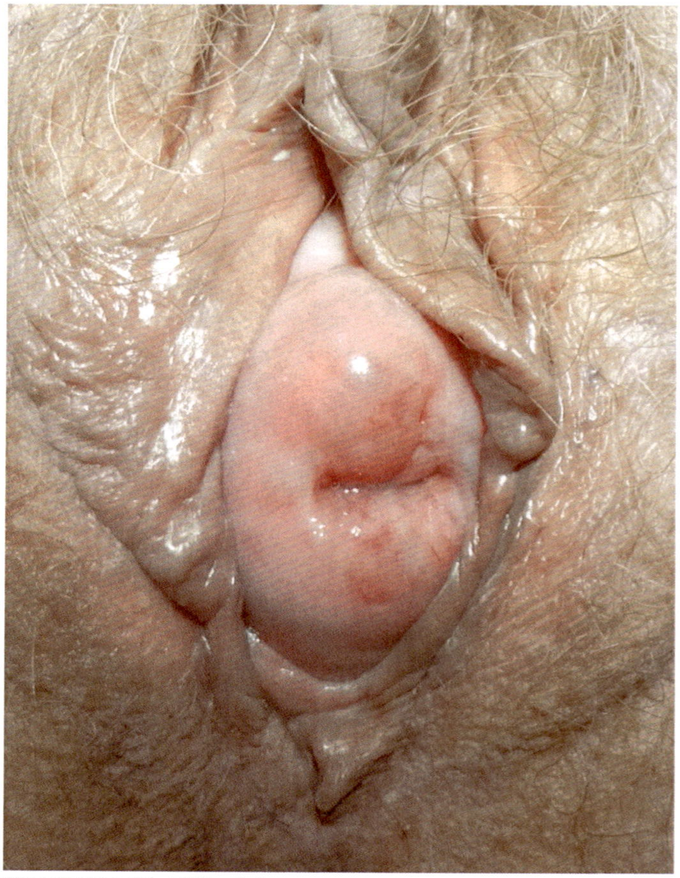

Mikael Häggström, CC0, via Wikimedia Commons

FIGURE 17.2.28 - Uterine Prolapse

1. Pelvic Organ Prolapse: Differential Diagnosis
D. Prolapsed uterine leiomyoma
E. Urethral diverticulum
F. Imperforate hymen
G. Prolapsed uterine leiomyoma; "aborting intracavitary leiomyoma"
    1. Labor-like pains
    2. Firm, smooth, round mass in vagina; dilated cervix
    3. Irregularly enlarged uterus
    4. History of heavy menstrual bleeding
H. Urethral diverticulum: herniation of urethral mucosa
    1. Mid to distal ⅔ of urethra
    2. Similar risk factors to pelvic organ prolapse
    3. Presents with urinary symptoms (stress incontinence, post-void dribbling), dysuria, dyspareunia
    4. Physical exam will reveal a tender anterior vaginal wall mass
    5. Conservative (mild symptoms), surgical (suspicion of malignancy)
I. Imperforate hymen
    1. Hymen completely obstructing vagina
    2. Adolescent female
    3. Primary amenorrhea
    4. Cyclical abdominal pain
    5. Blue-tinged bulge from the vagina (hematocolpos)

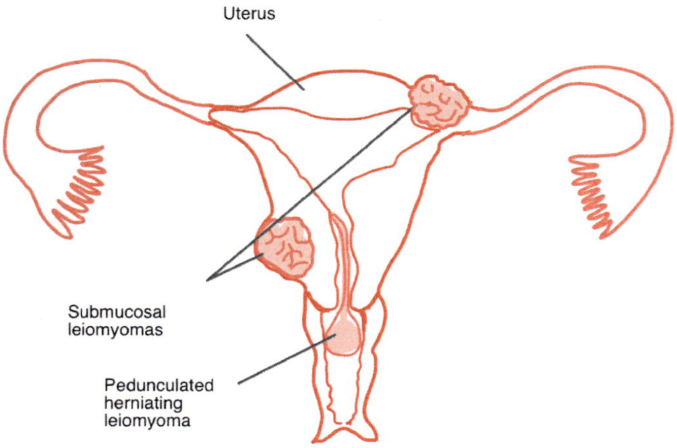

FIGURE 17.2.29 - Prolapsed Uterine Leiomyoma

2. Pelvic Organ Prolapse: Diagnosis
J. History
    1. Urinary, fecal, or sexual dysfunction
K. Pelvic physical exam
    1. Vaginal mass that increases in size with Valsalva maneuver
    2. Perform valsalva maneuver in lithotomy position: patient lying on back with hips and knees flexed and thighs apart
L. Digital rectal exam (DRE)
    1. Evaluation of anal sphincter tone: decreased (weak pelvic floor muscles)
M. Evaluate degree of prolapse by level of descent of the prolapsed organ

V. Pelvic Organ Prolapse: Management
A. Asymptomatic: reassurance and observation
B. Symptomatic: conservative or surgical
C. Conservative treatment
    1. Weight loss
    2. High fiber diet: decrease straining from constipation
    3. Pelvic floor (Kegel) exercises
    4. Vaginal pessary: chronically ill patients or patients with contraindications to surgery
D. Surgical treatment
    1. Indication: no improvement of symptoms or declined with conservative treatment
    2. Anterior/posterior vaginal wall repair: colporrhaphy
    3. Apical prolapse: hysterectomy with suspension of vaginal apex
    4. Decision of conservative vs. surgical treatment depends on patients' preferences and surgical risk assessment

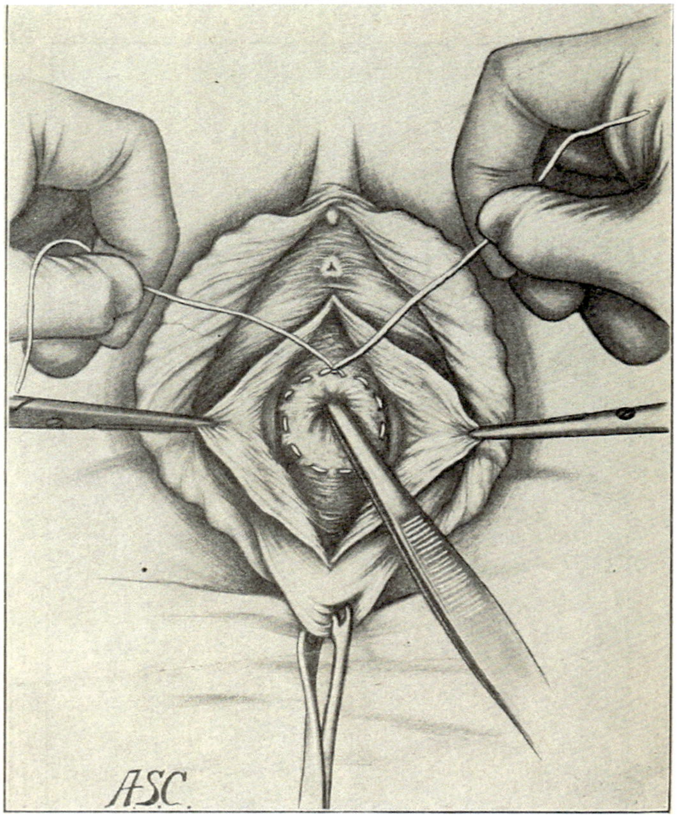

Internet Archive Book Images, No restrictions, via Wikimedia Commons

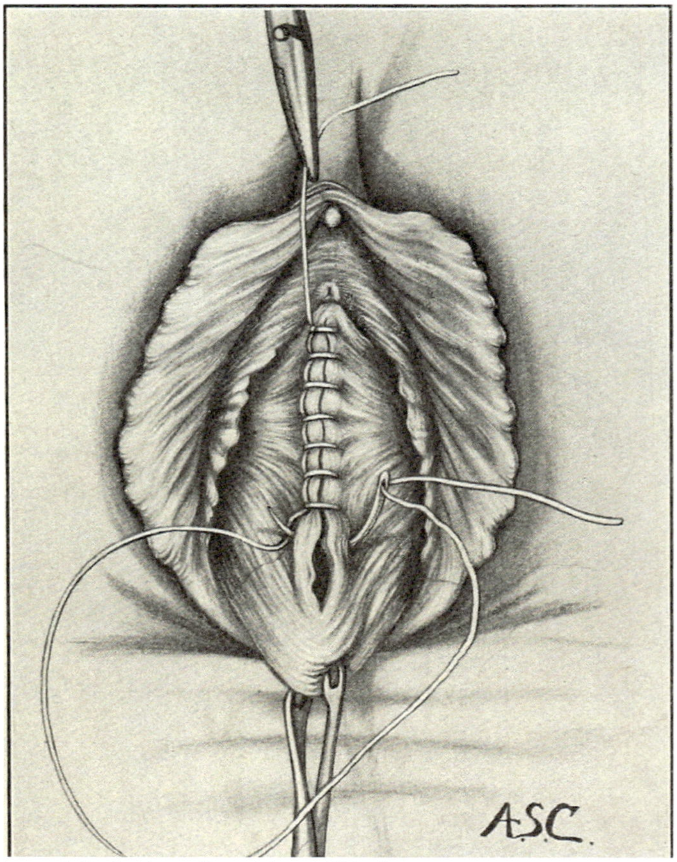

Internet Archive Book Images, No restrictions, via Wikimedia Commons

FIGURE 17.2.30 - Colporrhaphy

Condition	Etiology	Key Features
Pelvic organ prolapse	- Anterior vaginal wall prolapse (cystocele) - Posterior vaginal wall prolapse (rectocele, enterocele) - Apical vaginal wall prolapse (uterine prolapse) - Uterine procidentia	- Anterior, posterior, or apical vaginal mass ↑ in size with Valsalva maneuver - Urinary symptoms (stress incontinence, urinary retention); bowel symptoms (constipation); dyspareunia
Aborting intracavitary leiomyoma	- Prolapsed uterine leiomyoma	- Labor-like pains - Irregular and enlarged uterus - Heavy menstruation
Imperforate hymen	- Complete vaginal obstruction	- Primary amenorrhea in adolescent girls - Cyclic abdominal pain - Blue-tinged vaginal bulge (hematocolpos)
Urethral diverticulum	- Urethral mucosal herniation	- Urinary symptoms (stress incontinence, post-void dribbling); dysuria, dyspareunia - Tender anterior vaginal wall mass

TABLE 17.2.4 - Overview of Pelvic Organ Prolapse and Differential Diagnosis

REVIEW QUESTIONS ?

1. A 55-year-old woman comes to her primary care physician because of a vaginal bulge that she has noticed of the past few months. She mentions that the budge increases in size with coughing and sneezing. On examination, when she is asked to cough, a posterior vaginal budge is seen. What is the most likely diagnosis?
   - **The most likely diagnosis is a rectocele.**
   - Posterior vaginal bulge that increases in size with coughing and sneezing, which increases intraabdominal pressure, should raise suspicion for rectocele.
   - Rectocele is a prolapse of the rectum, while an enterocele means prolapse of the small intestines. Both can be due to weakness of the rectovaginal fascia.
   - Rectocele is far more common than enterocele
2. A 29-year-old African American woman comes to the emergency department because of severe lower abdominal pain. She has a past medical history of chronic pelvic and back pain, as well as heavy menstrual bleeding. She is not currently sexually active. Pelvic examination shows a firm, smooth, round mass in the vagina and a dilated cervix. A pregnancy test is obtained, and the results are negative. What would most likely be present on further examination in this patient?
   - **On further examination of this patient, an irregularly enlarged uterus would most likely be present.**
   - This African American patient presents with severe lower abdominal pain.
   - Given her history of chronic pelvic and back pain as well as heavy menstrual bleeding, we should have a strong suspicion of uterine fibroids.
   - Physical examination showing a firm, smooth, round vaginal mass further supports that diagnosis of fibroids, specifically an aborting intracavity leiomyoma
   - Pelvic ultrasound is confirmatory and will show an irregularly enlarged uterus with well-circumscribed hypoechoic masses.
3. A 34-year-old woman comes to her primary care physician because of urinary incontinence for the past 2 months. She reports small amounts of urine leakage after voiding. She denies urine leakage with coughing or sneezing. She also mentions that over this same time period, she has felt discomfort during intercourse. Physical examination shows a tender anterior vaginal wall mass that does not enlarge with the Valsalva maneuver. Post-void residual volume is increased. What is the most likely diagnosis?
   - **The most likely diagnosis is urethral diverticulum.**
   - She presents with post-void leakage for 2 months and dyspareunia.
   - Physical examination shows a tender anterior vaginal wall mass that does not enlarge with Valsalva maneuver. Meaning increasing the intra-abdominal pressure does not affect the size of the mass.
   - This is most likely consistent with urethral diverticulum.
   - Urethral diverticulum is most commonly acquired secondary to recurrent periurethral gland infections, vaginal delivery, gynecological surgery, or pelvic trauma

REVIEW QUESTIONS

4. A 50-year-old G3P3 woman comes to her primary care physician because of involuntary urine leakage for the past 3 weeks. She notes a feeling of fullness in her pelvis. She had a total abdominal hysterectomy 5 years ago. She does not smoke or drink alcohol. Pelvic examination shows an anterior vaginal bulge that increases in size with the Valsalva maneuver and some clear vaginal discharge. Which of the following is the most likely diagnosis?

   A. Neurogenic bladder
   B. Cystocele
   C. Atrophic vaginitis
   D. Bartholin gland cyst
   E. Rectocele

- **The correct answer is option B.**
- This 50-year-old multigravid woman presents with symptoms of urinary incontinence and feeling of fullness in her pelvis.
- She has a past surgical history of total abdominal hysterectomy.
- Pelvic examination shows an anterior bulge that increases in size with the Valsalva maneuver, concerning for a cystocele.
- Cystocele is herniation of the bladder and causes prolapse of the anterior wall of the vagina vs posterior wall, which is caused by rectocele.
- Option A is incorrect because the neurogenic bladder causes urinary incontinence due to a spinal cord or nerve injury, which is not present in this patient.
- Option C is incorrect as this patient does not complain of vaginal dryness or irritation, which are characteristic of atrophic vaginitis.
- Option D is incorrect because Bartholin gland cyst presents as a soft, painful mass at the vaginal vestibule that does not increase in size with the Valsalva.
- Option E is incorrect because rectocele results in a posterior wall prolapse rather than an anterior vaginal wall.

Gynecology | Section 8: Transient Urinary Incontinence

I. Urinary Incontinence: Definition
   A. The role of the bladder is to accumulate and release urine appropriately
   B. Urinary incontinence occurs when this function is impaired

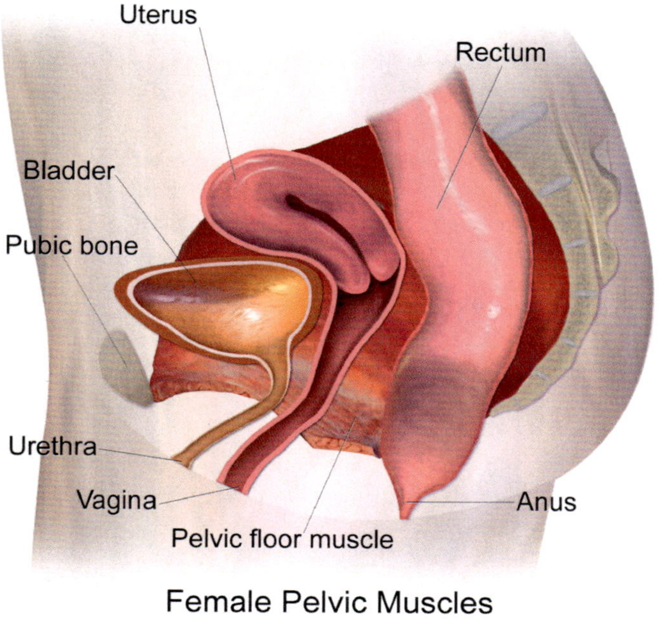

FIGURE 17.2.31 - Sagittal View of the Female Pelvis

Causes of Transient Incontinence

- **D**elirium
- **I**nfections of the urinary tract
- **A**trophic urethritis and vaginitis
- **P**harmaceuticals
  - (e.g. prazosin, furosemide)
- **P**sychological diagnoses
  - (e.g. depression)
- **E**xcessive urine output
  - (e.g. diabetes mellitus, congestive heart failure)
- **R**estricted mobility
  - (e.g. post-surgery)
- **S**tool impaction

FIGURE 17.2.32 - Causes of Transient Incontinence

II. Transient Incontinence: Urinary Tract Infection
   A. Symptoms may include frequency, urgency, dysuria, hematuria
   B. All patients with urinary incontinence should have a urinalysis performed
      1. Leukocyte esterase (+) on urine dipstick or ≥ 10 leukocytes/μL microscopically is essentially diagnostic
   C. First-line treatment options include nitrofurantoin, trimethoprim-sulfamethoxazole, fosfomycin, and pivmecillinam

III. Transient Incontinence: Genitourinary Syndrome of Menopause
   A. Low levels of estrogen (e.g. menopausal female) can lead to atrophy of the urogenital tissues
      1. Urinary symptoms: urgency incontinence, recurrent urinary tract infections
      2. Vaginal symptoms: dryness, pruritus, dyspareunia, bleeding

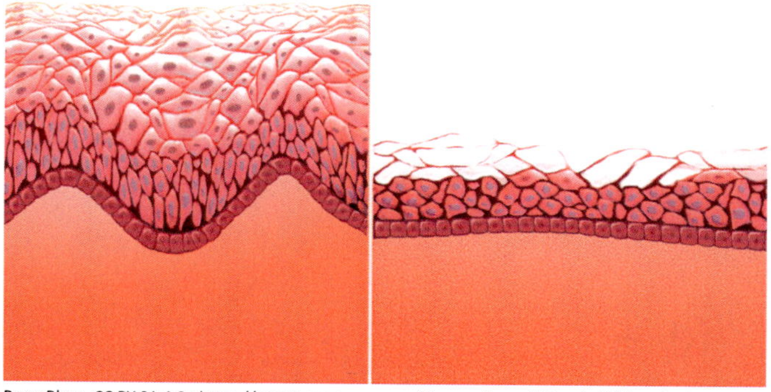

FIGURE 17.2.33 - Normal Vaginal Mucosa and Menopausal Vaginal Mucosa

IV. Transient Incontinence: Genitourinary Syndrome of Menopause
   A. Physical exam shows decreased vaginal rugae, thinned vulvar epithelium, reduced elasticity, and petechiae
   B. Treat with vaginal lubricants initially and then consider topical estrogen

V. Transient Incontinence: Functional Incontinence
   A. Inability to properly void despite the presence of intact urinary system functions
   B. Usually the result of physical or psychological impairment (e.g. restricted mobility, dementia)
   C. Treatment includes the reversal of the underlying condition where possible and supportive care if the cause is irreversible

Condition	Etiology	Key Features
Urinary tract infection	- Bacterial infection of the urinary tract - Most common pathogen is *E. Coli*	- Dysuria, urgency, frequency, hematuria, suprapubic pain - More common in sexually active females, pregnant women, and individuals with an indwelling catheter
Genitourinary syndrome of menopause	- Decreased estrogen levels in association with aging and menopause leading to atrophy of the urogenital tissues	- Urgency incontinence, recurrent urinary tract infections, vaginal dryness, pruritus, dyspareunia, bleeding - Physical exam shows decreased vaginal rugae, thinned vulvar epithelium, reduced elasticity, and petechiae
Functional incontinence	- Physically or psychologically unable to properly void even with intact bladder and urinary sphincter functions	- Urine loss without making it to the toilet - More common in post-surgical patients, elderly women, and patients with dementia

TABLE 17.2.5 - Transient Urinary Incontinence

REVIEW QUESTIONS

1. An 82-year-old woman is brought to the Emergency department via ambulance from her long-term care facility. The staff stated that she woke up confused and had wet herself. On arrival she is more oriented and is able to answer questions appropriately. She has a past medical history of hypertension, hyperlipidemia, and type 2 diabetes. She states that for the past few days, she has been urinating more frequently and has been having pain during urination. Vitals signs are significant for a temperature of 100.6° F (38.1° C). What is the next best step in management?

- **The next best step in management is to order a urinalysis to assess for a possible urinary tract infection.**
- The elderly woman is a resident of a long-term care facility who woke up confused and had wet herself.
- Vitals are significant for a low-grade fever, 100.6° F (38.1° C).
- While there are multiple causes of transient urinary incontinence, she has also been having increased frequency as well as dysuria.
- Given her low-grade fever and symptoms, UTI is likely, and it is a large cause of delirium in the elderly.
- Therefore the best next step in management would be to order a urinalysis to assess for a possible UTI.

Gynecology | Section 9: Stress Incontinence

I. Stress Urinary Incontinence: Definition
   A. Urine loss with elevated intra-abdominal pressure (e.g. coughing, sneezing, lifting, laughing, having intercourse)

II. Stress Urinary Incontinence: Pathophysiology
   A. Occurs when intravesical pressure > intraurethral pressure
      1. Urethral hypermobility
      2. Sphincter insufficiency

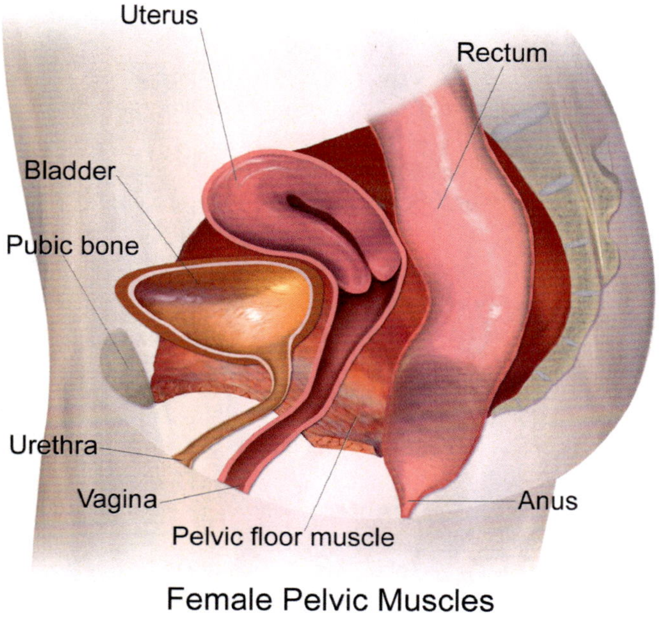

FIGURE 17.2.31 - Sagittal View of the Female Pelvis

III. Stress Urinary Incontinence: Risk factors
   A. Urethral hypermobility
      1. Multiple vaginal deliveries
      2. Obesity
      3. Sustained high-impact activity (e.g. running)
      4. Chronic cough
   B. Sphincter insufficiency
      1. Neuromuscular damage (e.g. multiple pelvic surgeries)

IV. Stress Urinary Incontinence: Clinical Presentation
   A. Leakage of urine occurs during activities that increase the intra-abdominal pressure (e.g. coughing, sneezing, lifting, laughing, having intercourse)
   B. No nocturia, urgency, or frequency

V. Stress Urinary Incontinence: Diagnosis
   A. The cough stress test is positive
   B. Urinalysis is normal
   C. Post-void residual volume is normal (< 150 mL in females and < 50 mL in males)

VI. Stress Urinary Incontinence: Management
   A. First-line therapy is Kegel exercises and weight loss
   B. Incontinence pessaries can be helpful
   C. Periurethral bulking agents can be used, particularly for stress incontinence caused by sphincter insufficiency
   D. Surgical placement of a mid-urethral sling is the definitive management

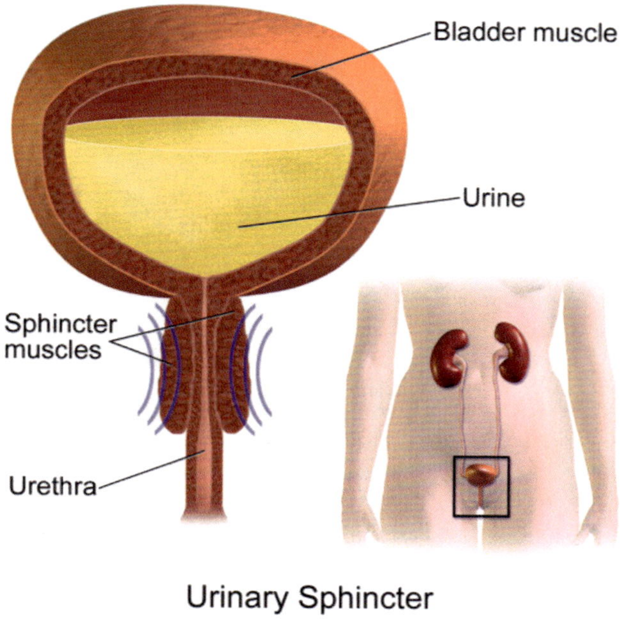

FIGURE 17.2.34 - Urinary Sphincter

Condition	Etiology	Key Features
Urinary tract infection	- Bacterial infection of the urinary tract - Most common pathogen is *E. Coli*	- Dysuria, urgency, frequency, hematuria, suprapubic pain - More common in sexually active females, pregnant women, and individuals with an indwelling catheter
Genitourinary syndrome of menopause	- Decreased estrogen levels in association with aging and menopause leading to atrophy of the urogenital tissues	- Urgency incontinence, recurrent urinary tract infections, vaginal dryness, pruritus, dyspareunia, bleeding - Physical exam shows decreased vaginal rugae, thinned vulvar epithelium, reduced elasticity, and petechiae
Functional incontinence	- Physically or psychologically unable to properly void even with intact bladder and urinary sphincter functions	- Urine loss without making it to the toilet - More common in post-surgical patients, elderly women, and patients with dementia
Stress incontinence	- Urethral hypermobility from a weakened pelvic floor or urethral sphincter insufficiency as a result of neuromuscular damage	- Urine loss with increased intra-abdominal pressure (e.g. laughing, coughing, lifting, sneezing) - More common in those with multiple vaginal deliveries, obesity, or a history of pelvic surgeries

TABLE 17.2.6 - Overview of Differential Diagnoses of Urinary Incontinence

REVIEW QUESTIONS ?

1. A 37-year-old woman presents to her primary care provider because she has been having urinary incontinence as well as constipation for the past 4 months. History also reviews she has heavy periods and severe cramps during her cycle. She is sent for a transvaginal ultrasound which shows and an irregularly shaped uterus. What is the most likely cause for this patients symptoms?
   - **The most likely cause for this patient's symptoms is uterine fibroids**
   - The combination of urinary incontinence, constipation, and irregularly shaped uterus is most consistent with fibroids.
   - Uterine fibroids can increase the pressure on the bladder, causing stress incontinence

2. A 39-year-old G5P5 woman comes to her primary care physician because of intermittent involuntary urinary incontinence. She first noticed urinary incontinence 1 year ago, and it has recently become more frequent. She notes that she has urinary leakage every time she laughs or sneezes. Her vital signs include a temperature of 98.6° F (37° C), blood pressure of 110/80 mmHg, heart rate of 87 beats/min, and respiratory rate of 15 breaths/min. Physical examination shows a post-void residual volume of 100 mL. Urinalysis is normal. Which of the following is the next best step in the management?

   A. Kegel exercises
   B. Antimuscarinic agents
   C. Intermittent catheterization
   D. Mid-urethral sling procedure

- **The correct answer is option A.**
- This patient has an intermittent involuntary loss of urine associated with laughing and sneezing; which are both actions that increase intraabdominal pressure.
- Therefore, the most likely diagnosis in this patient is stress urinary incontinence.
- Stress incontinence is further supported by the fact that she has had 5 successful vaginal deliveries, as multiple vaginal deliveries contribute to pelvic floor instability.
- The best next step in management is to strengthen the pelvic floor muscles, which can be accomplished with Kegel exercises.
- Option B is incorrect because antimuscarinic agents are used for urgency incontinence.
- Option C is incorrect because intermittent catheterization is performed by patients with overflow incontinence.
- Option D is incorrect because a mid-urethral sling procedure is the last resort for treatment of stress incontinence. Kegel exercises should be attempted before an invasive surgical procedure.

Gynecology | Section 10: Urgency, Mixed, and Overflow Incontinence

I. Urgency Incontinence: Definition
   A. A strong urge to void that is unrelated to an activity or anatomical position

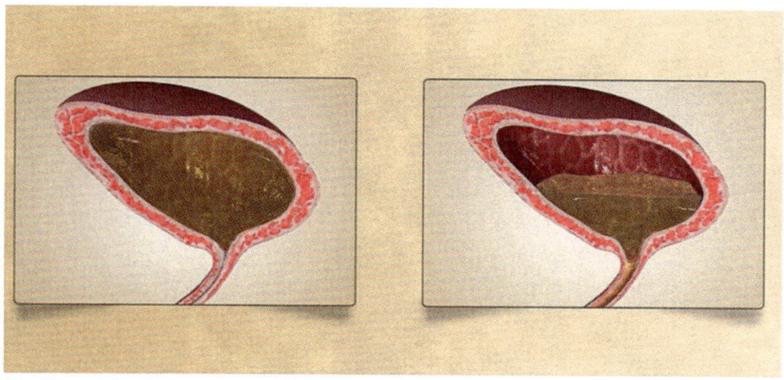

FIGURE ### - Urgency Incontinence

II. Urgency Incontinence: Risk Factors
   A. Frequently idiopathic
   B. Age > 40
   C. Neurologic disease (e.g. multiple sclerosis)
   D. Inflammatory conditions (e.g. urinary tract infection)
   E. Previous pelvic surgery

III. Urgency Incontinence: Clinical Presentation
   A. Unable to make it to the bathroom in time
   B. Increased nighttime voids
   C. It may be triggered by the sight of a bathroom or the sound of running water

IV. Urgency Incontinence: Diagnosis
   A. Clinical history is the most important part of this diagnosis
   B. Urinalysis is normal
   C. Post-void residual is normal (< 150 mL in females and < 50 mL in males)

V. Urgency Incontinence: Management
   A. Initial treatment is pelvic floor exercises and bladder training
   B. Pharmacologic agents can also be useful
      1. Anticholinergic medications are first-line (e.g. oxybutynin)
      2. Mirabegron is a beta-agonist that is a second-line option
      3. Both classes of medication have the potential to result in urinary retention
   C. Botulinum toxin or sacral neuromodulation are last resort options

VI. Mixed Incontinence
   A. Symptoms of both urgency incontinence and stress incontinence
   B. Start with a voiding diary to delineate the primary type

VII. Overflow Incontinence: Definition
   A. Excessive accumulation of urine within the bladder
      1. Malfunctioning nerves
      2. Physical obstruction

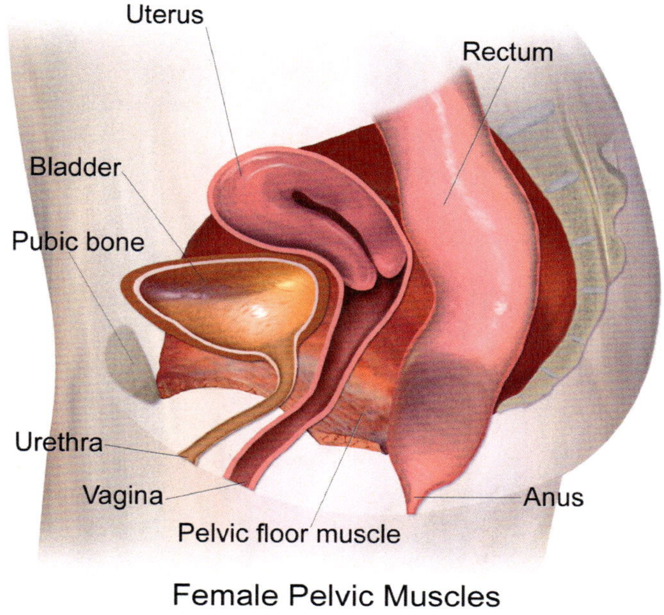

FIGURE 17.2.31 - Sagittal View of the Female Pelvis

VIII. Overflow Incontinence: Risk Factors
   A. Malfunctioning nerves
      1. Diabetes
      2. Alcoholism
      3. Epidural anesthesia
      4. Spinal cord damage (e.g. cauda equina syndrome, multiple sclerosis)
   B. Physical obstruction
      1. Pelvic organ prolapse
      2. Fibroids
      3. Urethral obstruction after surgery

IX. Overflow Incontinence: Clinical Presentation
   A. Lower abdominal pressure
   B. Suprapubic fullness
   C. Dribbling, hesitancy, weak stream of urine

X. Overflow Incontinence: Diagnosis
   A. Post-void residual volume > 150 mL
   B. Urodynamic testing may be performed in complicated cases

XI. Overflow Incontinence: Management
   A. Urethral catheterization
   B. Timed voiding
   C. Identify and treat the underlying pathology

Condition	Etiology	Key Features
Urinary tract infection	- Bacterial infection of the urinary tract - Most common pathogen is *E. Coli*	- Dysuria, urgency, frequency, hematuria, suprapubic pain - More common in sexually active females, pregnant women, and individuals with an indwelling catheter
Genitourinary syndrome of menopause	- Decreased estrogen levels in association with aging and menopause leading to atrophy of the urogenital tissues	- Urgency incontinence, recurrent urinary tract infections, vaginal dryness, pruritus, dyspareunia, bleeding - Physical exam shows decreased vaginal rugae, thinned vulvar epithelium, reduced elasticity, and petechiae
Functional incontinence	- Physically or psychologically unable to properly void even with intact bladder and urinary sphincter functions	- Urine loss without making it to the toilet - More common in post-surgical patients, elderly women, and patients with dementia
Stress incontinence	- Urethral hypermobility from a weakened pelvic floor or urethral sphincter insufficiency as a result of neuromuscular damage	- Urine loss with increased intra-abdominal pressure (e.g. laughing, coughing, lifting, sneezing) - More common in those with multiple vaginal deliveries, obesity, or a history of pelvic surgeries
Urgency incontinence	- Underactive detrusor muscle, which can be due to damage to the bladder or nervous system, secondary to a systemic process, or idiopathic	- Strong urge to void regardless of activity or body position, nocturia, unable to make it to the bathroom in time - More common in patients with multiple sclerosis, urinary tract infection, or a prior pelvic surgery
Overflow incontinence	- Inability to adequately void urine due to detrusor muscle underactivity, bladder outlet obstruction, or medication side effects	- Dribbling of urine, hesitancy, weak stream, lower abdominal pressure, suprapubic fullness - More common in those with diabetes, spinal cord damage, fibroids, or pelvic organ prolapse

TABLE 17.2.7 - Overview of Urinary Incontinence

REVIEW QUESTIONS

1. A 72-year-old woman presented to her primary care provider to discuss medical management of her urgency incotinence. She has a past medical history of first-degree AV heart block, COPD, and angle-closure glaucoma. Which aspect of her past medical history precludes her from the first-line medication used to treat urgency incontinence?

   - **This patient's history of angle-closure glaucoma precludes her from use of anticholinergic medications.**
   - Anticholinergic medications are the first-line treatment of urgency incontinence.
   - Common side effects of anticholinergic medications include flushing, urinary retention, constipation, dry mouth, tachycardia, and myadriasis.
   - Myadriasis (pupillary dilation) worsens angle closure glaucoma because as the aqueous humor drains from the anterior chamber gets blocked by the iris which would further increase the intraocular pressure.
   - First degree AV heart block is incorrect as this is not a contraindication to anticholinergic use as they do not block the AV node.
   - COPD is also incorrect. Recall that severe COPD treatment often involves the use of anticholinergic drugs such as tiotropium and ipratropium.

2. A 52-year-old woman comes to a primary care provider for the first time in 10 years. 10-years ago she was noted to have symptoms of polyuria and polydipsia per chart review and an A1C of 7.2. Over the past few years she reports a tingling sensation in her feet. She also notes a decrease in her urine output of the past 1-2 years. A post-void residual is performed and shows a volume of 400 mL. What is the most likely underlying diagnosis which has caused this patients symptoms?

   - **The most likely underlying diagnosis is uncontrolled diabetes.**
   - She was lost to follow-up after initially being found to be diabetic associated with symptoms of polyuria and polydispsai.
   - Now, 10 years later, she is have signs of peripheral neuropathy as well as nephropathy caused by years of uncontrolled blood sugar levels.
   - Post-void residual volume of 400 mL is consistent with overflow incontinence. This can be seen in the later stages of diabetes as the nerve supply to the bladder is compromised.

Gynecology | Section 11: Total Urinary Incontinence and Urethral Diverticulum

I. Total Incontinence: Definition
   A. Continuous urine loss at all times and in all positions
      1. Vesicovaginal fistula
      2. Non-functional urethral sphincter

II. Total Incontinence: Risk Factors
   A. Vesicovaginal fistula
      1. Pelvic surgery
      2. Pelvic radiotherapy
      3. Childbirth
   B. Non-functional urethral sphincter
      1. Pelvic surgery
      2. Nerve damage
      3. Infiltrative malignancy

III. Total Incontinence: Clinical Presentation
   A. Leakage of urine that is constant and unprovoked
   B. The patient usually wears a pad or diaper to catch the urine

IV. Total Incontinence: Diagnosis
   A. Urine in the vagina on pelvic exam
   B. Positive dye test
   C. Urinalysis is normal
   D. Post-void residual is normal (< 150 mL in females and < 50 mL in males)
   E. Voiding cystourethrogram can make a definitive diagnosis

V. Total Incontinence: Management
   A. For a fistula or a non-functional urethral sphincter, surgery is the treatment of choice

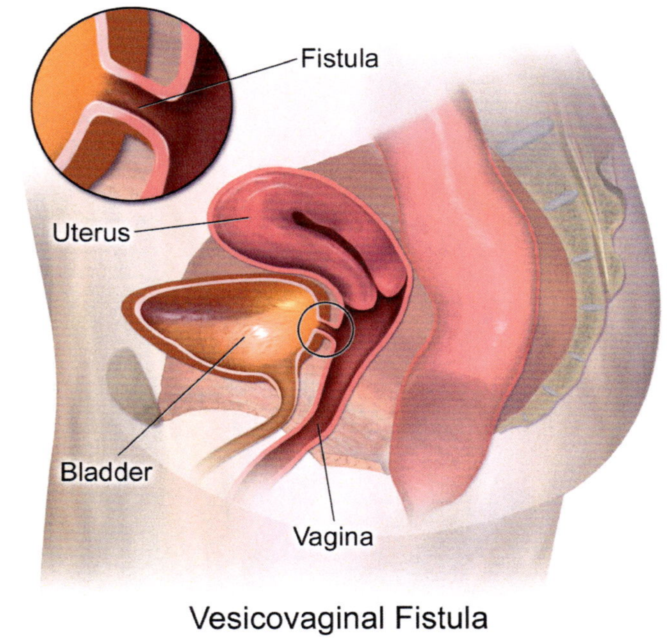

FIGURE 17.2.36 - Vesicovaginal Fistula

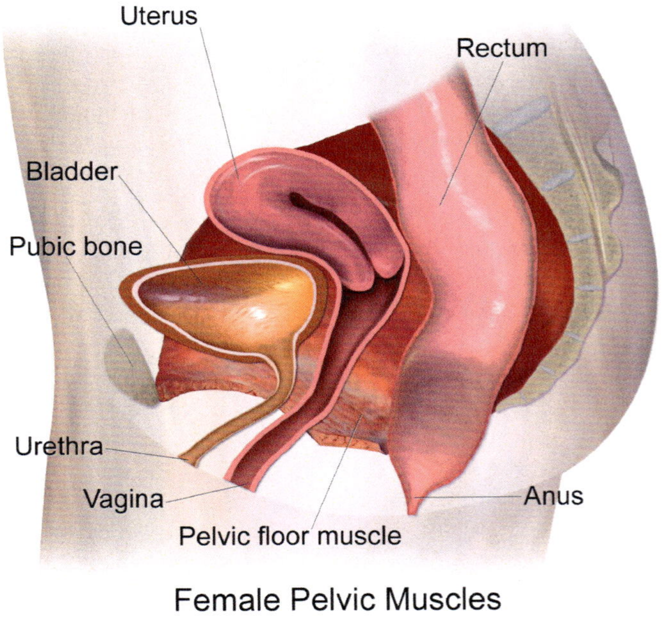

FIGURE 17.2.31 - Sagittal View of the Female Pelvis

VI. Urethral Diverticulum
   A. Caused by repeated urethral tissue infections
   B. Pelvic trauma and periurethral procedures may increase the risk
   C. Symptoms include dribbling of urine after voiding, dysuria, purulent discharge, dyspareunia
   D. A physical exam will show a mass in the anterior vaginal wall that is tender to palpation
   E. Diagnosis is made with an MRI of the pelvis
   F. Definitive treatment is with surgery

Condition	Etiology	Key Features
Urinary tract infection	- Bacterial infection of the urinary tract - Most common pathogen is *E. Coli*	- Dysuria, urgency, frequency, hematuria, suprapubic pain - More common in sexually active females, pregnant women, and individuals with an indwelling catheter
Genitourinary syndrome of menopause	- Decreased estrogen levels in association with aging and menopause leading to atrophy of the urogenital tissues	- Urgency incontinence, recurrent urinary tract infections, vaginal dryness, pruritus, dyspareunia, bleeding - Physical exam shows decreased vaginal rugae, thinned vulvar epithelium, reduced elasticity, and petechiae
Functional incontinence	- Physically or psychologically unable to properly void even with intact bladder and urinary sphincter functions	- Urine loss without making it to the toilet - More common in post-surgical patients, elderly women, and patients with dementia
Stress incontinence	- Urethral hypermobility from a weakened pelvic floor or urethral sphincter insufficiency as a result of neuromuscular damage	- Urine loss with increased intra-abdominal pressure (e.g. laughing, coughing, lifting, sneezing) - More common in those with multiple vaginal deliveries, obesity, or a history of pelvic surgeries
Urgency incontinence	- Underactive detrusor muscle, which can be due to damage to the bladder or nervous system, secondary to a systemic process, or idiopathic	- Strong urge to void regardless of activity or body position, nocturia, unable to make it to the bathroom in time - More common in patients with multiple sclerosis, urinary tract infection, or a prior pelvic surgery
Overflow incontinence	- Inability to adequately void urine due to detrusor muscle underactivity, bladder outlet obstruction, or medication side effects	- Dribbling of urine, hesitancy, weak stream, lower abdominal pressure, suprapubic fullness - More common in those with diabetes, spinal cord damage, fibroids, or pelvic organ prolapse
Total incontinence	- Vesicovaginal fistula or non-functioning urinary sphincter	- Urine loss at all times and in all positions - More common in those who have had pelvic surgery, pelvic radiotherapy or obstructed labor
Urethral diverticulum	- Repeated urethral tissue infections causing an outpouching of the urethral mucosa	- Dribbling of urine after voiding, dysuria, purulent discharge, tender mass along the anterior vaginal wall - More common in those with a history of pelvic trauma or periurethral procedure

TABLE 17.2.8 - Types of Urinary Incontinence and Urethral Diverticulum

REVIEW QUESTIONS

1. A 45-year-old woman comes to her primary care physician because of continuous urinary leakage for the past 3 weeks. She had pelvic surgery 4 months ago. Speculum examination shows the pooling of a clear liquid in the vagina. What would be seen on a voiding cystourethrogram in this patient?
   - **On the cystourethrogram, contrast dye would be seen moving from the bladder to the vaginal canal**
   - This patient has a history of recent pelvic surgery and is suffering from continuous urinary leakage.
   - Speculum examination shows the pooling of a clear liquid in the vagina, which should raise a strong suspicion of vesicovaginal fistula.

2. Why are patients affected by a urethral diverticulum susceptible to recurrent urinary tract infections?
   - **Patients affected by a urethral diverticulum are susceptible to recurrent urinary tract infections because the outpouching of urethral mucosa creates a space for urine to pool and become stagnant. As urine is chronically retained within this area, infectious organisms can accumulate.**

3. A 66-year-old postmenopausal woman comes to OB/GYN clinic for "problems with peeing my pants." Over the past year, she has experienced moments of sudden urinary urgency along with occasional instances of wetting herself. Initially, this occurred a few times a month, but now is happening almost daily. She has had two urinary tract infections in the past year. She had one pregnancy over 10 years ago, which was uncomplicated. On pelvic examination, the vagina appears pale, and there is mild labial retraction. Cough stress test is negative. The remainder of the physical examination is unremarkable. Urinalysis is normal. What would be the preferred initial therapy for this patient?

   A. Antibiotics
   B. Pelvic floor exercises
   C. Urethral catheterization
   D. Vaginal lubricants

   - **The preferred initial therapy is vaginal lubricants, option D.**
   - This patient has urinary urgency in addition to having had two urinary tract infections in the past year.
   - Physical examination shows a vagina that appears pale and mild labial retraction.
   - Given her genital and urinary symptoms in the context of being post-menopausal, she is most likely suffering from the genitourinary syndrome of menopause as a result of decreased estrogen.
   - Option A is incorrect; antibiotics would be the treatment of choice for a urinary tract infection, but in this patient, the urinalysis was normal.
   - Option B is incorrect because her urgency incontinence seems to be best explained by the genitourinary syndrome of menopause and should be treated accordingly. Also, her cough stress test was negative, which essentially rules out stress incontinence, for which pelvic floor exercises would be the first-line treatment.
   - Option C is incorrect because of urethral catheterization for patients with overflow incontinence. Here, the patient is struggling from overly frequent urination and not the inability to urinate.

Gynecology | Section 12: Menstrual Cycle And Menopause

I. Menstrual Cycle
   A. Consists of ovarian and uterine cycles
      1. Ovarian cycle: follicular phase and luteal phase
      2. Uterine cycle: proliferative phase and secretory phase
   B. Follicular phase: variable length
   C. Luteal phase: always 14 days
   D. Menstruation: sloughing off of stratum functionalis due to estrogen and progesterone withdrawal

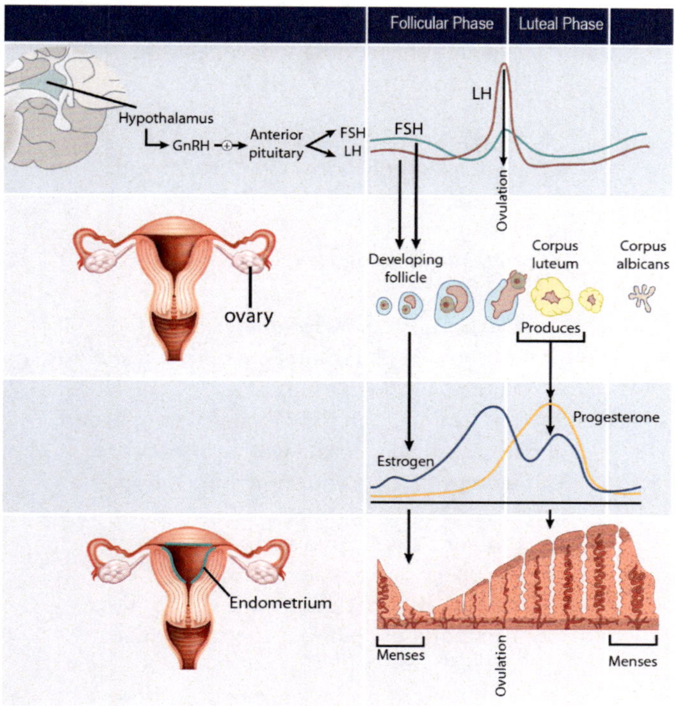

FIGURE 17.2.37 - The Menstrual Cycle

II. Menopause: Definition
   A. Menopause
      1. Amenorrhea for at least 12 months
      2. Average age: 49 - 52 years (earlier in smokers)
   B. Perimenopause
      1. Time from first appearance of menopausal symptoms to one year after menopause
      2. Average duration: 4 years

III. Menopause: Pathophysiology
   A. Number of ovarian follicles decrease with age
   B. Low estrogen and progesterone levels
   C. Signs and symptoms mostly due to estrogen deficiency
   D. Loss of negative feedback on GnRH and FSH/LH
   E. High GnRH, FSH and LH

IV. Menopause: Clinical Presnetation
   A. Psychological symptoms
      1. Mood swings, irritability, anxiety, insomnia
   B. Autonomic symptoms
      1. Hot flashes, heat intolerance, increased sweating
   C. Hyperthyroidism should be ruled out with TSH due to similarity of symptoms
   D. Genitourinary syndrome of menopause (atrophic vaginitis)
      1. Vulva, vagina, cervix, and urethral epithelium are responsive to estrogen
      2. Atrophy of vulva, vagina, and cervix resulting in dyspareunia
      3. Atrophy or urinary epithelium resulting in increased urinary frequency, urgency, dysuria, incontinence
   E. Osteoporosis
      1. Due to decreased osteoblastic activity and increased osteoclast activity caused by low estrogen levels
      2. Screen women ≥ 65 years old for osteoporosis via DEXA scan
   F. Coronary artery disease
      1. Increased LDL and decreased HDL caused by low estrogen

V. Menopause: Diagnosis
   A. Mostly clinical diagnosis
   B. Serum estrogen and FSH levels
   C. Serum total cholesterol, LDL and HDL to screen for hypercholesterolemia
   D. Serum TSH to rule out hyperthyroidism

VI. Menopause: Management
   A. Treatment only for
      1. Severe symptoms and decreased quality of life
      2. Premature menopause
      3. Surgical menopause
   B. Types of therapy
      1. Lifestyle modifications; topical estrogen
      2. Non-hormonal therapy; hormone replacement therapy
   C. Lifestyle modifications
      1. Impaired sleep: exercise, relaxation techniques
      2. Osteoporosis prevention: vitamin D and calcium intake, weight-bearing exercise
      3. Bisphosphonates initiated after diagnosis of osteoporosis
   D. Topical estrogen for atrophic vaginitis
      1. Cream or vaginal ring
   E. Non-hormonal therapy
      1. Raloxifene (SERM) to treat osteoporosis
   F. Adverse effects
      1. Exacerbation of hot flashes
      2. Increased thromboembolic risk (DVT/PE, stroke)

G. Advantage
   1. No increase in the risk for endometrial carcinoma (vs. tamoxifen)
H. Hormone replacement therapy (HRT)
   1. Short-term treatment of menopausal symptoms
I. Types
   1. Estrogen only HRT: for women who have had a hysterectomy
   2. Estrogen and progestin HRT: for women with intact uterus
J. Risks of HRT
   1. Estrogen only HRT: endometrial cancer in women with intact uterus
   2. Estrogen and progestin HRT: breast cancer
K. Contraindications
   1. Undiagnosed vaginal bleeding; breast and endometrial cancers
   2. Chronic liver disease; history of DVT, PE, or stroke

REVIEW QUESTIONS

1. A 70-year-old woman is brought to her primary care physician by her family because of upper back pain that started 3 days ago. She has a past medical history of a left distal radius fracture 3 years ago that was casted for several weeks. Her family has noticed that her height has decreased over the last 4 years. A DEXA scan reveals a T-score of -3.0. Physical examination shows tenderness at the level of the T8 spinous process. What is the first-line treatment option for this patient's condition?
   - **The first-line treatment option for this patient's condition is a bisphosphonate.**
   - This patient presents with acute upper back pain that started 3 days ago.
   - She had a distal radius fracture, also known as Colles fracture, three years ago.
   - Her height has decreased over the last 4 years.
   - DEXA scan reveals a T-score of -3.0. A T-score of less than -2.5 is diagnostic for osteoporosis.
   - Acute upper back pain, along with the patient's hx, is most likely due to an acute vertebral compression fracture.
   - A decrease in height is caused by multiple acute and chronic vertebral compression fractures over time.
   - The first-line treatment option for osteoporosis patients is bisphosphonate,s like alendronate, risedronate, and pamidronate.
   - Bisphosphonates inhibit osteoclast activity in the bone matrix, preserving bone mineral density.

REVIEW QUESTIONS

2. A 53-year-old woman comes to her primary care physician because of pain during sexual intercourse. Her last menstrual period was two years ago. Past medical history is significant for a deep venous thrombosis 5 years ago. She has no past surgical history. She notes that sometimes she feels intense heat arising from her chest and spreading to her face. Vital signs include a temperature of 96.8° F (36° C), blood pressure of 135/80 mmHg, heart rate of 85 beats/min, and respiratory rate of 15 breaths/min. Genitourinary examination shows a dry mucosa of t he vagina.. Which of the following is the best treatment option for this patient?

   A. Vaginal estrogen cream
   B. Estrogen-only hormone replacement therapy
   C. Tamoxifen
   D. Weight-bearing exercise

   - **The correct answer is option A.**
   - This patient presents with pain during sexual intercourse and hot flashes.
   - Physical examination shows vaginal driness and her last menstrual period was two years ago.
   - This along with her symptoms should trigger a suspicion for menopause.
   - The patient's chief complaint is dyspareunia, which is likely due to vaginal atrophy.
   - The best treatment option for genitourinary syndrome of menopause is topical vaginal estrogen cream.
   - Option B is incorrect because estrogen-only hormone replacement therapy is contraindicated in women with an intact uterus due to the risk for endometrial carcinoma. This patient has not undergone any surgeries, suggesting that she likely has an intact uterus. Additionally, she has a past medical history of deep venous thrombosis, which is another contraindication for hormone replacement therapy.
   - Option C is incorrect because tamoxifen is indicated for the prevention and treatment of estrogen receptor-positive breast cancer rather than for menopause. Additionally, tamoxifen can exacerbate hot flashes, predispose this patient to another episode of deep venous thrombosis, and even increase her risk of endometrial adenocarcinoma.
   - Option D is incorrect because although weight-bearing exercise is recommended to prevent osteoporosis in postmenopausal women, weight-bearing exercise is not effective for vaginal atrophy, which causes dyspareunia.

Gynecology | Section 13: Primary Amenorrhea

I. Primary Amenorrhea: Definition
   A. Absence of menses by age 16, normal growth and secondary sexual characteristics
   B. Absence of menses by age 13, no secondary sexual characteristics (e.g. pubic hair, breasts)

II. Primary Amenorrhea: Pathophysiology and Etiologies
   A. Outflow-tract anomalies
      1. Imperforate hymen
      2. Transverse vaginal septum
      3. Androgen insensitivity syndrome (defect in androgen receptor)
      4. Mullerian agenesis with 46 XX chromosome
   B. Ovarian pathology
      1. Turner syndrome (45 X)
      2. Gonadal dysgenesis (46 XY)
   C. Hypothalamic amenorrhea
      1. Functional hypothalamic amenorrhea: excessive exercise, anorexia nervosa, stress → ↓ GnRH cycles
      2. Antipsychotics: inhibition D2 receptors → ↑ prolactin → ↓ GnRH
      3. Kallmann syndrome: absence of GnRH neuron migration
   D. Pituitary amenorrhea
      1. Prolactinoma (suppressed GnRH)
      2. Craniopharyngioma (reduced FSH and LH)
   E. Thyroid amenorrhea
      1. Hypothyroidism: ↑ TRH → ↑ prolactin → ↓ GnRH
      2. Hyperthyroidism: ↑ SHBG → ↓ free estradiol → ↑ LH → amenorrhea

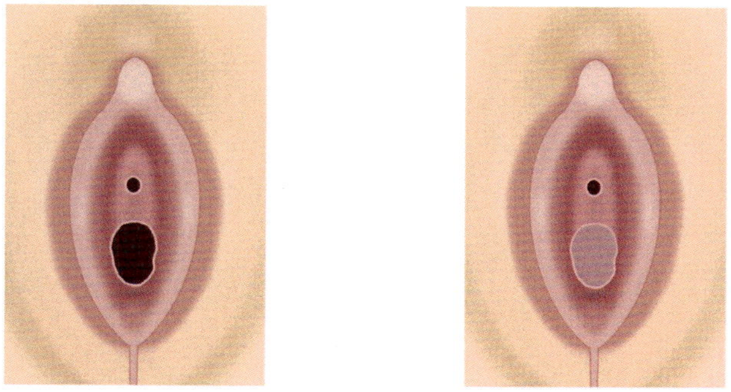

Normal Imperforate hymen

FIGURE 17.2.38 - Imperforate Hymen

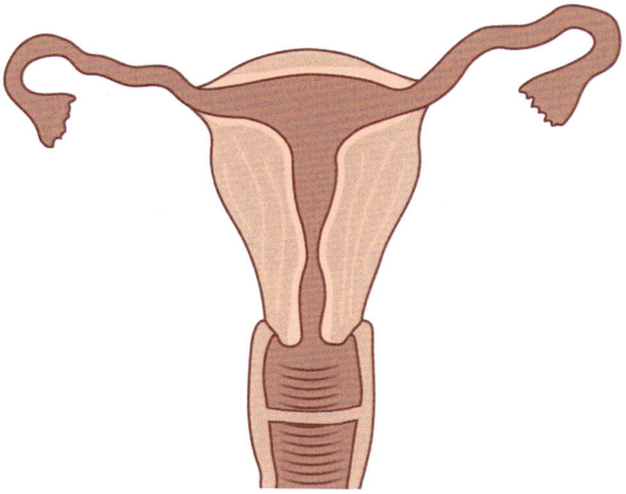

Transverse Vaginal Septum

FIGURE 17.2.39 - Transverse Vaginal Septum

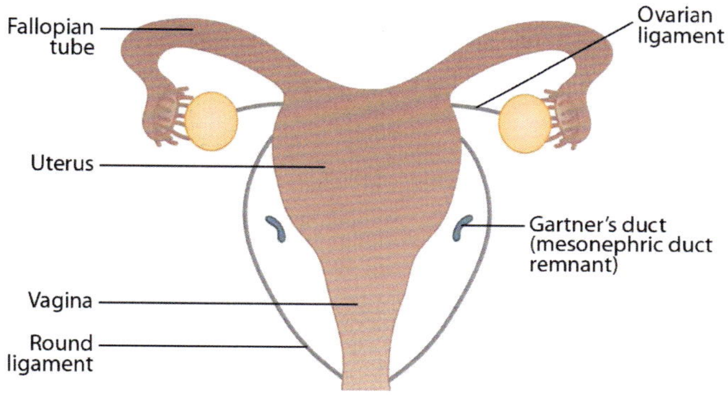

FIGURE 17.2.40 - Normal Anatomy of Female Genital Tract

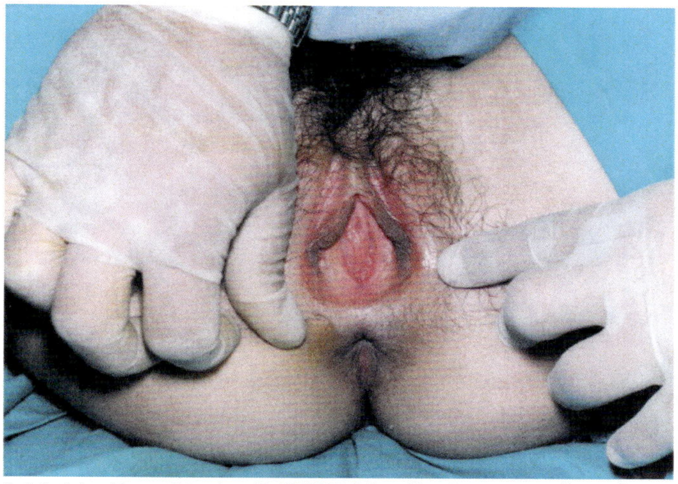

FIGURE 17.2.41 - Vaginal Agenesis

III. Primary Amenorrhea: Clinical Features
   A. Imperforate hymen
      1. Bulging, bluish translucent membrane, hematocolpos
      2. Urinary retention, bulges with valsalva
   B. Transverse vaginal septum
      1. Pelvic pain, hematocolpos
      2. No bulging with valsalva
   C. Androgen insensitivity
      1. Normal breast development, female external genitalia
      2. Absent pubic and axillary hair, absent uterus and cervix
   D. Mullerian agenesis
      1. Normal secondary sexual characteristics and breast development
      2. Normal external genitalia
      3. Absence of fallopian tubes, uterus, upper vagina
   E. Turner syndrome
      1. Rudimentary ovaries, no menstruation, poor breast development
   F. Gonadal dysgenesis, 46 XY
      1. Streak gonads, normal uterus, fallopian tubes, vagina
   G. Hypothalamic amenorrhea
      1. Eating disorders, stress, female athletes
      2. Long distance running, amenorrhea, osteoporosis
   H. Kallmann syndrome
      1. Hypogonadotropic hypogonadism
      2. Anosmia, midline facial defect, renal agenesis
      3. Absence of pubertal development and menses
   I. Pituitary amenorrhea
      1. Amenorrhea, headache, vision problems, bilateral nipple discharge
   J. Thyroid amenorrhea
      1. Hypothyroidism (amenorrhea, weight gain, constipation, cold intolerance)

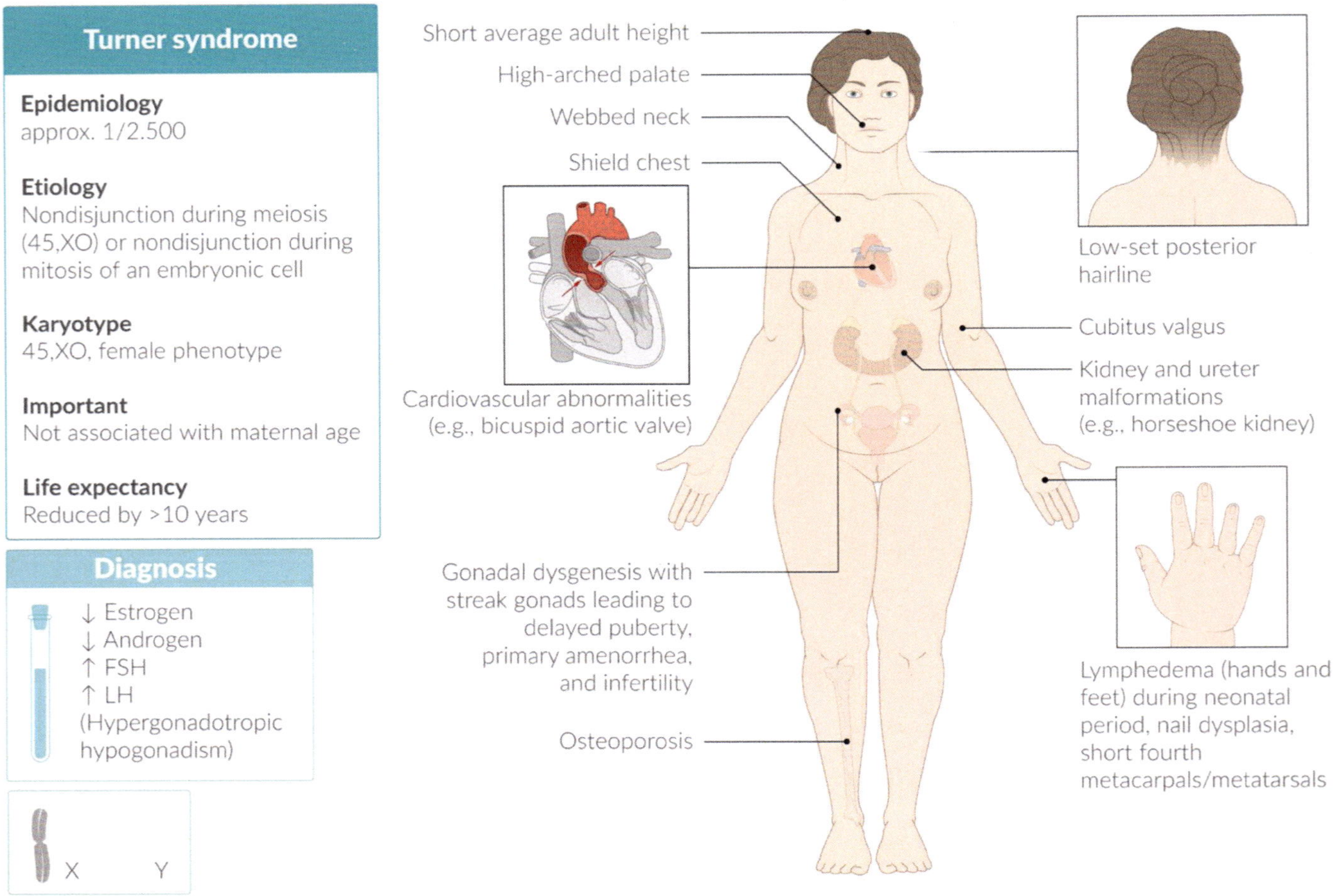

FIGURE 17.2.42- Turner Syndrome

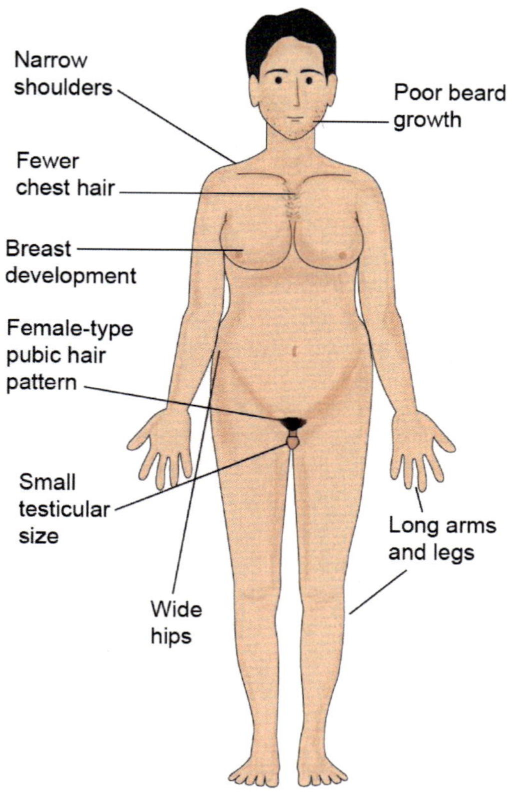

FIGURE 17.2.43 - Swyer Syndrome

IV. Primary Amenorrhea: Diagnosis
   A. History and physical exam
   B. Beta-hCG serum or urine qualitative
   C. Pelvic ultrasound
   D. LH, FSH, prolactin, TSH
   E. May require testosterone levels, sex-hormone binding globulin, MRI brain or pelvis, dehydroepiandrostenedione levels, or chromosomal analysis based on initial tests

V. Primary Amenorrhea: Treatment
   A. Mullerian agenesis: vaginal elongation by dilators, surgical creation of neovagina
   B. Imperforate hymen: hymenotomy
   C. Transverse vaginal septum: surgery followed by vaginal dilators
   D. Androgen insensitivity: removal of gonads, hormone replacement
   E. Turner syndrome: estrogen therapy, IVF if interested in pregnancy
   F. Gonadal dysgenesis, 46 XY: removal of streak gonads
   G. Kallmann syndrome: hormone replacement therapy, IM gonadotropins
   H. Treat underlying conditions (e.g. hypothyroidism, prolactinoma, anorexia nervosa, etc.)

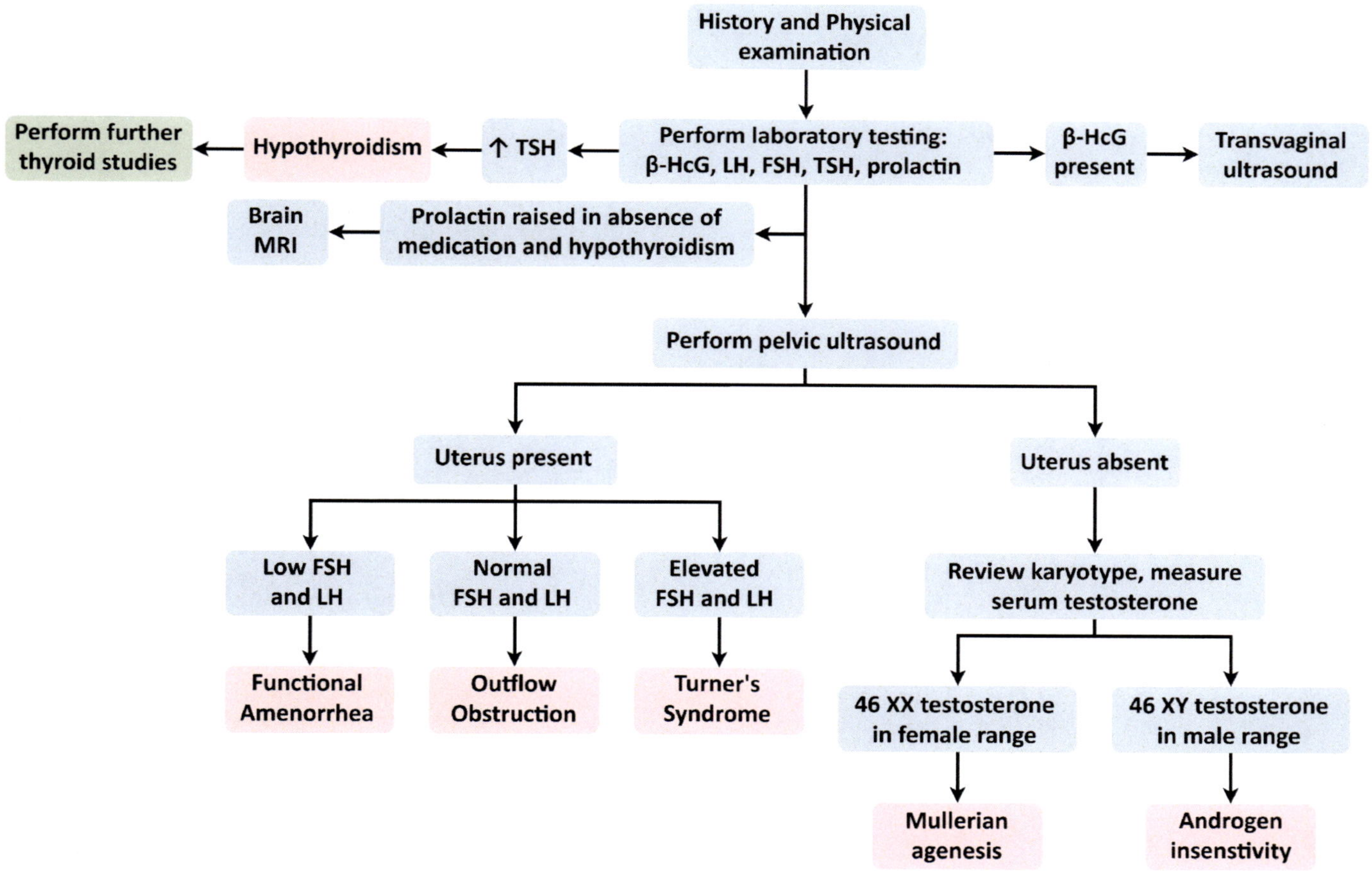

FIGURE 17.2.44 - Evaluation of Primary Amenorrhea

REVIEW QUESTIONS

1. A 14-year-old girl is brought to her primary care physician by her mother because she is concerned her daughter has not had her first period. Physical examination shows Tanner stage I breasts, genitalia, and pubic hair. FSH, LH, and estrogen levels are low. The patient reports a poor appetite because she cannot smell or taste anything. What is the most likely pathophysiology of this patient's underlying condition?

    - **The most likely pathophysiology of this patient's underlying condition is defective migration of GnRH-producing neurons from the olfactory pit to the preoptic nucleus of the hypothalamus.**
    - This 14-year-old girl presents with absent menses and Tanner stage I breasts, genitalia, and pubic hair.
    - These findings indicate primary amenorrhea and secondary hypogonadism.
    - The patient reports a poor appetite because she cannot smell or taste anything.
    - Primary amenorrhea, secondary hypogonadism, and anosmia are the classic findings of Kallmann syndrome, which is caused by defective migration of GnRH-producing neurons from the olfactory pit to the preoptic nucleus of the hypothalamus.
    - Patients with Kallmann syndrome have underdeveloped olfactory bulbs resulting in anosmia and an underdeveloped preoptic nucleus resulting in secondary hypogonadism and primary amenorrhea.

2. A 15-year-old girl is brought to her primary care physician by her mother because she is concerned her daughter has not had her first period. The daughter's height is at the 3rd percentile for her age. Physical examination shows a flat chest with widely spaced nipples along with bilateral neck swellings. Laboratory studies show low estrogen and high LH, and FSH levels. Which two cardiovascular comorbidities may accompany this patient's underlying condition?

    - **Cardiovascular comorbidities that may accompany this patient's underlying condition are bicuspid aortic valve and coarctation of the aorta.**
    - This 15-year-old girl with primary amenorrhea, short stature and flat chest with widely spaced nipples should raise suspicion for Turner Syndrome.
    - Bilateral neck swellings is due to defective lymphatic drainage.
    - Turner syndrome is further supported by low estrogen and high LH and FSH.
    - The two cardiovascular comorbidities that may accompany Turner syndrome include bicuspid aortic valve and coarctation of the aorta.

3. A 16-year-old girl comes to her primary physician with her mother because of absent menses. Physical exam shows Tanner stage V breasts, genitalia, and pubic hair. Genital examination reveals a dark blue bulge between the labia minora. What is the best next step in the management of this patient?

    - **The next best step in the management of this patient is a hymenotomy.**
    - This 16-year-old patient has no menses; however she has Tanner stage V breasts, genitalia, and pubic hair.
    - There is a dark blue bulge between the labia minora which is a classic description of an imperforate hymen.
    - The bulge is blue due to blood accumulated in the vagina.
    - Imperforate hymen, as the name implies, is the persistence of the hymenal membrane.
    - The best next step in the management of an imperforate hymen is a hymenal incision, also known as hymenotomy, which restores the normal passage of menstrual blood.

REVIEW QUESTIONS

4. A 15-year-old girl is brought to her primary care physician by her mom because of absent menses. Physical examination shows Tanner stage V breasts and genitalia. Pubic and axillary hair are absent. Physical exam also shows circular masses in the labia majora. LH, FSH, testosterone, and estrogen levels are high. Pelvic ultrasound is performed and shows an absence of the uterus and fallopian tubes. What is the best next step in management?

- **The best next step in the management is the removal of the mass (testicles) after completion of puberty to prevent testicular cancer.**
- This 15-year-old girl has not had her menses and is found to have an absence of the uterus and fallopian tubes.
- The physical exam shows Tanner stage V breasts and genitalia. However, pubic and axillary hair are absent.
- This classic description indicates estrogen is exerting its physiologic effects; however androgens are ineffective.
- High androgen levels, along with androgen ineffectiveness, is consistent with androgen insensitivity syndrome.
- The best next step in the management of this patient is to remove the testicles after completion of puberty. This is because intra-abdominal retention of testicles at high temperatures predisposes the patient to testicular cancer, especially seminomas.

5. A 16-year-old girl is brought to her primary care physician by her mom because of absent menses. Physical exam shows Tanner stage V breasts, genitalia, and pubic hair. Further genitourinary examination shows the vagina ends in a blind pouch. Vital signs are within normal limits. Laboratory studies show normal levels of LH, FSH, estrogen, and testosterone. Pelvic ultrasound shows normal-sized ovaries, but an absent uterus and fallopian tubes. Which of the following is the most likely diagnosis in this patient?

   A. Mullerian agenesis
   B. Androgen insensitivity syndrome
   C. Turner syndrome
   D. Kallmann syndrome

- **The correct answer is option A.**
- This 16-year-old girl has not yet had her period.
- Physical examination shows Tanner stage V breasts, genitalia, and pubic hair, indicating both estrogen and androgens are exerting their physiological effects.
- Levels of LH, FSH, estrogen, and testosterone levels are all within the normal range, indicating a normal hypothalamic-pituitary-ovarian axis.
- The vagina ends in a blind pouch and ultrasound reveals an absence of a uterus and fallopian tubes.
- Normal hypothalamic-pituitary-ovarian axis, along with absent uterus and fallopian tubes is consistent with the diagnosis of Mullerian agenesis.
- The Mullerian duct is the embryologic structure responsible for the development of the fallopian tubes, uterus, and the upper vagina. Mullerian agenesis results in the absence of these structures.
- Option B is incorrect because androgen insensitivity syndrome is associated with high LH, FSH, estrogen, and testosterone levels. Additionally, the patients with androgen insensitivity syndrome have testes rather than ovaries.
- Option C is incorrect because Turner syndrome is associated with high FSH, high LH, and low estrogen. Additionally, this patient has no physical characteristics of Turner syndrome, like a webbed neck or shield chest.
- Option D is incorrect because Kallmann syndrome is associated with low FSH, LH, estrogen, and testosterone levels. Additionally, patients with Kallmann syndrome have anosmia, which is absent in this patient.

Gynecology | Section 14: Secondary Amenorrhea

I. Secondary Amenorrhea: Definition
   A. Absence of menses for 3 months in a woman with previously regular menses or 6 months in a woman with previously irregular menses
   B. Normal genital tract

II. Secondary Amenorrhea: Pathophysiology and Etiologies
   A. Anatomic abnormalities (e.g. Asherman syndrome, cervical stenosis)
      1. Development of adhesions after procedures (e.g. D&C, myomectomy, C-section, infections, pelvic irradiation, cone biopsy)
   B. Premature ovarian failure
      1. Decreased primordial follicles, increased apoptosis, impaired maturation and recruitment of follicles
      2. Idiopathic, autoimmune, chemotherapy
   C. Polycystic ovarian syndrome
      1. Ovarian hyperandrogenism → ↑ LH → ↑ LH:FSH ratio → anovulation
      2. Excessive testosterone production
      3. Hyperinsulinemia
      4. Obesity and insulin resistance
   D. Hyperprolactinemia-associated amenorrhea
      1. Inhibition of GnRH release by increased prolactin levels

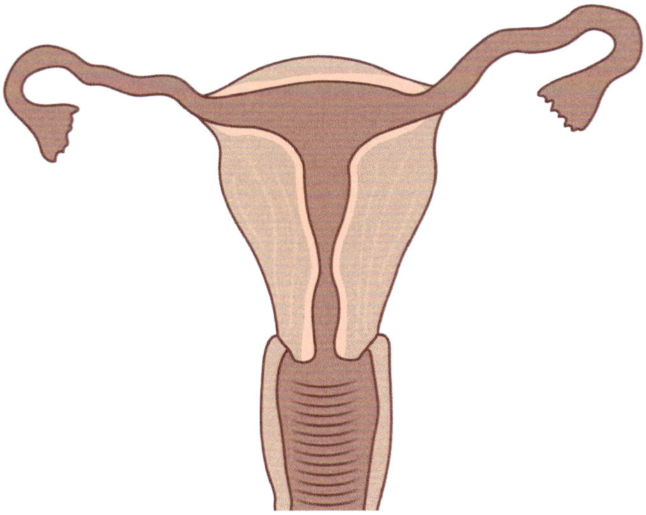

FIGURE 17.2.45 - Normal Uterus

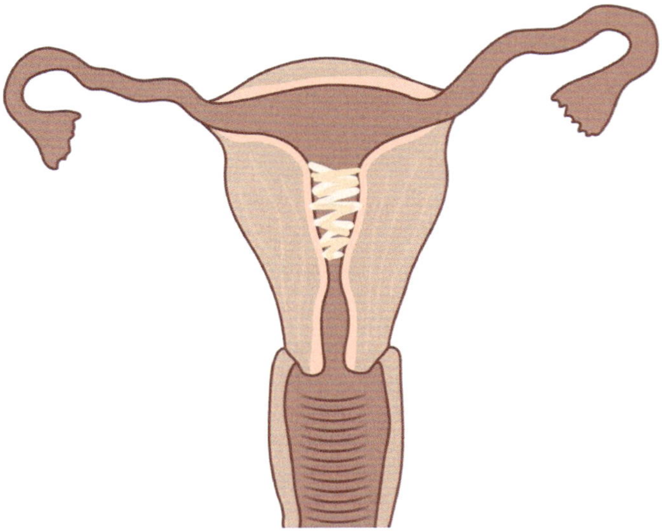

FIGURE 17.2.46 - Uterine Adhesions in Asherman Syndrome

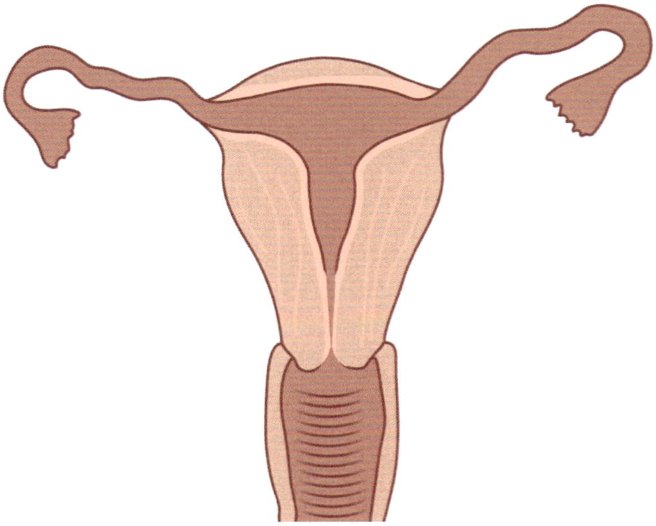

FIGURE 17.2.47 - Cervical Stenosis

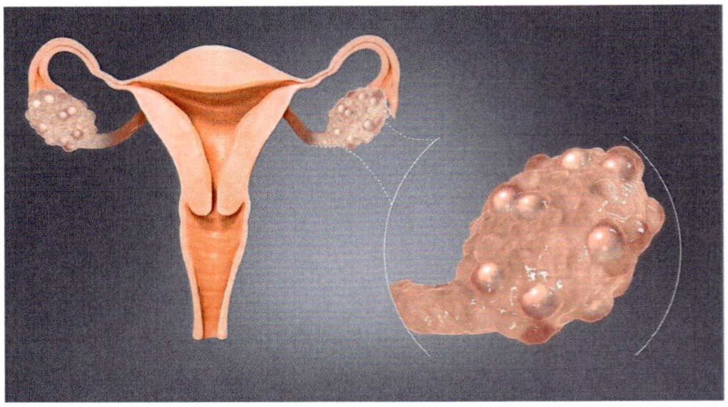

FIGURE 7.2.48 - Polycystic Ovaries

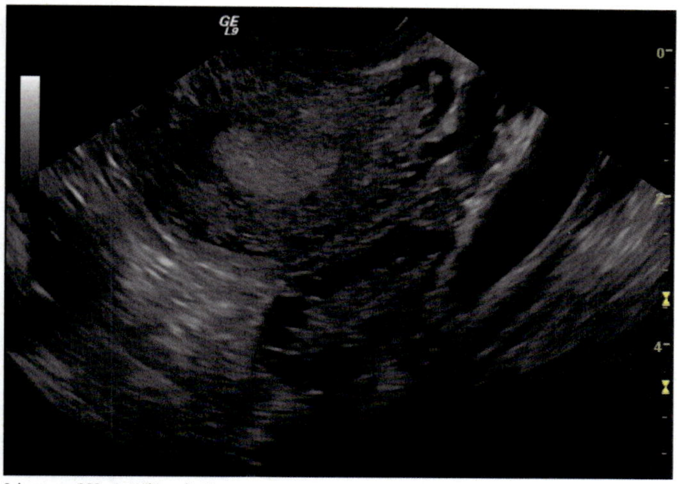

Schomynv, CC0, via Wikimedia Commons

FIGURE 17.2.49 - Transvaginal Ultrasound: Polycystic Ovaries

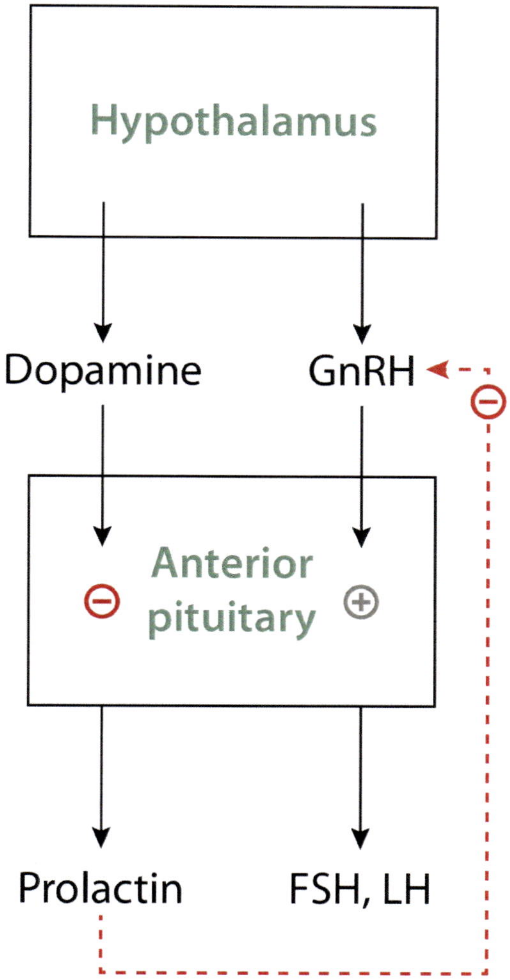

FIGURE 17.2.50 - Hypothalamic-Pituitary Axis

III. Secondary Amenorrhea: Clinical Features
   A. Asherman syndrome
      1. Absence of menstrual bleeding, infertility
      2. Pelvic pain during menses (e.g. cervical adhesions)
   B. Premature ovarian failure
      1. Irregular or skipped periods
      2. Hot flashes, night sweats, vaginal dryness
   C. Polycystic ovarian syndrome
      1. Amenorrhea, infertility
      2. Acne, hirsutism (e.g. chest, chin)
      3. Androgenic alopecia
      4. Metabolic syndrome (e.g. central obesity)
      5. Comorbidities (e.g. diabetes mellitus, OSA, Dyslipidemia, endometrial hyperplasia or cancer)
   D. Hyperprolactinemia-associated amenorrhea
      1. Absence of menses, neurological signs (e.g. headache, vision problems), galactorrhea

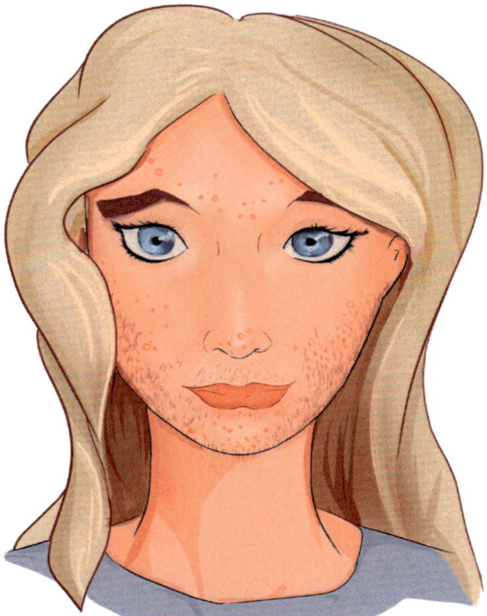

FIGURE 17.2.51 - Facial Features in Polycystic Ovarian Syndrome

IV. Secondary Amenorrhea: Diagnosis
   A. History and physical exam
   B. B-hCG, TSH, FSH, LH, prolactin
   C. Progestin challenge test
   D. If clinically indicated perform pelvic ultrasound, MRI, karyotype, testosterone, DHEA-S, hysteroscopy

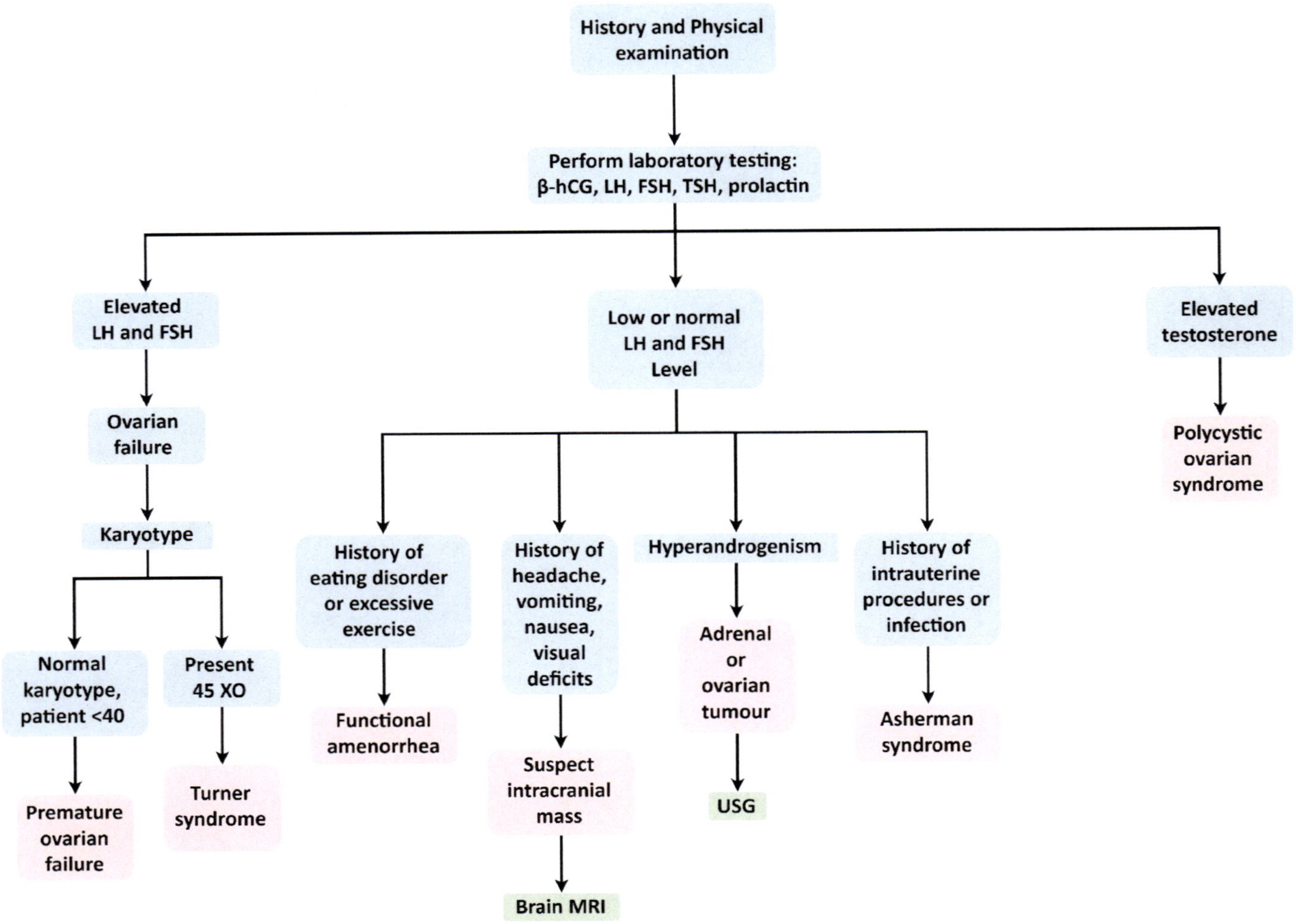

FIGURE 17.2.52 - Evaluation of Secondary Amenorrhea

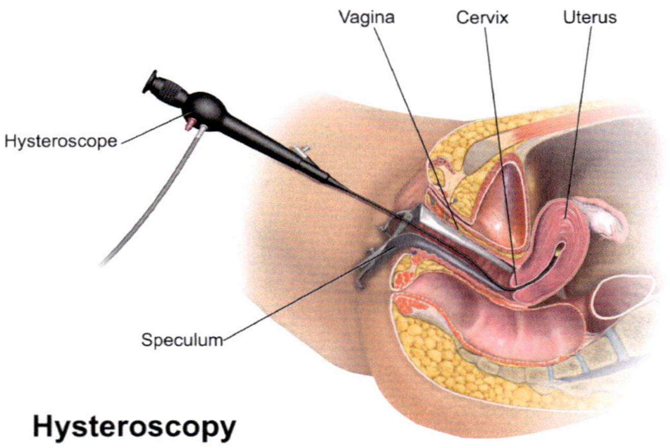

FIGURE 17.2.53 - Hysteroscopy

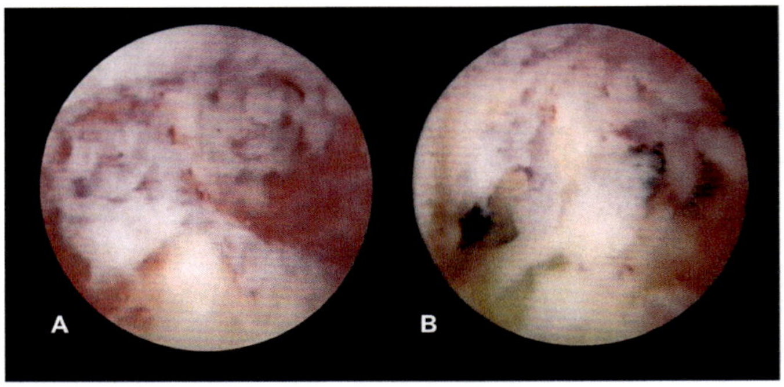

FIGURE 17.2.54 - Hysteroscopy: Uterine Adhesions in Asherman Syndrome

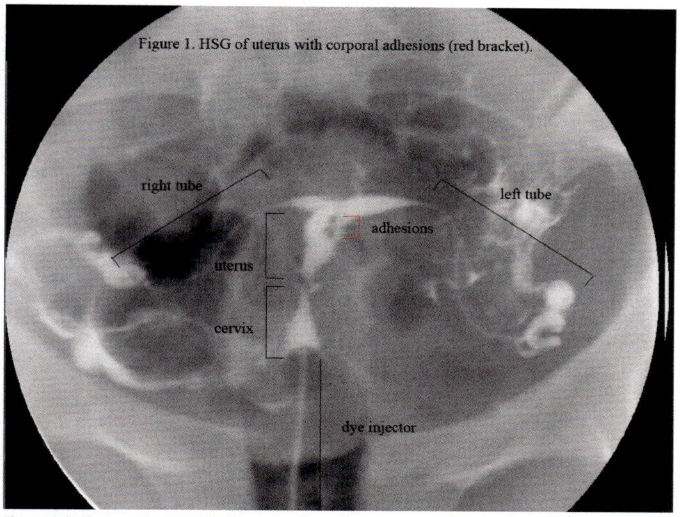

FIGURE 17.2.55 - Hysterosalpingography: Intrauterine Adhesions in Asherman Syndrome

V. Secondary Amenorrhea: Management
   A. Asherman syndrome
      1. Remove adhesions
      2. Cyclic estrogen and progesterone therapy
   B. Premature ovarian failure
      1. Estrogen therapy
      2. Vitamin D and calcium
   C. Polycystic ovarian syndrome
      1. Weight loss
      2. OCPs (e.g. for hyperandrogenism and menstrual abnormalities)
      3. Metformin (e.g. coexisting DM type 2)
      4. Clomiphene (e.g. ovulation induction)
   D. Hyperprolactinemia-induced amenorrhea
      1. Bromocriptine, cabergoline

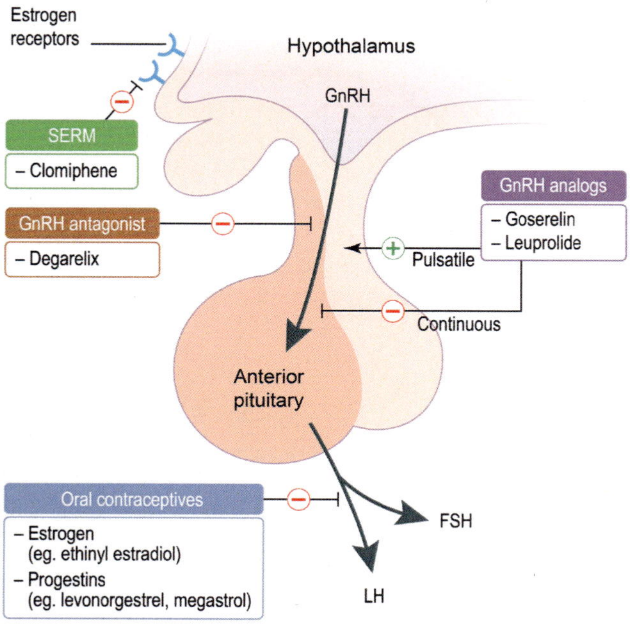

FIGURE 17.2.56 - Mechanism of Action of Certain Medications

REVIEW QUESTIONS

1. A 31-year-old woman comes to her primary care physician because of absent menses for the last 6 months. She has a past medical history of a molar pregnancy treated with dilation and curettage. Laboratory studies show a normal serum prolactin level. A progesterone challenge test results in no bleeding. What is the most likely underlying cause of this patient's complaint?

   - **The most likely underlying cause is Asherman syndrome.**
   - This patient presents with absent menses for the last 6 months.
   - She has a medical history of a molar pregnancy treated with dilation and curettage.
   - Her serum prolactin levels are normal, indicating that hyperprolactinemia is not the cause of her secondary amenorrhea.
   - A progesterone challenge test results in no bleeding. This suggests that the cause of secondary amenorrhea is not anovulation.
   - Dilation and curettage likely caused scarring of the endometrium, which is most likely responsible for this patient's secondary amenorrhea.
   - Scarring of the endometrial lining leading to secondary amenorrhea after a gynecological procedure is called Asherman syndrome.

2. A 28-year-old woman comes to her primary care physician because of absent periods for the last 4 months. She also complains of severe episodic headaches. Ophthalmologic examination shows vision loss in the temporal visual fields of both eyes. Which laboratory test should be ordered next to confirm this patient's underlying condition?

   - **The next laboratory test that should be ordered to confirm this patient's underlying condition is serum prolactin.**
   - This patient presents with absent menses for the last 4 months.
   - She also complains of severe episodic headaches.
   - Ophthalmologic exam shows vision loss in the temporal visual fields of both eyes. This description is consistent with the bitemporal hemianopsia due to optic chiasm compression.
   - Secondary amenorrhea, headache, and bitemporal hemianopsia suggest the diagnosis of prolactinoma.
   - The laboratory test that should be ordered next is serum prolactin.

REVIEW QUESTIONS

3. A 32-year-old woman comes to her primary care physician because of absent menses for the last 6 months. She occasionally feels intense heat spreading from her chest all the way to her face. Recently, she has been experiencing pain during sexual intercourse. Her family history is significant for fragile X syndrome in her brother. Laboratory studies show low levels of estrogen and high levels of FSH and LH. What is the most likely cause of her current symptoms?

- **The most likely cause of her current symptoms is premature ovarian failure.**
- This patient presents with absent menses for the last 6 months and hot flashes.
- Recently, she has been experiencing pain during sexual intercourse, which is consistent with dyspareunia.
- Estrogen is low, while FSH and LH are high, consistent with primary hypogonadism.
- All of these symptoms in a woman less than 40 years of age indicate premature ovarian failure, also known as primary ovarian insufficiency.
- This patient's family history is significant for the fragile X syndrome in her brother. Therefore, she may be a premutation carrier of the FMR1 gene.
- Premutation in the FMR1 gene predisposes women to primary ovarian insufficiency.

4. A 45-year-old G2P2 woman comes to her primary care physician because of vaginal spotting and an unintentional loss of 14 kg over the past 4 months. Her last menstrual period was 10 years ago. Her BMI is 32 kg/m^2. Physical examination shows dark hair on the upper lip, chin, and upper back. Pelvic ultrasound shows bilateral enlarged ovarian follicles. Laboratory findings are significant for high LH and FSH with an LH:FSH ratio of 3. Estrogen and testosterone levels are high as well. Which of the following is the best next step in the management of this patient's condition?

   A. Pelvic MRI
   B. Pelvic X-ray
   C. Endometrial biopsy
   D. Complete blood count

- **The correct answer is option C.**
- This patient's last menstrual period was 10 years ago.
- Physical examination shows dark hair on the upper lip, chin, and upper back, consistent with hyperandrogenism.
- High testosterone levels confirm hyperandrogenism.
- LH and FSH are high, with LH:FSH ratio of 3.
- All these findings are consistent with the diagnosis of polycystic ovarian syndrome.
- However, this patient currently presents with vaginal spotting and an unintentional loss of 14 kg over the past 4 months.
- Since patients with polycystic ovarian syndrome are at high risk for endometrial hyperplasia and cancer due to high estrogen levels, she should undergo endometrial biopsy to exclude the malignancy.
- Option A, pelvic MRI, and option B, pelvic X-ray, are incorrect because they are not sensitive enough to diagnose endometrial cancer. Additionally, pelvic MRI and X-ray may not differentiate endometrial hyperplasia from endometrial cancer.
- Option D, complete blood count, is incorrect because it cannot help with the diagnosis of endometrial cancer.

Gynecology | Section 15: Primary Dysmenorrhea, Premenstrual Syndrome & Premenstrual Dysphoric Disorder

I. Primary Dysmenorrhea
   A. Pathophysiology
      1. Excessive prostaglandin production (e.g. PGE_2, PGF_{2a}) increases uterine contractions during menstrual period
   B. Risk factors
      1. Age < 30; BMI < 20 kg/m^2
      2. Menarche at < 12 years of age; tobacco use
      3. Heavy menstrual periods; sexual abuse
   C. Clinical features
      1. Pain during first 2 to 3 days of menses
      2. Nausea, vomiting, and possible diarrhea
      3. Normal pelvic exam (diagnosis of exclusion)
   D. Management
      1. Exercise and heat application
      2. NSAIDs or OCPs based on patient's preference

II. Premenstrual Syndrome
   A. Pathophysiology
      1. Hormonal fluctuations in luteal phase result in physical and affective symptoms
      2. Symptoms are cyclical and occur only during luteal phase
   B. Clinical features
      1. Physical symptoms:
         a) Fatigue, bloating, hot flashes
         b) Headache, breast tenderness
         c) Affective symptoms:
         d) Irritability and mood swings
   C. Diagnosis
      1. Menstrual diary
      2. Exclusion of other causes of physical and affective symptoms
   D. Treatment
      1. Relaxation technique and yoga
      2. Avoidance of chocolate and tobacco
      3. SSRIs in severe cases

III. Premenstrual Dysphoric Disorder
   A. Pathophysiology
      1. Hormonal fluctuations in luteal phase result in physical and affective symptoms
      2. Symptoms are cyclical and occur only during luteal phase
   B. Physical symptoms: fatigue, bloating, hot flashes, breast tenderness
   C. Affective symptoms: irritability, mood swings, anxiety, low interest in previously enjoyable activities
   D. Diagnosis
      1. Menstrual diary
      2. Exclusion of other causes of physical and affective symptoms
   E. Treatment
      1. SSRIs
      2. Behavioral modifications unlikely to be effective

REVIEW QUESTIONS ?

1. A 22-year-old woman comes to her primary care physician because of lower abdominal pain for the last 3 days. She is currently on her period, which started 3 days ago. She is sexually active with her boyfriend, and she wants to start birth control. She notes she experiences severe cramps every time she has a period. Pelvic examination is unremarkable. Her vital signs are all within normal limits. What is the best treatment option for this patient?
   - **The best treatment option for this patient is oral contraceptive pills.**
   - This woman presents with lower abdominal pain for the last 3 days, which recurs every time she has menses.
   - Given that her pelvic examination is unremarkable and the pain only occurs during her menses, the most likely diagnosis in this patient is primary dysmenorrhea.
   - Since this patient needs treatment for primary dysmenorrhea and also wants to start birth control, the best treatment option for her is oral contraceptive pills.

2. A 29-year-old woman comes to her primary care physician because she has felt depressed for the past week. She has a regular menstrual cycle of 28 days, and her last period was 18 days ago. She also complains of fatigue, bloating, and breast tenderness; However, she is more concerned about her mood changes. She says her moods change before her periods, and it is severe enough to cause serious conflict with her family and partner. Which findings best differentiate whether this patient has premenstrual syndrome or premenstrual dysphoric disorder?
   - **The findings that best differentiate whether this patient has premenstrual syndrome or premenstrual dysphoric disorder is the presence of severe mood symptoms that disturb personal life.**
   - This woman presents with a depressed mood for the last week. She also complains of fatigue, bloating, and breast tenderness.
   - Her mood disturbances are so severe that she frequently has conflicts with her family and partner, disrupting her life.
   - These physical and affective symptoms occur regularly before her periods.
   - Since she has mood symptoms affecting her personal life, this patient's condition is most likely to be a premenstrual dysphoric disorder.

Gynecology | Section 16: Abnormal Uterine Bleeding

I. Abnormal Uterine Bleeding
  A. Classified according to:
    1. Duration of menstrual cycle
    2. Amount of menstrual blood flow
    3. Timing of vaginal bleeding across the menstrual period
    4. Structural causes ("PALM")
    5. Non-structural causes ("COEIN")
  B. Polymenorrhea
    1. Menstrual cycle lasting less than 21 days
    2. Increased total number of menstrual cycles
  C. Oligomenorrhea
    1. Menstrual cycle lasting more than 35 days
    2. Decreased total number of menstrual cycles
  D. Abnormal uterine bleeding/heavy menstrual bleeding (AUB/HMB)
    1. Also known as menorrhagia
    2. Menstrual period lasting more than 7 days
    3. Menstrual pad is fully saturated with blood in roughly 1 hour
  E. Vaginal spotting
    1. Scant bleeding with less than 1 inch of menstrual pad saturated with blood
  F. Structural causes of abnormal uterine bleeding ("PALM")
    1. Endometrial **P**olyp
    2. **A**denomyosis
    3. **L**eiomyoma (fibroid)
    4. Endometrial **M**alignancy or hyperplasia
  G. Abnormal uterine bleeding / intermenstrual bleeding (AUB/IMB)
    1. Also known as metrorrhagia
    2. Woman has normal menstrual periods and intermenstrual spotting
    3. Called menometrorrhagia if accompanied by heavy menstrual bleeding
  H. Non-structural causes of abnormal uterine bleeding ("COEIN")
    1. **C**oagulopathy
    2. **O**vulatory dysfunction
    3. **E**ndometrial causes
    4. **I**atrogenic causes
    5. **N**ot yet classified

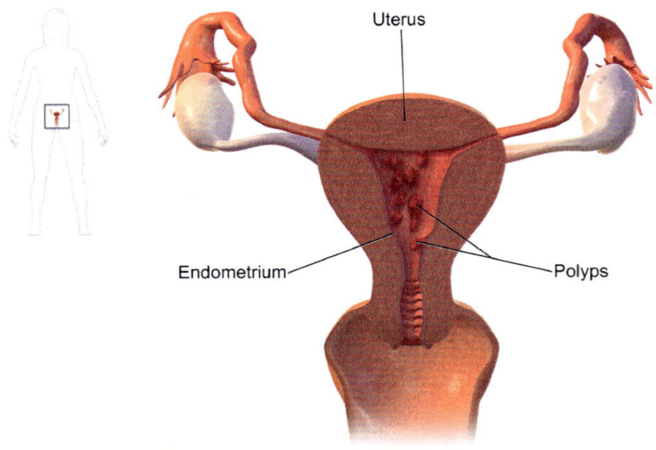

Uterine Polyps

FIGURE 17.2.57 - Uterine Polyps

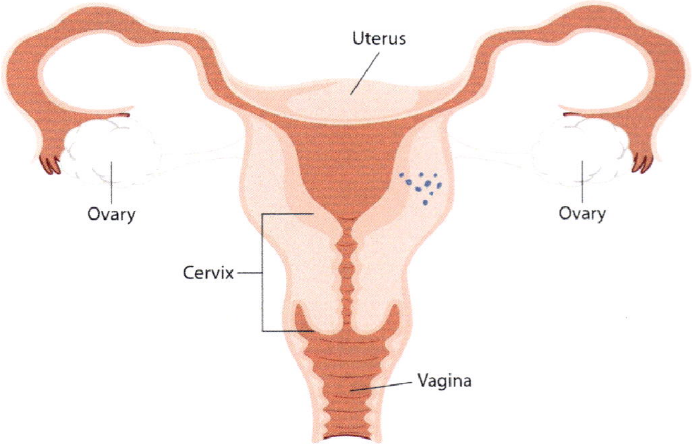

FIGURE 17.2.58 - Adenomyosis

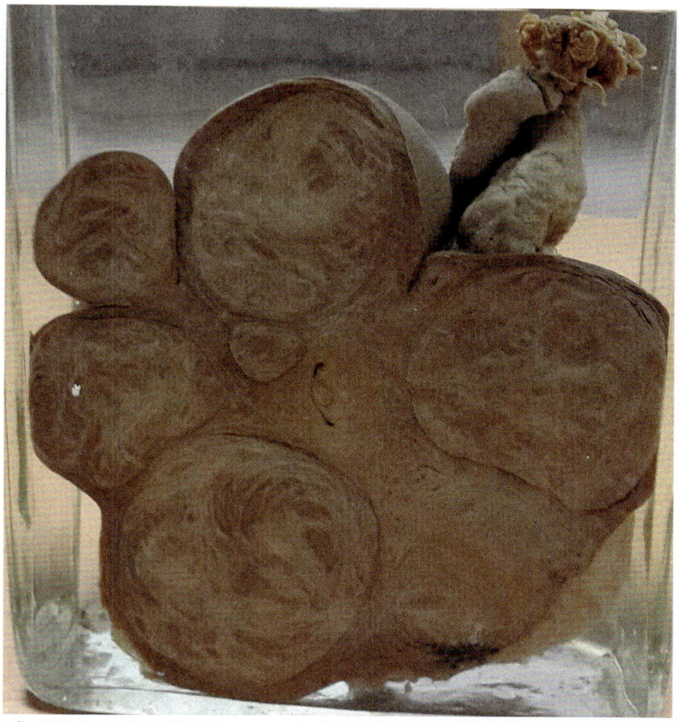

FIGURE 17.2.59 - Uterine Leiomyomas

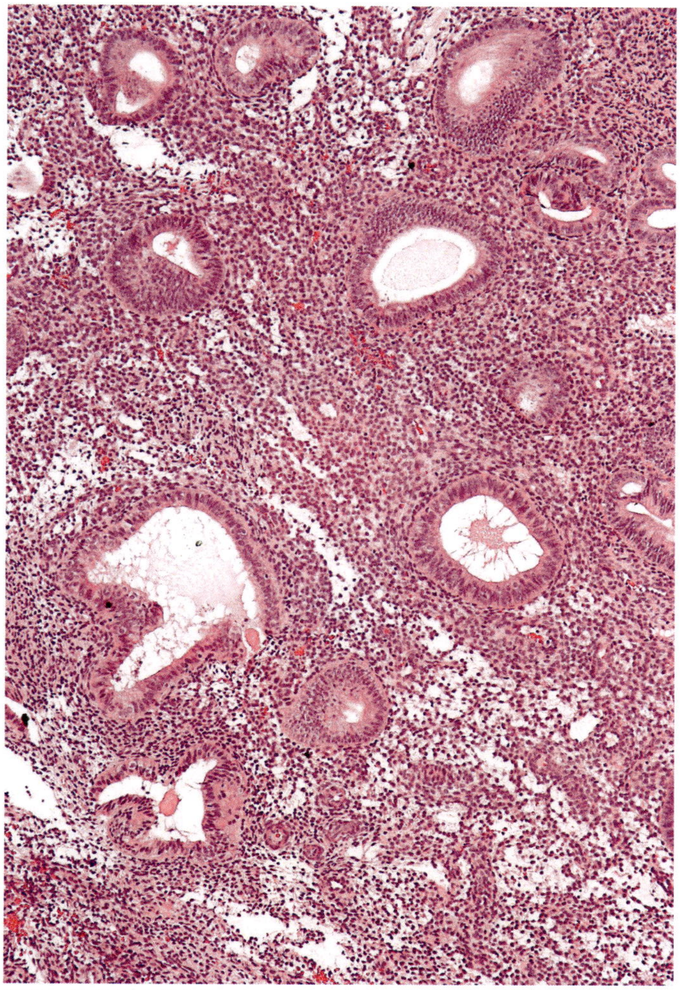

FIGURE 17.2.60 - Light Microscopy: Endometrial Hyperplasia

REVIEW QUESTIONS

6. A 37-year-old woman comes to her primary care physician because of lower abdominal pain and heavy vaginal bleeding for the last 7 days. Her last menstrual period started a week ago. She experiences similar pain at the beginning of her periods. She and her husband have been trying to conceive for the last year but have been unsuccessful. Her vital signs include a temperature of 98.6° F (37° C), blood pressure of 110/80 mmHg, heart rate of 110 beats/min, and respiratory rate of 19 breaths/min. Her laboratory studies show low ferritin and low serum iron concentrations. Her BMI is 22 kg/m^2. Physical examination shows an asymmetrically enlarged, irregularly shaped uterus with palpable masses. Which of the following is the most likely diagnosis?

   A. Endometrial polyp
   B. Adenomyosis
   C. Leiomyoma
   D. Endometrial adenocarcinoma

- **The correct answer is option C.**
- This woman presents with heavy menstrual bleeding for the last seven days. She complains of regular lower abdominal pain during her periods and has been unsuccessful with conception for 1 year.
- She is slightly tachycardia, and laboratory studies show low ferritin and low serum iron concentrations consistent with iron deficiency anemia.
- Physical examination shows an asymmetrically enlarged uterus with palpable masses. This description is classic for leiomyomas, also known as fibroids.
- Option A is incorrect because although an endometrial polyp can cause abnormal uterine bleeding, it does not result in an asymmetrically enlarged uterus with palpable masses.
- Option B is incorrect because although adenomyosis can cause abnormal uterine bleeding, it is characterized by a symmetrically, rather than asymmetrically, enlarged uterus with no discrete palpable masses.
- Option D is incorrect because she is a relatively young woman with a normal BMI. Endometrial adenocarcinoma, on the other hand, is usually seen in middle-aged obese women.

Gynecology | Section 17: Hirsutism And Virilism

I. Hirsutism and Virilism: Definitions
   A. Hirsutism
      1. Excessive terminal hair growth
      2. Male pattern: chin, upper lip, abdomen, back
   B. Virilization
      1. More extensive evidence of masculinization
      2. Increased muscle mass, deepening of the voice, acne, balding, clitoral hypertrophy

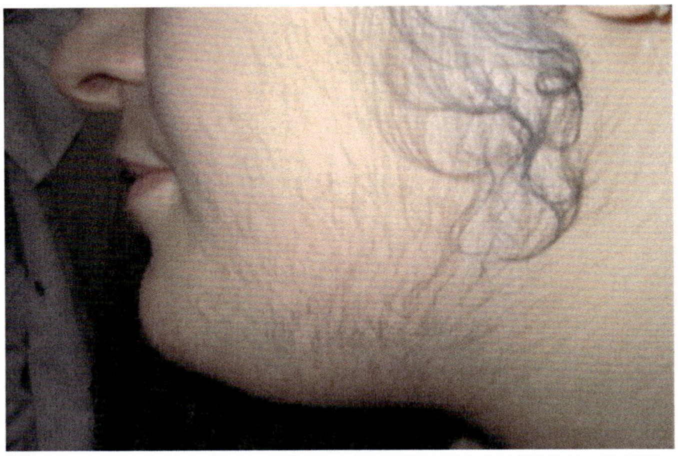

FIGURE 17.2.61 - Hirsutism

II. Hirsutism and Virilism: Etiology and Pathophysiology
   A. Cushing syndrome
      1. Most commonly secondary to Cushing syndrome due to adrenal carcinomas
         a) ↑ ↑ androgenic precursors with a inability to convert all of them to cortisol → hirsutism and potential virilization
      2. ACTH-dependent Cushing syndrome can lead to hirsutism
   B. Congenital adrenal hyperplasia
      1. 21β-hydroxylase and 11β-hydroxylase deficiencies → ↑ androgens, ↓ cortisol and aldosterone
      2. XX infants may have clitoromegaly, male external genitalia, and signs of virilization; non-classic type may present in childhood
      3. Will not see signs of hyperandrogenism in 17α-hydroxylase deficiency
   C. Polycystic ovarian syndrome
      1. Most common cause of hirsutism
      2. Exact cause unknown
      3. Functional ovarian hyperandrogenism leads to classic features such as hirsutism, acne, and polycystic ovaries
   D. Gestational hyperandrogenism
      1. Luteoma: benign solid mass of hyperplastic lutein cells secondary to hCG; if active can cause virilization of mother and fetus
      2. Theca lutein cysts: luteinized and hypertrophied theca interna cells secondary to hCG; more common in multiples and gestational trophoblastic disease
      3. Typically regress after pregnancy
      4. Placental aromatase deficiency: inability for the placenta to convert increased androgens during pregnancy to estrogen
         a) Leads to virilization of the fetus the the mother
   E. Ovarian hyperthecosis
      1. Severe hyperandrogenism and insulin resistance in a postmenopausal woman
      2. Ovarian interstitial cells differentiate into luteinized stromal cells that produce steroids
      3. Gradual onset of hirsutism, acne, and virilization

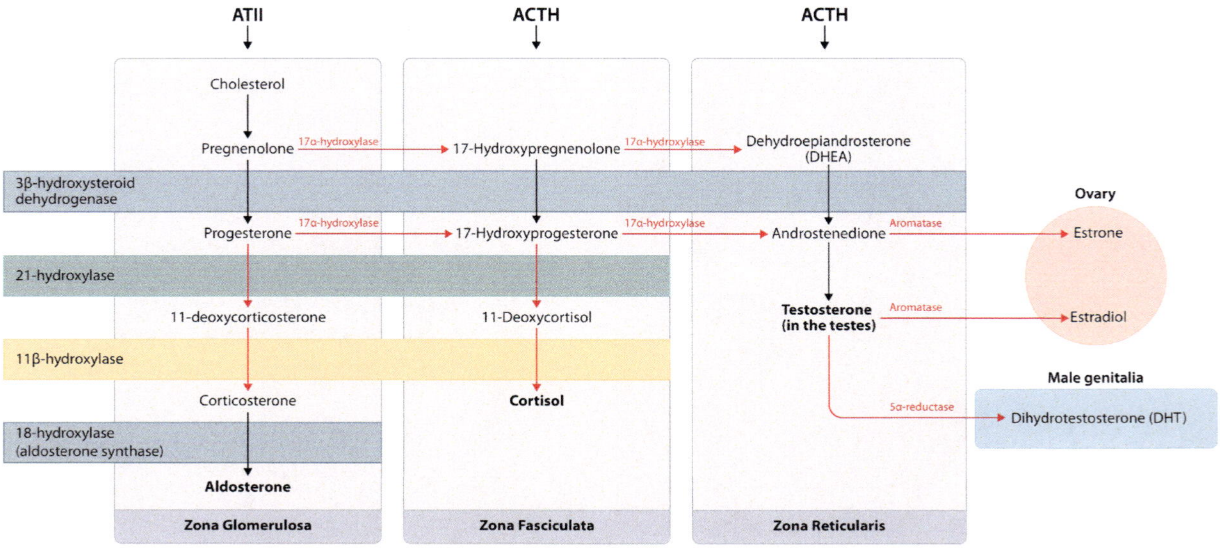

FIGURE 17.2.62 - Androgen Synthesis Pathway

F. Androgen-secreting ovarian tumors
  1. Sertoli-Leydig: sex-cord stromal tumor that is typically benign; common to have androgenic effects
  2. Granulosa-theca: potentially malignant sex-cord stromal tumor; theca cells may produce androstenedione; estrogenic effects more common

G. Medications
  1. Corticosteroids
  2. Minoxidil
  3. Phenytoin
  4. Cyclosporine

H. Exogenous hormones

III. Hirsutism and Virilism: Diagnosis
  A. History and physical; review medication list carefully
  B. CAH detected on newborn screening
  C. Cortisol, total testosterone, DHEA-S, LH, FSH, 17-hydroxyprogesterone, prolactin, TSH
  D. Pelvic ultrasound, adrenal imaging with CT or MRI

IV. Hirsutism and Virilism: Management
  A. Management of the underlying medical condition
  B. Oral contraceptives
  C. Antiandrogen (spironolactone)
  D. Direct hair removal
  E. Virilizing symptoms such as clitoromegaly and deepening of the voice are irreversible

REVIEW QUESTIONS ?

1. A 27-year-old woman comes to her primary care physician because of excessive hair growth, deepening of her voice, and cessation of menstrual cycle for the past 2 months. Past medical history is significant for type 2 diabetes mellitus. Family history reveals hirsutism in her mother. Her vital signs are unremarkable. BMI is 32 kg/m^2 (19 kg/m^2 - 25 kg/m^2). Physical examination shows hair growth on her upper lip, chin, chest, and back. On genitourinary examination, clitoromegaly is noted. Laboratory findings show FSH level of 2 IU/L (3 IU/L - 10 IU/L), LH of 1 IU/L (2 IU/L - 8 IU/L), total testosterone of 80 ng/dL (15 ng/dL - 70 ng/dL), and DHEA level of 900 mcg/dL (65 mcg/dL - 380 mcg/dL). Which of the following is the most likely cause of this patient's current complaints?

   A. Ovarian Sertoli-Leydig cell tumor
   B. Adrenal tumor
   C. Polycystic ovarian syndrome
   D. Idiopathic hirsutism

REVIEW QUESTIONS ?

- **The correct answer is option B.**
- This young woman presents with excessive hair growth, deepening of her voice, and cessation of her menstrual cycle for the past 2 months.
- Physical examination is consistent with hirsutism and virilism.
- Laboratory findings reveal low levels of FSH and LH, likely due to negative feedback from androgens.
- While total testosterone slightly increased at 80 ng/dL, DHEA levels are significantly high at 900 mcg/dL.
- When virilization develops rapidly, there is a high index suspicion for either ovarian or adrenal tumors.
- Ovarian tumors causing virilization typically produce testosterone, while adrenal tumors causing virilization produce DHEA. Therefore, this patient most likely has an adrenal tumor.
- Option A is incorrect because ovarian Sertoli-Leydig cell tumors predominantly produce testosterone rather than DHEA. Although testosterone is slightly increased in this patient, it is probably due to increased conversion of DHEA to androstenedione and then testosterone.
- Option C is incorrect because although polycystic ovarian syndrome is characterized by amenorrhea and hyperandrogenism, it usually presents with high LH and high or normal FSH with LH:FSH ratio more than 2:1. This patient has low FSH and LH.
- Option D is incorrect because idiopathic hirsutism is a diagnosis of exclusion characterized by normal levels of androgen, FSH, and LH. Although this patient has a family history of hirsutism, her hormone levels are abnormal, which excludes idiopathic hirsutism.

Gynecology | Section 18: Natural Method of Contraception, Barriers & Spermicides

I. Natural Methods of Contraception
   A. Least effective methods of preventing pregnancy
   B. Do not protect patients against sexually transmitted diseases
   C. Options
      1. Periodic abstinence
      2. Coitus interruptus
      3. Lactational amenorrhea

II. Natural Methods of Contraception: Periodic Abstinence
   A. Track the menstrual cycle and avoid intercourse during ovulation
      1. Woman needs to have predictable, regular menstrual cycles
   B. Supplementary ovulation tracking methods (e.g. ovulation kits)
   C. Advantage: no need for mechanical or chemical barriers
   D. Disadvantages:
      1. High effort, low reliability
      2. May warrant prolonged periods of abstinence

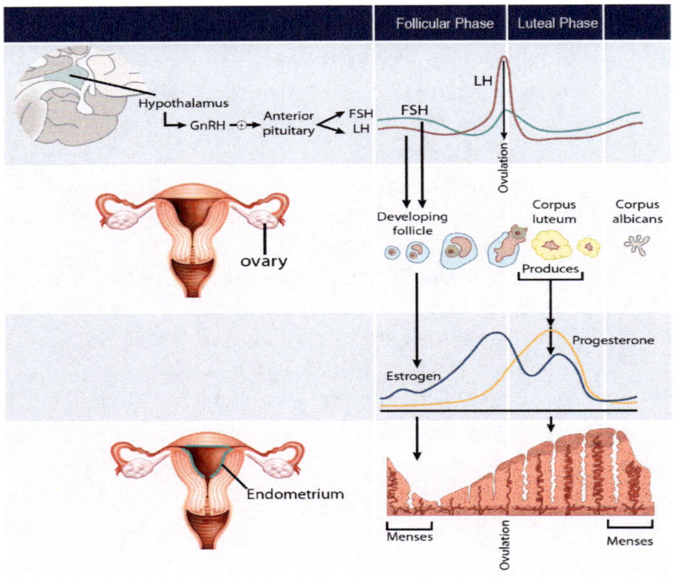

FIGURE 17.2.37 - The Menstrual Cycle

III. Natural Methods of Contraception: Coitus Interruptus
   A. Withdrawal of the penis from the vagina prior to ejaculation
   B. Advantage: no need for mechanical or chemical barriers
   C. Disadvantages
      1. Low reliability
      2. Does not prevent deposition of pre-ejaculate into the vagina

IV. Natural Methods of Contraception: Lactational Amenorrhea
   A. Temporary state of infertility during the breastfeeding period
      1. Prolactin inhibits release of GnRH from the hypothalamus
      2. ↓ GnRH → ↓ FSH and LH → no ovulation
   B. Advantage: no need for mechanical or chemical barriers
   C. Disadvantages
      1. Low reliability
      2. Cannot be used beyond the first six months postpartum

V. Barriers: Male Condom
   A. A thin latex sheath placed over an erect penis prior to intercourse
   B. Prevents the ejaculate from entering the female reproductive tract
   C. Advantages
      1. Cheap and highly effective, if used properly
      2. Protects against sexually transmitted infections (e.g. HIV)
   D. Disadvantage
      1. Decreases sensation during intercourse

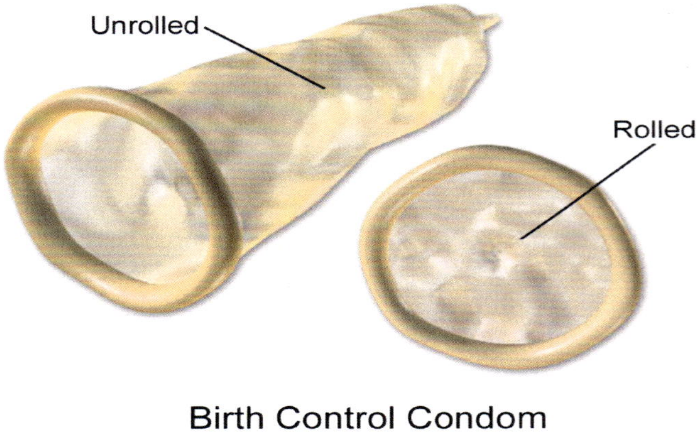

FIGURE 17.2.63 - Male Condom

VI. Barriers: Female Condom
   A. A soft pouch inserted into the vagina prior to intercourse
   B. Prevents the ejaculate from entering the uterus
   C. Advantage
      1. Protects against sexually transmitted infections
   D. Disadvantages
      1. More expensive and less straightforward than the male condom
      2. Decreases sensation during intercouse

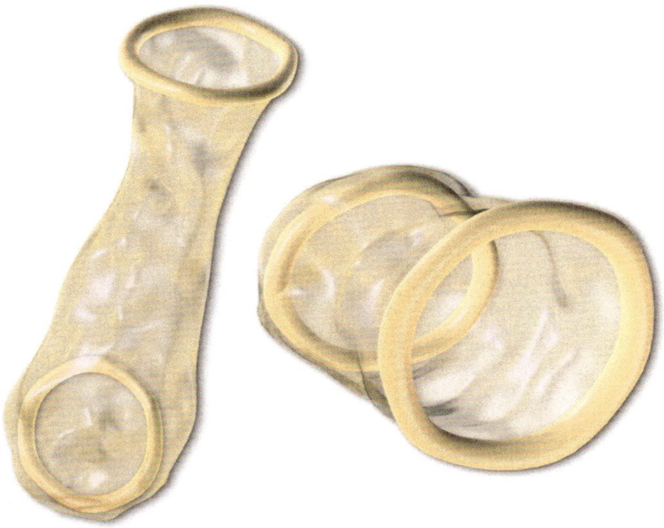

FIGURE 17.2.64 - Female Condom

VII. Barriers: Contraceptive Diaphragm
   A. Reusable dome-shaped rubber or silicone cup that covers the cervix
      1. Inserted into the vagina prior to intercourse
      2. Used in combination with spermicide cream, foam, or gel
   B. Advantage: more effective than the female condom
   C. Disadvantages
      1. Requires proper fitting by an experienced clinician
      2. Requires replacement every two years
      3. May no longer fit after a significant change in weight
      4. Must be left in place for at least six hours following intercourse
      5. May be colonized by *Staphylococcus aureus* and predispose to toxic shock syndrome

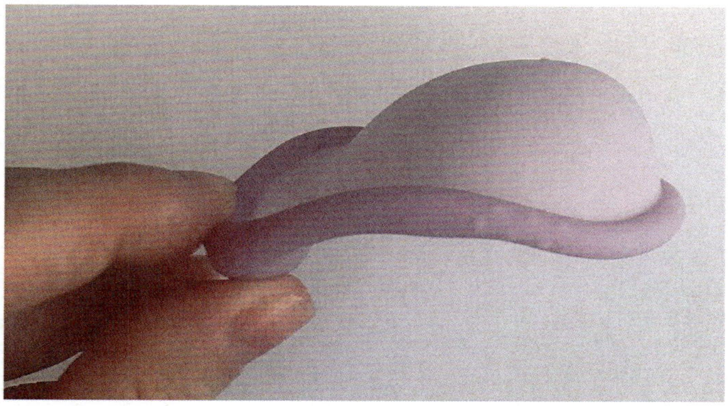

FIGURE 17.2.65 - Contraceptive Diaphragm

VIII. Barriers: Cervical Cap
   A. A small cap that covers the cervix
   B. Prevents entry of sperm into the uterus
   C. Used in combination with spermicide cream, foam, or gel
   D. Requires proper fitting by an experienced clinician
   E. Advantages
      1. May be placed up to 6 hours prior to intercourse
      2. May be left in place for one to two days
   F. Disadvantages
      1. Difficult for patients to place and remove the cap
      2. Frequently dislodges

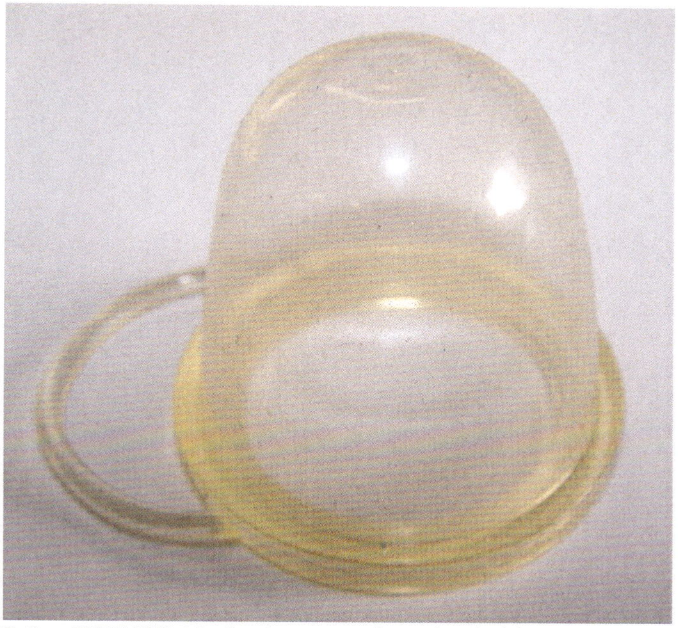

FIGURE 17.2.66 - Cervical Cap

IX. Spermicides
   A. Products designed to disrupt cell membranes of sperm cells and create a barrier to entry into the uterus (e.g. creams, foams, gels)
   B. Often used in combination with barriers (e.g. cervical cap)
   C. Advantage
      1. Cheap and easily available
   D. Disadvantages
      1. Must be placed into the vagina at least 30 minutes prior to intercourse
      2. Thought to increase risk of contracting sexually transmitted infections

REVIEW QUESTIONS

1. A 25-year-old woman comes to her primary care physician for a routine examination with no complaints. She has a history of gonorrhea treated with ceftriaxone and azithromycin 5 years ago. She has recently learned that her new male partner is HIV-positive. Physical examination is unremarkable. Her vital signs include a temperature of 98.6° F (37° C), blood pressure of 115/80 mmHg, heart rate of 90 beats/min, and respiratory rate of 16 breaths/min. Which of the following contraceptive methods best protects this patient from contracting her partner's infection?

    A. Coitus interruptus
    B. Cervical diaphragm
    C. Cervical cap
    D. Male condom

- **The correct answer is option D.**
- This patient found out that her new male partner is HIV positive.
- HIV is a sexually transmitted disease.
- From the given options, a male condom is the only contraceptive method that protects the patient from contracting sexually transmitted infections. This is because a male condom prevents direct contact between mucosal surfaces during sexual intercourse.
- Option A is incorrect because coitus interruptus is when the man withdraws the penis from the vagina immediately before ejaculation. This does not protect against sexually transmitted diseases.
- Option B, cervical diaphragm, and option C, cervical cap, are incorrect because they do not cover the vaginal mucosa. Therefore, a woman using either of these contraceptive methods are still at risk for contracting sexually transmitted diseases.

Gynecology | Section 19: Hormonal Contraception & Intrauterine Devices

I. Oral Contraceptive Pills
   A. Highly effective oral medications designed to prevent pregnancy
      1. Estrogen-progesterone pills (combination pills)
      2. Progesterone-only pills (minipills)
   B. Exogenous estrogen inhibits FSH and suppresses follicle maturation
   C. Exogenous progesterone
      1. Inhibits LH, thereby suppressing ovulation
      2. Thickens cervical mucus and thins endometrial lining
   D. Common reasons for discontinuation
      1. Breakthrough bleeding
      2. Dyspepsia (e.g. bloating, nausea)
      3. Requirement to take a pill every day

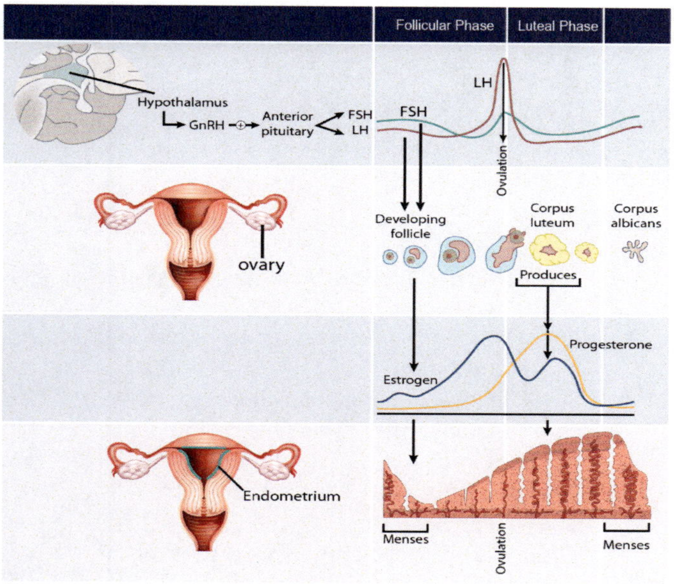

FIGURE 17.2.37 - The Menstrual Cycle

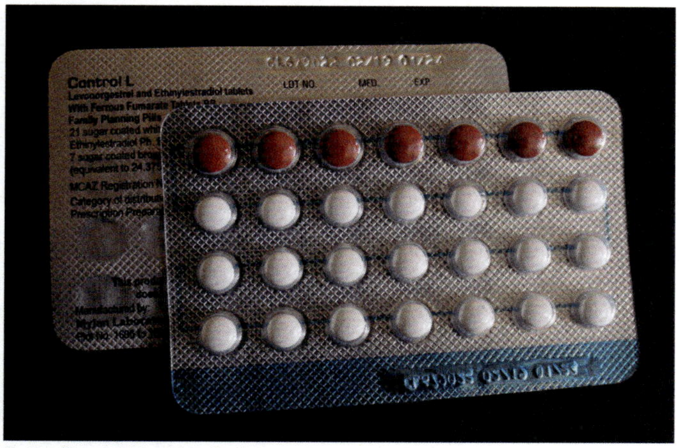

Photo by Stewart Mukonzi from Pexels

FIGURE 17.2.67 - Oral Contraceptive Pills

II. Oral Contraceptive Pills: Combination Pills
   A. Therapeutic indications
      1. Primary dysmenorrhea
      2. Anovulation (e.g. women with polycystic ovarian syndrome)
      3. Anemia (e.g. due to menorrhagia)
      4. Cancer risk reduction (e.g. endometrial cancer)
      5. Acne, hirsutism
      6. Ovarian cysts
   B. Adverse effects of hormonal therapy are largely attributed to estrogen
      1. Hypertension
      2. Hypercoagulability (e.g. stroke, MI, DVT, PE)
      3. Benign hepatic tumors (e.g. hepatic adenoma)
      4. Increased risk for gallbladder disease (e.g. cholelithiasis)
      5. Increased risk for cervical cancer

III. Oral Contraceptive Pills: Progesterone-Only Pills
   A. Unlike a combination pill, a progesterone-only pill:
      1. Does not contain estrogen
      2. Has a more favorable side effect profile
      3. Has a higher failure rate than a combination pill
      4. Requires a more punctual schedule for maximum efficacy
      5. Worsens acne

IV. Contraceptive Patch
   A. A patch that continuously delivers estrogen and progesterone through the skin
      1. Each patch lasts only a week
      2. Common placements: upper arm, back, abdomen, buttock
   B. As effective as oral contraceptive pills (OCPs)
      1. Less effective in women who weigh > 90 kg (198 lbs)
   C. Associated with a higher risk of venous thromboembolism than OCPs

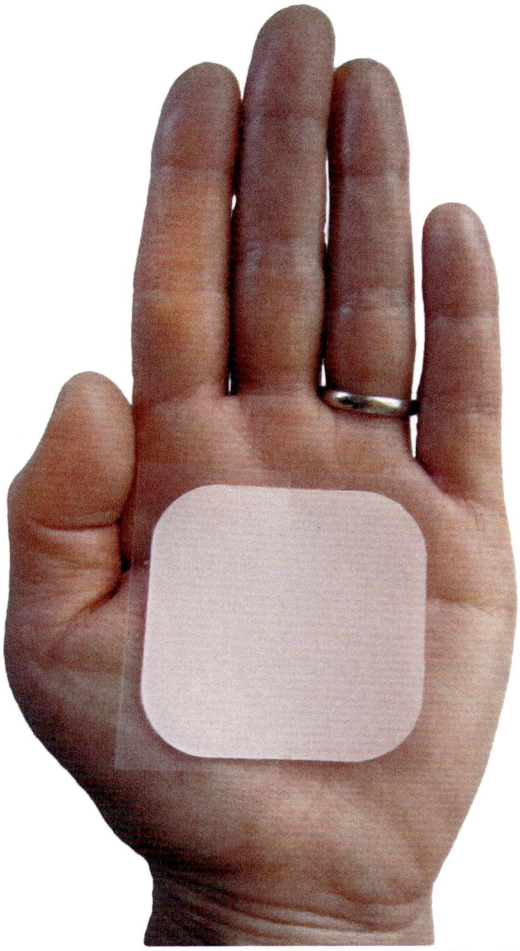

James Heilman, MD, CC BY-SA 3.0 <https://creativecommons.org/licenses/by-sa/3.0>, via Wikimedia Commons

FIGURE 17.2.68 - Contraceptive Patch

V. Nuvaring
   A. A vaginal ring that continuously releases estrogen and progesterone
      1. One-size-fits-all
      2. Each ring lasts one month
   B. Remains in place during intercourse
      1. If removed for intercourse, must be placed back within 3 hours
   C. As effective as oral contraceptive pills
   D. May lead to increased vaginal discharge

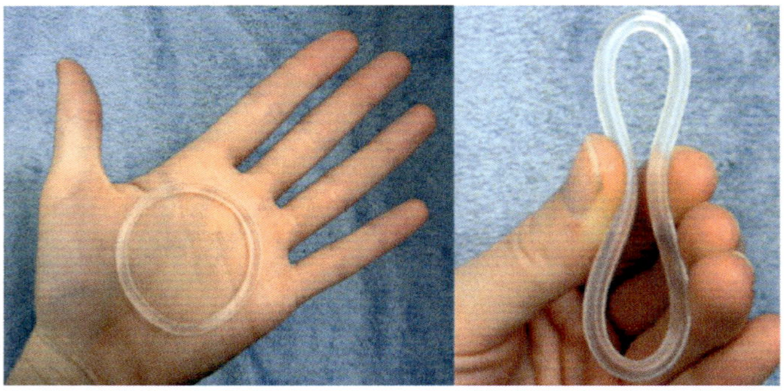

User:Sakky, Public domain, via Wikimedia Commons

FIGURE 17.2.69 - NuvaRing

VI. Depo Shot
   A. An intramuscular injection of progestin given once every 3 months
      1. Each shot prevents pregnancy for 14 weeks
   B. About half of women will experience amenorrhea after one year of use
      1. There may be a delay in ovulation following cessation of use
   C. May lead to decreased bone mineral density after two years of use
      1. The effect is reversible with discontinuation of the depo shot
   D. Weight gain is a common side effect

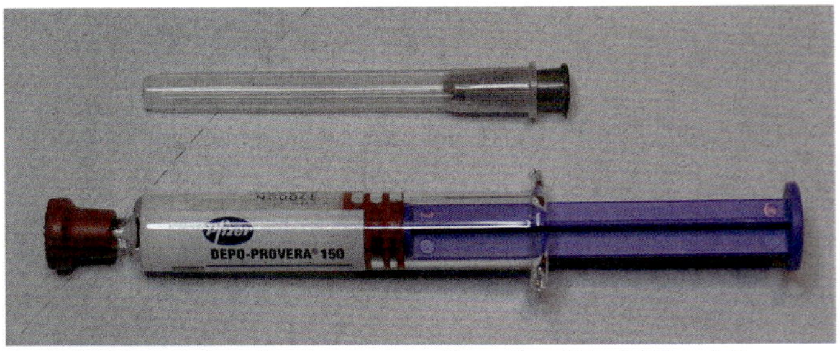

User:Ciell, CC BY-SA 2.5 <https://creativecommons.org/licenses/by-sa/2.5>, via Wikimedia Commons

FIGURE 17.2.70 - Depo Shot

VII. Nexplanon Implant
   A. A plastic rod placed under the skin by a clinician (e.g. upper arm)
      1. Continuously releases progesterone into the bloodstream
      2. Effective 24 hours following placement
      3. Lasts up to three years (no maintenance required)
   B. The most effective method of reversible contraception
   C. Often causes irregular menstrual spotting
   D. Must be removed by a clinician

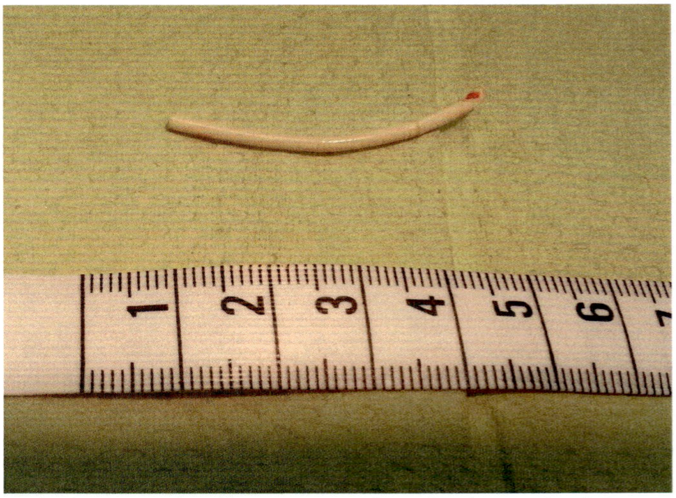

Vera de Kok, CC BY-SA 4.0 <https://creativecommons.org/licenses/by-sa/4.0>, via Wikimedia Commons

FIGURE 17.2.71 - Nexplanon Implant

Absolute Contraindications to Estrogen-Containing Contraceptives
Hypertension (≥ 160/100 mmHg)
Age ≥ 35 and smoking ≥ 15 cigarettes daily
Migraine with aura
Antiphospholipid syndrome
History of venous thromboembolism (e.g. DVT, PE)
History of stroke
Early postpartum period (< 3 weeks)
Breast or endometrial cancer
Surgery with subsequent prolonged immobilization
Liver cancer or cirrhosis
Diabetes mellitus with end-organ damage

TABLE 17.2.9 - Absolute Contraindications to Estrogen-Containing Contraceptives

VIII. Intrauterine Devices
- A. Two main types
  - 1. Levonorgestrel intrauterine devices (e.g. Mirena)
  - 2. Copper intrauterine devices (e.g. ParaGard)
- B. Require placement by a clinician
- C. Prevent pregnancy largely by:
  - 1. Eliciting a sterile inflammatory response that kills sperm cells
  - 2. Impairing tubal motility

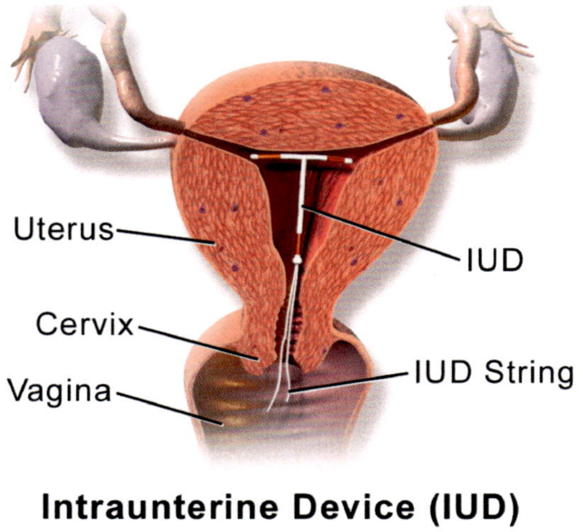

FIGURE 17.2.72 - Intrauterine Device

IX. Intrauterine Devices: Levonorgestrel IUDs
- A. Cause thickening of the cervical mucus and atrophy of the endometrium
- B. Generally, approved for use up to 5 years
- C. Non-contraceptive clinical indications
  - 1. Dysmenorrhea
  - 2. Menorrhagia
  - 3. Postmenopausal women on estrogen therapy

X. Intrauterine Devices: Copper IUDs
- A. Cause impaired sperm motility and capitation
- B. Approved for use up to 10 years
- C. Adverse effects
  - 1. Menorrhagia
  - 2. Dysmenorrhea

XI. Intrauterine Devices: Complications of IUDs
- A. Pelvic pain/cramps
- B. Device expulsion
- C. Perforation
- D. Ectopic pregnancy

Contraindications to Intrauterine Devices (IUDs)	
Pregnancy (known or suspected)	
Infection of the reproductive tract (e.g. pelvic inflammatory disease)	
Unexplained vaginal bleeding	
Abnormal uterine anatomy (e.g. large intrauterine fibroids)	
Gestational trophoblastic disease (e.g. hydatidiform mole)	
Endometrial cancer	
Cervical cancer	
Levonorgestrel IUDs	**Copper IUDs**
Current breast cancer	Wilson disease
Current liver disease	Copper allergy
	Active menorrhagia
	Active dysmenorrhea

TABLE 17.2.10 - Contraindications to Intrauterine Devices

Method of Contraception	Typical Use Failure Rate (%)	Duration of Effect	Key Point(s)
Oral contraceptive pills	7	1 day	- May worsen hypertension - Increase hypercoagulability
Contraceptive patch	7	1 week	- Less effective in women > 90 kg (198 lbs) - Higher risk of blood clots than OCPs
Nuvaring	7	1 month	- May lead to increased vaginal discharge
Depo shot	4	3 months	- Amenorrhea after 1 year - Reversible osteopenia after 2 years - Weight gain
Nexplanon implant	0.1	3 years	- The most effective method of contraception - Causes irregular menstrual spotting
Intrauterine devices	0.1 - 0.8	5 - 10 years	- The most popular form of reversible contraception

TABLE 17.2.11 - Overview of Hormonal Contraception

REVIEW QUESTIONS

1. A 24-year-old woman comes to her primary care physician because her blood pressure was noted to be elevated during a clinical skills class. Her history is unremarkable, and her only medication is a combination oral contraceptive pill. Today, her blood pressure is 140/90 mmHg, and her BMI is 23 kg/m^2. What is the next best step in management?

    - **The next best step in management is discontinuation of her combination oral contraceptive pills and considering an alternative method of contraception.**
    - This 24-year-old woman has noticed that her blood pressure is elevated.
    - Her only medication is a combination oral contraceptive pill.
    - Today, her blood pressure is 140/90 mmHg.
    - Combination oral contraceptive pills are known to increase a woman's risk of developing secondary hypertension if used for a long period of time.

2. What is the most effective form of reversible contraception?

    - **The most effective form of reversible contraception is the Nexplanon implant.**
    - It is also hassle-free because once the implant is in place, it can stay there for up to 3 years.

3. A 23-year-old woman comes to her primary care physician because she wants to discuss birth control options. She says she is getting married soon and does not want to become pregnant for the first several years of her marriage. Her past medical history is notable for heavy periods, for which she takes oral iron pills. The patient says she often forgets to take her iron supplements. She denies tobacco and alcohol use. Vital signs are unremarkable. Physical examination, including a full breast and pelvic exam, is unremarkable. Which of the following options should the clinician recommend for this patient?

    A. Copper IUD
    B. Levonorgestrel IUD
    C. Progesterone-only pill
    D. Female condom
    E. Cervical cap
    F. Tubal ligation

    - **The correct answer is option B.**
    - This is a case of a young woman asking about birth control options to prevent pregnancy for a few years.
    - Notably, she has a history of heavy periods, for which she often forgets to take her iron supplements.
    - This makes levonorgestrel IUD the best option for her because it is highly efficacious in preventing pregnancy, doesn't have the hassle of taking pills every day, and would likely improve her menorrhagia.
    - Option A is not ideal because a copper IUD would worsen her heavy periods.
    - Option C is not correct because progesterone-only pills require an extremely punctual schedule for maximum efficacy. Given that she often forgets to take her iron supplements, progesterone-only pills would not be the best option.
    - Options D and E are incorrect because both the female condom and the cervical cap are less effective than a levonorgestrel IUD in preventing pregnancy. They also tend to involve more hassle than an IUD would.
    - Option F, tubal ligation, is incorrect because this patient is very young and said nothing about her childbearing preferences.

Gynecology | Section 20: Emergency Contraception & Sterilization

I. Emergency Contraception: Indications
   A. Prevention of pregnancy following:
      1. Unprotected sex
      2. Failure of a contraceptive method (e.g. condom tear)
      3. Contraceptive negligence (e.g. missed pill or depo shot)

II. Emergency Contraception: Contraindications
   A. Known or suspected pregnancy

III. Emergency Contraception: Options
   A. Emergency contraceptive pills (morning-after pill)
   B. Emergency copper IUD
   C. Selective progesterone receptor modulators

IV. Emergency Contraception: Emergency Contraceptive Pills
   A. Pills containing high doses of estrogen and progesterone or progesterone alone
      1. Inhibit tubal transport and implantation of a fertilized egg
   B. Must be taken within 72 - 120 hours of unprotected intercourse
   C. No contraindications
   D. Will not harm an existing pregnancy

V. Emergency Contraception: Emergency Copper IUDs
   A. Elicits sterile inflammatory response
      1. Minimizes likelihood of fertilization
   B. The most effective form of emergency contraception
   C. Must be inserted within 120 hours of unprotected intercourse
   D. Will not harm an existing pregnancy
   E. Cannot be used in women with contraindications to IUD placement

VI. Emergency Contraception: Selective Progesterone Receptor Modulators
   A. Delay ovulation and inhibit implantation of a fertilized egg
   B. Ulipristal is the most commonly used agent
   C. Must be taken within 120 hours of unprotected intercourse
   D. Cannot be used in breastfeeding women
   E. Will harm an existing pregnancy
      1. Require a pregnancy test before administration

VII. Sterilization: Vasectomy
   A. Ligation of the vas deferens under local anesthesia
   B. Patients remain fertile for 6 - 8 weeks following the procedure
      1. Viable sperm remains distal to the ligation site
      2. Patients should use another form of contraception (e.g. condoms)
      3. Semen analysis can confirm azoospermia
   C. The procedure is considered permanent
      1. Reversal is possible, but unreliable

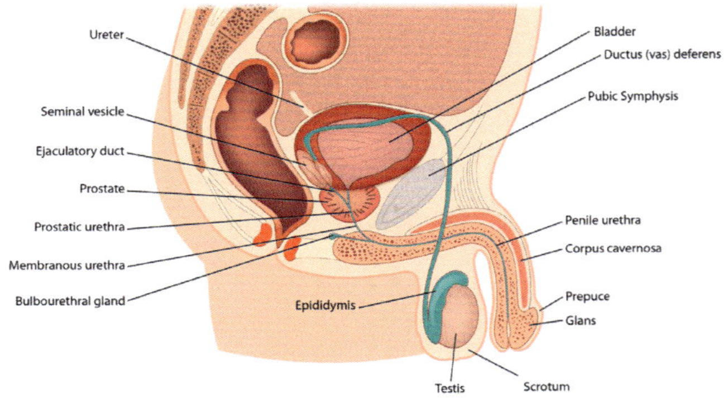

FIGURE 17.2.73 - Anatomy of Male Genital Tract

Emergency Contraception	Mechanism of Pregnancy Prevention	Time Frame Following Unprotected Intercourse	Will it Harm an Existent Pregnancy?
Emergency contraceptive pills	High doses of hormones interfere with tubal transport and implantation	72 - 120 hours	No
Emergency copper IUD	Elicits sterile inflammatory response which reduces likelihood of fertilization	120 hours	No
Selective progesterone receptor modulator (Ulipristal)	Inhibits fertilization and implantation	120 hours	Yes

TABLE 17.2.12 - Emergency Contraception

1. Sterilization: Tubal Ligation
    a. Ligation of the fallopian tubes
    b. Can be performed immediately postpartum
    c. Clinicians must counsel women about the risk of regret
        i. Regret is more likely in women younger than 30 years of age
    d. The procedure is considered permanent
        i. Reversal is possible, but unreliable

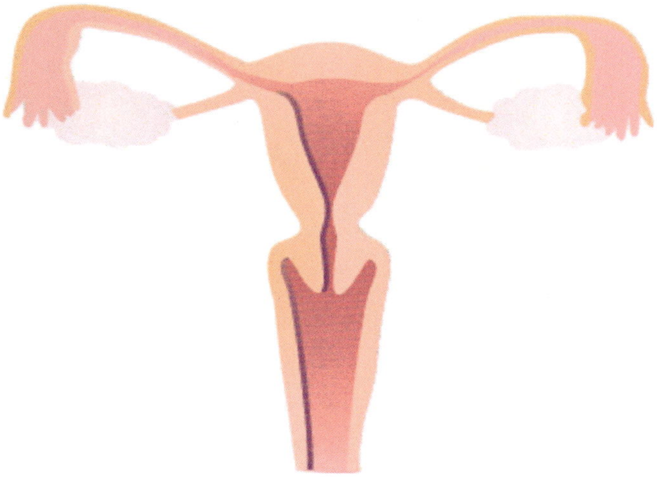

FIGURE 17.2.74 - Female Genital Tract

REVIEW QUESTIONS ?

1. What are the contraindications to placement of copper IUDs?
    - **Contraindications to placement of copper IUDs include Wilson disease, copper allergy, menorrhagia, and dysmenorrhea.**
    - Wilson disease is a genetic disorder characterized by excessive copper retention in the body, which means that copper-based IUDs could make symptoms a lot worse.
    - A copper allergy and a copper-based IUD are clearly not a good mix.
    - Menorrhagia and dysmenorrhea would get substantially worse after placement of a copper-based IUD.
2. What is the most effective form of emergency contraception?
    - **The most effective form of emergency contraception is the ParaGard copper IUD.**

REVIEW QUESTIONS ?

3. A 35-year-old man comes to the physician to discuss different forms of contraception. He has 5 sons, and he no longer wishes to father a child. The physician outlines different types of reversible and irreversible contraception and the patient decides to undergo vasectomy. He understands that the results of this procedure are permanent. After the procedure, which of the following is the best recommendation for this patient?

    A. Use condoms for at least 6 to 8 weeks after the procedure
    B. Resume unprotected sex immediately after the procedure
    C. Regular screening for chlamydia for the next 6 to 8 weeks
    D. Regular screening for syphilis for the next 6 to 8 weeks

    - **The correct answer is option A.**
    - This patient decides to undergo vasectomy.
    - Vasectomy is a permanent form of male contraception achieved by ligation of vas deferens.
    - Viable sperm still remain in the segment of the vas deferens distal to the point of the ligation 6 to 8 weeks after the procedure. This means that unprotected sexual intercourse during this time period can still result in pregnancy. Therefore, the patient should be advised to use condoms for at least 6 to 8 weeks after the procedure.
    - Option B is incorrect because if the patient resumes unprotected sex immediately after the procedure, this may result in unintended pregnancy.
    - Options C and D are incorrect because, as a general rule, patients do not have to undergo regular screening for chlamydia or syphilis after vasectomy unless there are specific indications for screening, and this patient doesn't have risk factors for either of these conditions.

Gynecology | Section 21: Pregnancy Termination

I. Background Information
  A. In the US, elective pregnancy termination laws vary state by state
  B. Common reasons for seeking elective termination of pregnancy
    1. Financial hardships
    2. Disruption of work or education
    3. Concerns over single parenting

II. Preparing for Pregnancy Termination
  A. Determine gestational age
    1. Last menstrual period
    2. Ultrasound (e.g. crown-rump length)
  B. Offer screening for sexually transmitted illnesses (e.g. chlamydia)
  C. Give RhoGAM shots to all Rh-negative women
  D. Offer counseling

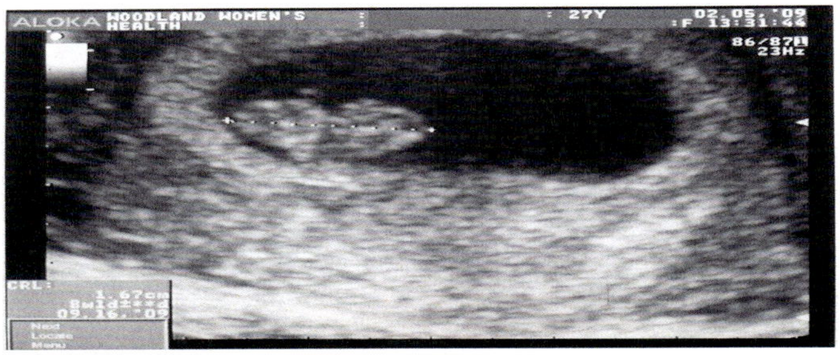

FIGURE 17.2.75 - Ultrasound of Fetus: Crown-to-Rump Length

III. Methods of Pregnancy Termination
  A. First trimester (up to 12 weeks gestation)
    1. Dilation and curettage
    2. Manual vacuum aspiration
    3. Medication abortion
  B. Second trimester (12-24 weeks gestation)
    1. Dilation and evacuation
    2. Induction of labor

IV. Methods of Pregnancy Termination: Dilation and Curettage (Suction Curettage)
  A. May be performed between 6 to 14 weeks of gestation
  B. The safest method of terminating a first trimester pregnancy
  C. Procedure
    1. Antibiotic prophylaxis (e.g. ceftriaxone, doxycycline)
    2. Dilation of the cervix
    3. Extraction of products of conception
    4. Sharp curettage
  D. Complications
    1. Infection
    2. Bleeding
    3. Perforation
    4. Asherman syndrome

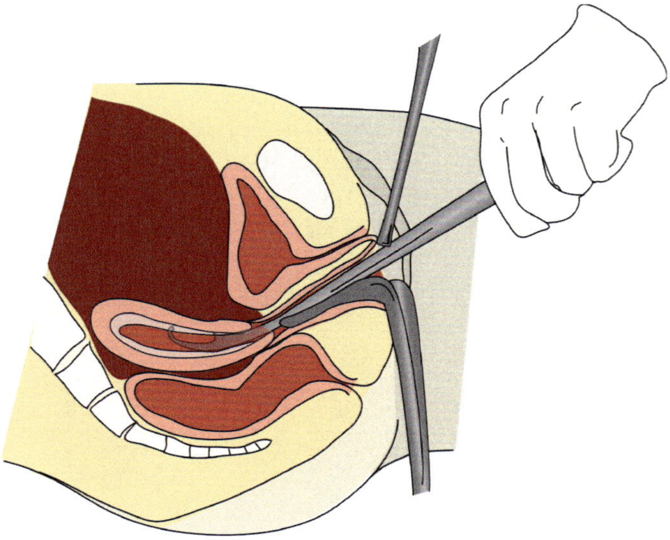

FIGURE 17.2.76 - Dilation and Curettage

V. Methods of Pregnancy Termination: Manual Vacuum Aspiration
  A. May be performed up to 12 weeks of gestation
  B. Procedure
    1. Placement of a cannula into the cervical os
    2. Extraction of uterine contents using a vacurette
    3. No curettage

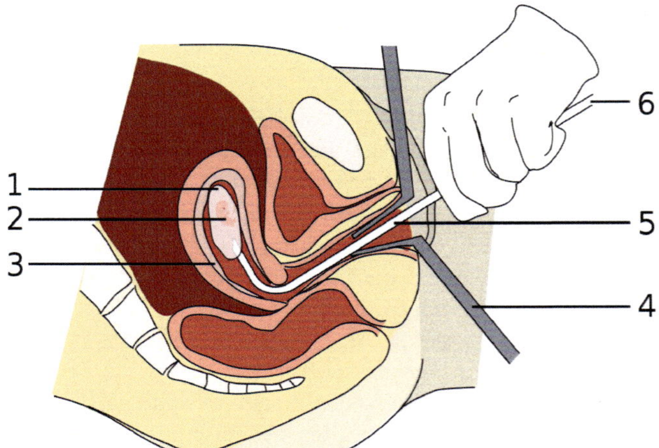

FIGURE 17.2.77 - Manual Vacuum Aspiration

VI. Methods of Pregnancy Termination: Medication Abortion
   A. Nonsurgical method of pregnancy termination
      1. Success rate is highest if performed before week 7 of gestation
   B. Options
      1. Mifepristone + misoprostol (gold standard)
      2. Methotrexate + misoprostol
         a) Misoprostol alone
   C. Patient experience is similar to a miscarriage
   D. Mifepristone is a progesterone receptor antagonist
      1. Causes detachment of the embryo from the uterine wall
   E. Methotrexate is a dihydrofolate reductase inhibitor
      1. Disrupts DNA synthesis
      2. Inhibits proliferation of placental villi
   F. Misoprostol is a prostaglandin analog
      1. Ripens the cervix and induces uterine contractions

Contraindications to Medication Abortion
Ectopic pregnancy
Allergy to abortifacients (e.g. mifepristone)
Bleeding disorder (e.g. hemophilia)
Cervical stenosis or obstruction
Gestational trophoblastic disease (e.g. hydatidiform mole)
In-place intrauterine device
Mifepristone specifically: chronic steroid use (e.g. patients with Crohn's disease), chronic adrenal failure (e.g. Addison's disease)

TABLE 17.2.13 - Contraindications to Medication Abortion

VII. Methods of Pregnancy Termination: Dilation and Evacuation
   A. May be performed between 14 to 24 weeks of gestation
   B. The safest method of terminating a second trimester pregnancy
   C. Procedure
      1. Antibiotic prophylaxis
      2. Dilation of the cervix
      3. Evacuation of products of conception (e.g. suction, forceps)
      4. Pelvic ultrasound to rule out retained products of conception
   D. Complications
      1. Infection
      2. Bleeding
      3. Perforation
      4. Asherman syndrome
      5. Retained products of conception
   E. Procedure does not allow for delivery of an intact fetus

VIII. Methods of Pregnancy Termination: Induction of Labor
   A. Induction of labor during second trimester using one of these options:
      1. Mifepristone + misoprostol (first-line)
      2. Misoprostol alone
      3. Intravenous oxytocin
   B. Procedure allows for delivery of an intact fetus
   C. Feticidal agents (e.g. digoxin) can be used to prevent a live birth
   D. Complications
      1. Infection
      2. Bleeding
      3. Retained products of conception

IX. Follow-Up Care
   A. Confirm completion of abortion
      1. Serum or urine β-hCG
      2. Pelvic ultrasound
   B. Offer emotional support and counseling
   C. Discuss contraceptive options

Abortion Method	Description	Take-Home Point(s)
Dilation and curettage	- Surgical extraction of products of conception	- The safest method of terminating a first trimester pregnancy
Manual vacuum aspiration	- Manual extraction of uterine contents using a vacuum syringe	- Does not involve sharp curettage
Medication abortion	- In essence, an iatrogenic miscarriage using mifepristone + misoprostol, methotrexate + misoprostol, or misoprostol alone	- Success rate is highest before 7 weeks of gestation
Dilation and evacuation	- Surgical extraction of products of conception	- The safest method of terminating a second trimester pregnancy - Impossible to deliver an intact fetus
Induction of labor	- Induction of labor in the second trimester using mifepristone + misoprostol, misoprostol alone, or IV oxytocin	- Possible to deliver an intact fetus - Live birth can be prevented with feticide agents

TABLE 17.2.14 - Methods of Pregnancy Termination

REVIEW QUESTIONS

1. What medication can be used to treat/terminate an early ectopic pregnancy?
   - **The medication that can be used to treat/terminate an early ectopic pregnancy is methotrexate.**
   - Unlike mifepristone and misoprostol, methotrexate can be used for both medical abortion and for treatment of ectopic pregnancies because it functions by disrupting fetal growth, eventually leading to fetal demise.
   - Mifepristone and misoprostol, on the other hand, work by affecting the environment of the fetus, specifically the uterus and the uterine cavity, instead of affecting the fetus itself.
   - Since an ectopic pregnancy is a pregnancy outside of the uterine cavity, mifepristone and misoprostol are unlikely to affect it.

2. A 29-year-old G1P0 woman comes to her primary care physician at 20 weeks gestation to discuss termination of pregnancy. Her history is notable for Addison's disease. She denies tobacco and alcohol use. Vitals include blood pressure of 121/76 mmHg, pulse of 72 beats/minute, and temperature of 97.7° F (36.5° C). Physical examination is notable for a smooth, firm uterus with a fundal height of 21 cm. Laboratory evaluation is unremarkable, and a pelvic ultrasound is consistent with a singleton intrauterine pregnancy. The patient does not express any preferences regarding the approach to termination of pregnancy. Which of the following methods of pregnancy termination should the clinician offer to this patient?

   A. Mifepristone and misoprostol
   B. Manual vacuum aspiration
   C. Dilation and evacuation
   D. Methotrexate

   - **The correct answer is option C.**
   - This is a case of a woman presenting to discuss options for termination of pregnancy.
   - She is at 20 weeks gestation, which is in her second trimester.
   - She has a history of Addison's disease.
   - Physical examination and pelvic ultrasound are both consistent with a singleton intrauterine pregnancy.
   - She does not express any preferences regarding the approach to termination of pregnancy.
   - Given all of these factors, dilation, and evacuation is the best possible option for this patient as it is considered to be the safest method of terminating a second-trimester pregnancy.
   - Option A, mifepristone and misoprostol, is incorrect because patients with Addison's disease should not be receiving mifepristone, which is a glucocorticoid receptor antagonist.
   - Option B, manual vacuum aspiration, is incorrect because it is an appropriate method of terminating a first-trimester pregnancy but not a second-trimester pregnancy.
   - Option D, methotrexate, is incorrect because methotrexate is used in the treatment of ectopic pregnancies, not intrauterine pregnancies. Since the pelvic ultrasound confirmed a singleton intrauterine pregnancy, methotrexate would not be an appropriate choice.

Gynecology | Section 22: Asherman Syndrome

I. Asherman Syndrome: Definition
   A. Formation of intrauterine synechiae (adhesions) as a result of damage to the endometrial lining of the uterus

II. Asherman Syndrome: Risk Factors
   A. Intrauterine procedures (e.g. dilation and curettage)
   B. Intrauterine inflammation (e.g. pelvic inflammatory disease)

III. Asherman Syndrome: Clinical Features
   A. Infertility or recurrent pregnancy loss
   B. Dysmenorrhea and/or cyclic pelvic pain
   C. Amenorrhea
   D. Abnormal vaginal bleeding

IV. Asherman Syndrome: Diagnosis
   A. Hysteroscopy

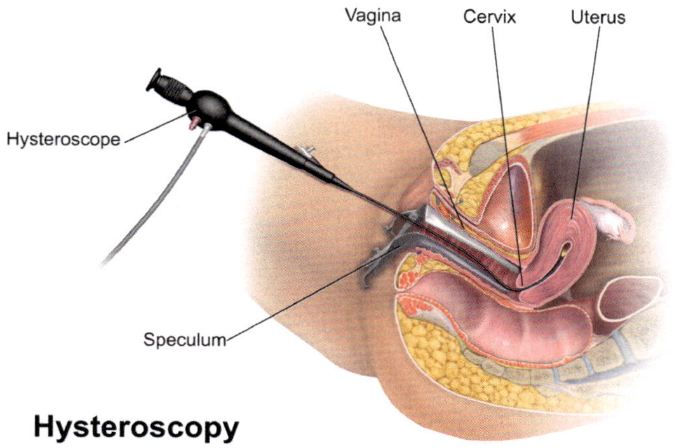

FIGURE 17.2.78 - Hysteroscopy

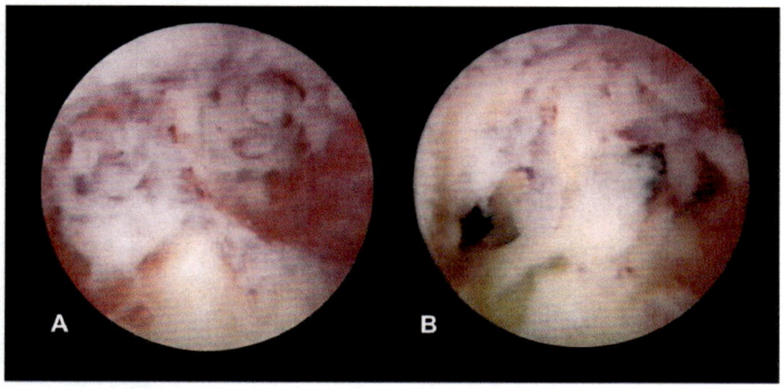

FIGURE 17.2.79 - Hysteroscopy: Intrauterine Adhesions in Asherman Syndrome

V. Asherman Syndrome: Management
   A. Lysis of adhesions

REVIEW QUESTIONS

1. How will patients with Asherman syndrome respond to a progesterone challenge test?
   - **Patients with Asherman syndrome will have no vaginal bleeding in response to the progesterone challenge test.**
   - In a progesterone challenge test, a dose of progesterone and monitored for subsequent vaginal bleeding.
   - Healthy patients will report vaginal bleeding within about 2 weeks of the progesterone challenge test. This is because, in the setting of normal estrogen levels and healthy endometrial lining, the endometrial lining will grow in response to the exogenous progesterone and then involute and slough off as soon as the progesterone runs out.
   - Patients with Asherman syndrome, however, will not have any vaginal bleeding in response to progesterone due to intrauterine adhesions and significant damage to the endometrial lining.

Gynecology | Section 23: Infertility and Assisted Reproductive Technologies

I. Infertility: General Information
   A. Failure to conceive despite having unprotected sexual intercourse for one year in females < 35 years and 6 months in females > 35 years
      1. Primary: infertility in nulliparous women
      2. Secondary: infertility in women who have conceived before
   B. Fecundability
      1. Probability of achieving pregnancy in single menstrual cycle
      2. Evaluates fertility potential
      3. 80% - 90% of couples conceive within one year
   C. Fecundity
      1. Probability of giving live birth in one menstrual cycle
      2. Lower than fecundability
   D. Infertility: Etiology
   E. Systemic diseases (e.g. diabetes mellitus, hypertension, obesity, chronic diseases)
   F. Endocrine disorders (e.g. thyroid disorders); hepatic and renal disease
   G. Infections (e.g. chlamydia, gonorrhea)
   H. Smoking, alcohol, drugs (e.g. antineoplastic agents)

II. Female Factor Infertility
   A. Advanced maternal age: ↓ decreased ovarian reserve in the 40s
   B. Ovarian causes (e.g. ovarian insufficiency, PCOS)
   C. Tubal causes (e.g. PID, endometriosis)
   D. Uterine causes (anatomical anomalies, Asherman's syndrome)
   E. Cervical causes (e.g. antisperm antibodies, ↓ mucus production)
   F. Endocrine causes (e.g. hyperprolactinemia, hypothalamic amenorrhea)
   G. Other causes: sexual dysfunction (e.g. genito-pelvic pain disorder)

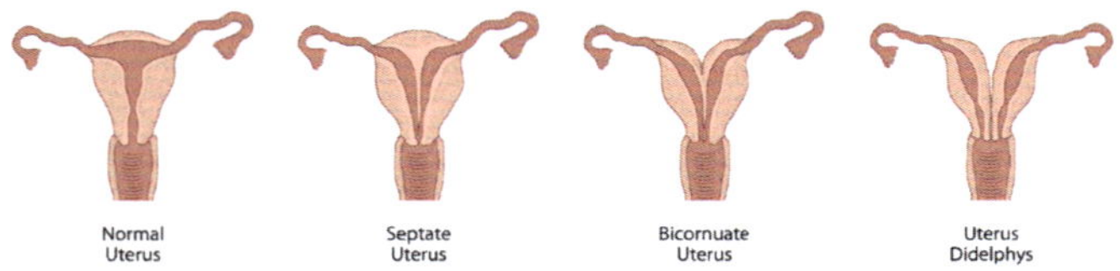

FIGURE 17.2.80 - Types of Anatomical Anomalies of the Uterus

III. Male Factor Infertility
   A. Sperm disorders: ↓ count, ↓ motility; anabolic steroid use
   B. Testicular: injury, infection (e.g. mumps)
   C. Scrotal: varicocele
   D. Psychiatric disorders: ↓ libido
   E. Medications (e.g. corticosteroids)
   F. Other: pituitary, thyroid, liver disease, Kallmann syndrome

IV. Unexplained Infertility
   A. When evaluation reveals no cause
   B. May be due to sperm transport abnormalities or antisperm antibodies

V. Infertility Work Up
   A. Start investigating after timed, unprotected sexual intercourse in:
      1. Women < 35 after 1 year
      2. Women > 35 after 6 months
   B. Initial screening in a couple: semen analysis
      1. Assess motility, concentration, morphology
      2. Identifies azoospermia, oligospermia, motility issues

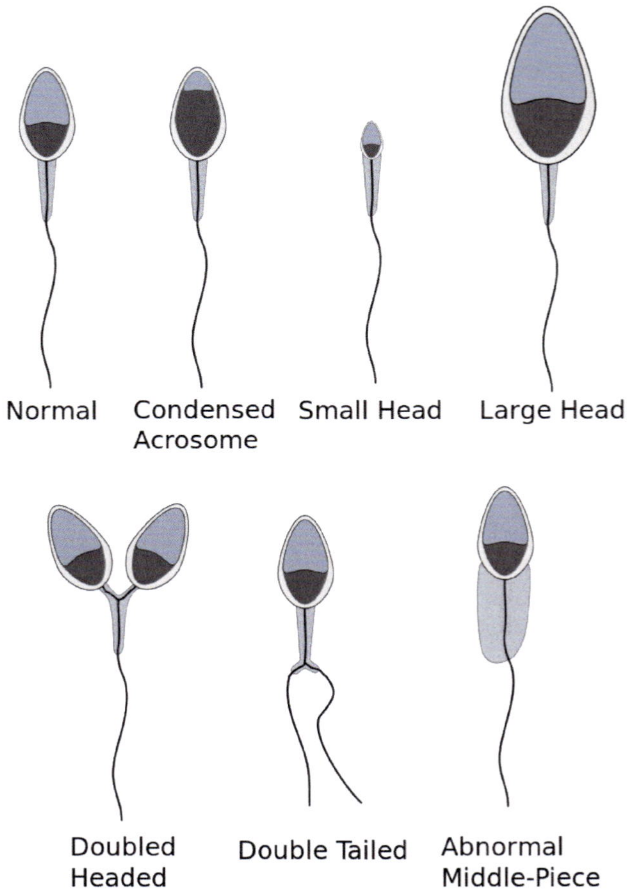

FIGURE 17.2.81 - Abnormal Morphologies of the Sperm

Condition		Diagnostics	Management
Female factors	Ovarian causes	- Basal body temperature - Hormone tests (e.g. mid-luteal progesterone, FSH)	- Ovulation induction - Intrauterine insemination - IVF
	Tubal causes	- Hysterosalpingography	- Treat underlying cause (e.g. resection/ ablation of endometriomas/fibroids) - IVF
	Uterine causes	- Ultrasound - Hysterosalpingogram - Sonohysterogram	- Treat underlying cause (e.g. surgical correction of structural abnormalities)
	Cervical causes	- Physical exam - Pap smear - Test for antisperm antibodies	- Intrauterine insemination with washed sperm - IVF
	Endocrine causes	- Hormone tests (e.g. prolactin, TSH, androgen levels)	- Treat underlying cause (e.g. levothyroxine, dopamine)
Male factors		- Semen analysis	- Intrauterine insemination - IVF - Donor insemination
Infertility due to aging		- Early follicular phase FSH - Clomiphene challenge test - Measure inhibin B levels	- Ovarian induction - Intrauterine insemination - IVF

TABLE 17.2.15 - Infertility Factors

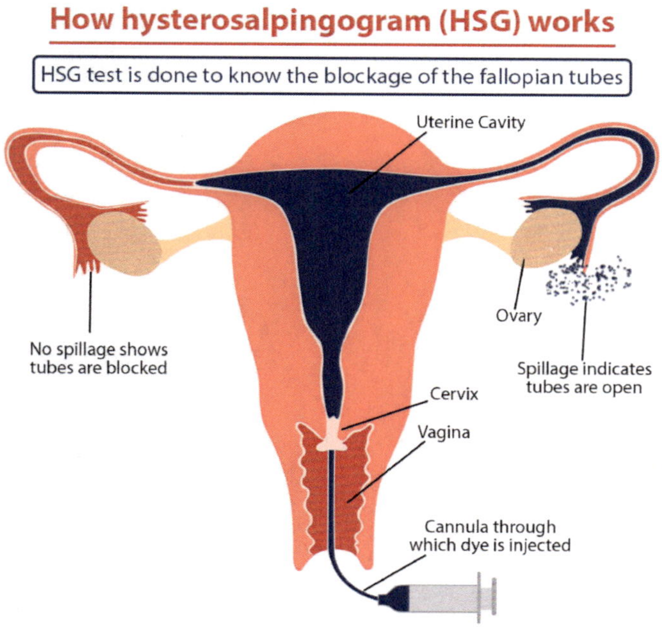

FIGURE 17.2.82 - Hysterosalpingogram

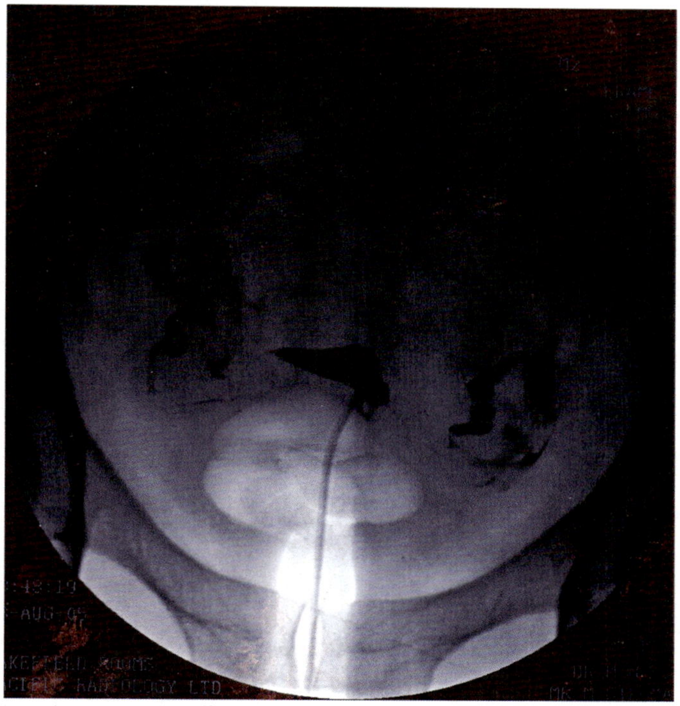

FIGURE 17.2.83 - Hysterosalpingography: Normal Findings

VI. Assisted Reproductive Techniques
    A. Ovulation induction
        1. Clomiphene citrate
        2. Tamoxifen
        3. Pulsatile GnRH
        4. Gonadotropins
        5. Side effects: multiple gestation pregnancy, ovarian hyperstimulation syndrome
    B. Advanced reproductive techniques
        1. IVF
        2. Intracytoplasmic sperm injection
    C. Intrauterine insemination

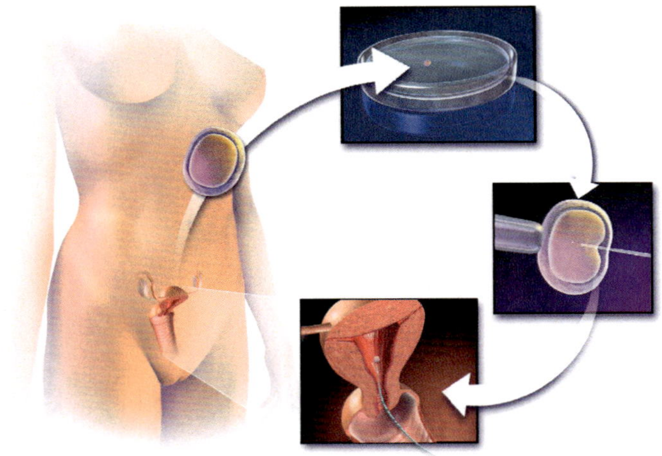

FIGURE 17.2.84 - In-Vitro Fertilization and Intracytoplasmic Sperm Injection

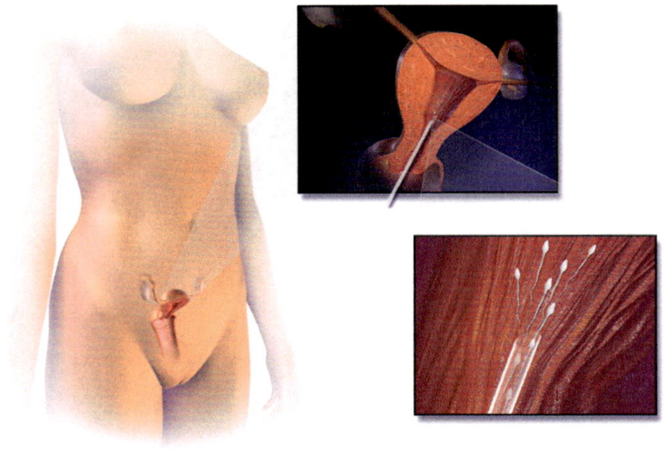

FIGURE 17.2.85 - Intrauterine Insemination

REVIEW QUESTIONS

?

1. A 45-year-old woman comes to an OBGYN because of inability to conceive for the past year. She does not currently take oral contraceptive pills, and she had her intrauterine device removed 2 years ago. Despite having regular unprotected sexual intercourse, she has been unsuccessful in conceiving. What is the most likely cause of this patient's chief complaint?
    - **The most likely cause of this patient's chief complaint is decreased ovarian reserve.**
    - This 45-year-old woman presents with an inability to conceive for the past year.
    - She has regular unprotected sexual intercourse, is not on any forms of birth control, and her UTD was removed over a year ago.
    - The most likely cause of this patient's inability to conceive is decreased ovarian reserve secondary to her age.
    - All women have a finite number of ovarian follicles, which decreases after every menstrual cycle.
    - Women in their 40s have a significantly lower number of follicles as they have had more menstrual cycles.

2. A 30-year-old woman comes to her primary care physician with her husband because of failure to conceive for the past 8 months. She has a regular 29-day menstrual cycle with moderate flow. She has no notable past medical history. Despite timed regular unprotected sexual intercourse, the couple is still unable to conceive. What is the next best step in the diagnosis of this couple's chief complaint?
    - **The next best step in the diagnosis of this couple's chief complaint is semen analysis.**
    - This 30-year-old woman with no pmhx reports failure to conceive for the past 8 months despite regular unprotected intercourse.
    - She has regular 29-day menstrual cycles with moderate flow, making menstrual disorders less likely causes of her infertility.
    - After a detailed menstrual, medical, surgical, and sexual history is obtained, the best next step is semen analysis, which can assess the motility, concentration, and morphology of sperm.

3. A 32-year-old woman comes to her primary care physician with her husband because of her inability to conceive for the past 2 years. She has a regular 28-day menstrual cycle with minimal flow. She has no history of sexually transmitted diseases or previous surgeries. Vital signs include a temperature of 98.6° F (37° C), blood pressure of 110/75 mmHg, heart rate of 84 beats/min, and respiratory rate of 15 breaths/min. Physical examination is unremarkable. A semen analysis of her partner was performed and was unremarkable. After a thorough discussion about assisted reproductive techniques, she agrees to undergo ovulation induction with clomiphene citrate. Which of the following complications should this patient be warned about?

    A. Gestational thrombocytopenia
    B. Eclampsia
    C. Placenta accreta
    D. Multiple gestation pregnancy

    - **The correct answer is option D.**
    - This 32-year-old woman reports inability to conceive for the past 2 years.
    - Semen analysis of her partner is normal.
    - She agrees to undergo ovulation induction with clomiphene citrate.
    - Clomiphene blocks estrogen receptors in the preoptic hypothalamic nucleus, causing a surge of GnRH. GnRH surge, in turn, will cause the surge of FSH and LH, leading to ovulation.
    - The most likely complication of ovulation induction is multiple gestational pregnancy. This is because multiple follicles may simultaneously undergo ovulation and release eggs.
    - Options A, B, and C are incorrect because ovulation induction has not been associated with gestational thrombocytopenia, eclampsia, and placenta accreta.

Gynecology | Section 24: Benign Dermatologic Conditions

I. Lichen Simplex Chronicus: General Characteristics
   A. Skin disorder secondary to chronic irritation
   B. Leads to lichenification and hyperplasia of the vulvar epithelium
   C. Scratch-itch cycle: initial irritant → scratching of the area → thickened skin → more itching → cycle repeats
   D. No increased risk of squamous cell carcinoma

II. Lichen Simplex Chronicus: Clinical Features
   A. Potential skin findings
      1. Excoriations and epidermal thickening
      2. May see accentuated skin markings
      3. Erythematous with hyperpigmented plaques

III. Lichen Simplex Chronicus: Diagnosis
   A. History and physical exam
   B. Typically a biopsy is not required unless lesion persists for > 3 months

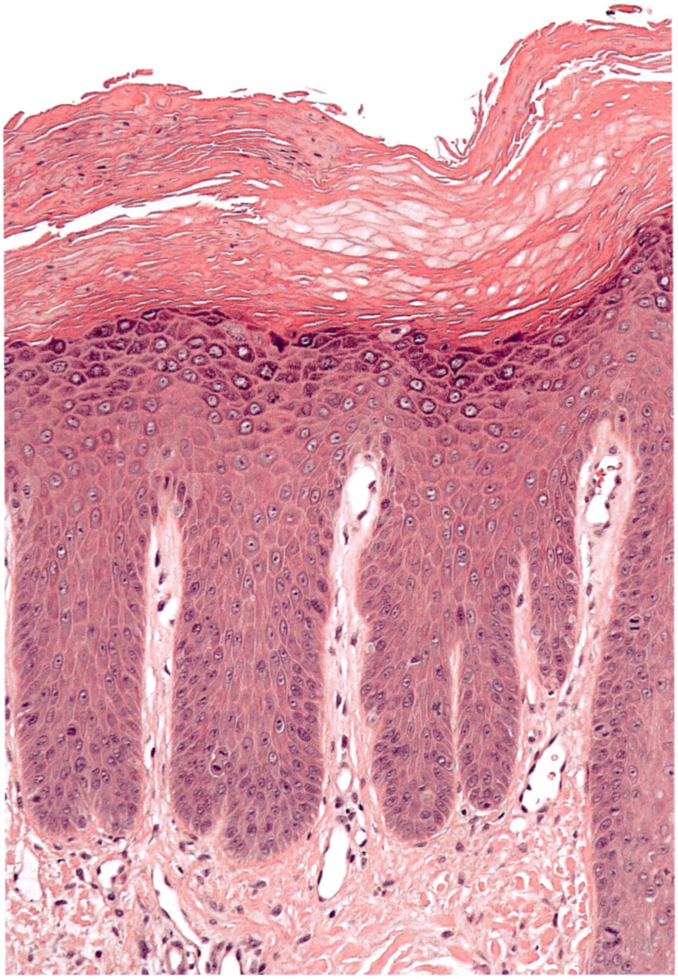

FIGURE 17.2.86 - Light Microscopy: Histopathological Findings of Lichen Simplex Chronicus

IV. Lichen Simplex Chronicus: Treatment
   A. Remove irritants
   B. Oral antihistamines
   C. Topical steroids
   D. Vulvar and vaginal hygiene
      1. Loose fitting clothing and underwear, cotton
      2. Avoid scented soaps, bubble baths, feminine sprays, douching

V. Lichen Sclerosus: General Characteristics
   A. Inflammatory dermatosis with unclear etiology
   B. Some familial association
   C. Can occur at any age, but most common in postmenopausal women
   D. Mild increase in risk for squamous cell carcinoma

VI. Lichen Sclerosus: Clinical Features
   A. Well demarcated thin skin
   B. Can involve vulva, labia majora or minora, clitoral and preclitoral skin, and perineum
      1. Sometimes described as a "figure of 8" pattern
   C. Pruritus, dyspareunia, bleeding with minimal trauma, painful defecation
   D. Atrophy can lead to labial fusion, contracture of the introitus, skin fragility

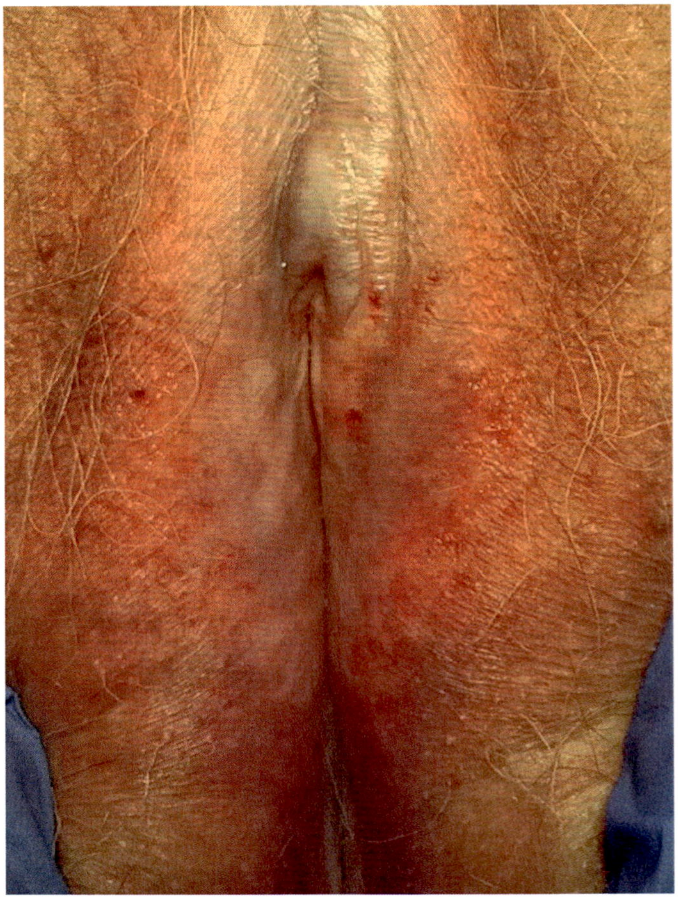

FIGURE 17.2.87 - Lichen Sclerosus

VII. Lichen Sclerosus: Diagnosis
   A. History and physical exam
   B. Punch biopsy to rule out carcinoma
   C. Histology: chronic inflammatory cells, thinning of the epithelium, sclerosis of the dermis, loss of rete pegs

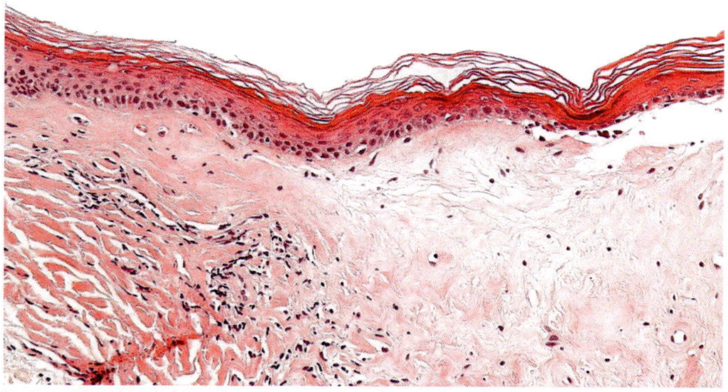

FIGURE 17.2.88 - Light Microscopy: Histopathological Findings of Lichen Sclerosus

VIII. Lichen Sclerosus: Treatment
   A. First line: high dose topical corticosteroids, followed by maintenance steroids
   B. Often persists after therapy
   C. Other potential treatments
      1. Topical tretinoin
      2. Pimecrolimus

IX. Lichen Planus: General Characteristics
   A. Often associated with autoimmune diseases and HCV
   B. Usually occurs at > 50 years of age
   C. Can be associated with drugs that cause lichenoid reactions
   D. Slightly increased risk of vulvar skin cancer

X. Lichen Planus: Clinical Features
   A. Shiny purple papules with white striae on the vulva
   B. Desquamative ulcers may be present
   C. Pruritus, burning, dyspareunia, vaginal discharge
   D. Can lead to vaginal adhesions and erosive vaginitis
   E. Associated with lichen planus in other locations
   F. "P's" of lichen planus: pruritic, polygonal, plantar, purple papules and plaques

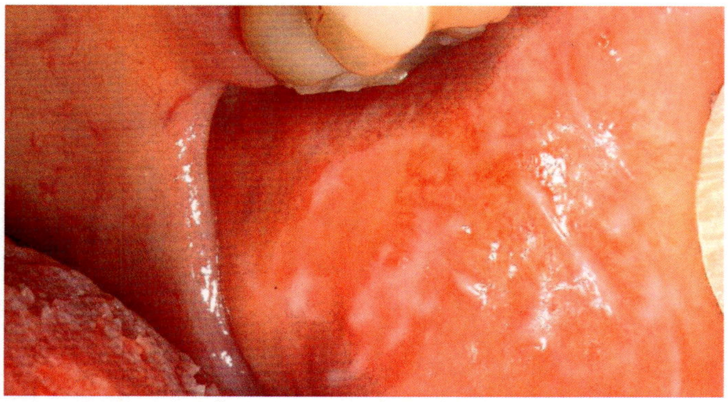

FIGURE 17.2.89 - Wickham Striae in Lichen Planus

XI. Lichen Planus: Diagnosis
   A. History and physical exam
   B. Histology: hyperkeratosis with basal layer destruction, lymphocytic infiltrate at the dermal-epidermal junction

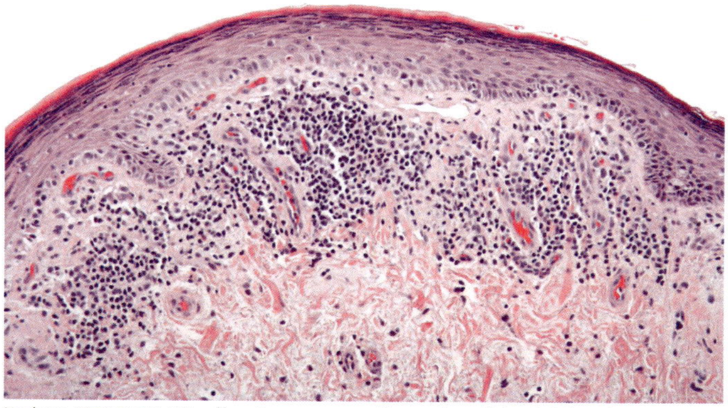

FIGURE 17.2.90 - Light Microscopy: Histopathological Findings of Lichen Planus

XII. Lichen Planus: Treatment
   A. Topical steroids and vaginal steroid suppositories
   B. Discontinue any medications associated with a lichenoid drug reaction

Condition	Etiology	Key Features
Lichen simplex chronicus	- Secondary to chronic irritation	- Hyperplasia and lichenification - May see excoriations - Remove irritants, oral antihistamines, topical steroids
Lichen sclerosus	- Inflammatory dermatosis with unclear etiology	- Well demarcated thin skin - "Figure of eight" pattern - Can be chronic - High dose topical steroids initially, then maintenance steroids
Lichen planus	- Associated with autoimmune diseases and HCV	- May be secondary to lichenoid drug eruption - Lichen planus on other parts of body - Topical steroids and cessation of any drugs that are associated with lichenoid eruptions

TABLE 17.2.16 - Overview of Benign Dermatologic Conditions

REVIEW QUESTIONS

1. A 25-year-old woman comes to her primary care physician because of vulvar irritation and itching. She is a dancer and frequently has to wear thick, tight polyester costumes. She enjoys taking bubble baths with scented soap at the end of the day. Physical examinations shows a thickened and lichenified vulva with multiple scratch marks. Topical application of which medication is most likely to resolve this patient's condition?

   - **Topical application of corticosteroids is most likely to resolve this patient's condition.**
   - This 25-year-old patient has vulvar irritation, itching, thickening, and lichenification.
   - Given her history of wearing thick, tight costumes and taking bubble baths with scented soap, this presentation is most consistent with the diagnosis of lichen simplex chronicus.
   - Topical application of corticosteroids has shown to be beneficial for patients with lichen simplex chronicus.

2. A 74-year-old woman comes to her primary care physician because of vulvar itching. She also reports pain during defecation for the last 6 months. Her last menstrual period was 20 years ago. Physical examination shows thin white skin around the vaginal introitus and the anus. Biopsy of the lesion reveals dermal fibrosis and epidermal atrophy with loss of epidermal ridges. How does this patient's condition differ from lichen simplex chronicus?

   - **This patient's condition differs from lichen simplex chronicus in the following ways: lichen sclerosus affects mainly postmenopausal and prepubertal women; it is associated with thin skin, epidermal atrophy, dermal fibrosis, and increased risk for vulvar SCC.**
   - This 74-year-old patient has vulvar itching, dyschezia, and thin white skin around vaginal introitus and the anus.
   - This presentation is consistent with the diagnosis of lichen sclerosus.
   - Lichen sclerosus is the disease of postmenopausal and prepubertal women while lichen simplex chronicus can occur at any age.
   - Secondly, lichen sclerosus is characterized by thin white skin, epidermal atrophy, and dermal fibrosis while lichen simplex chronicus is characterized by thick skin with epidermal hyperplasia.
   - Additionally, lichen sclerosus increases the risk for vulvar squamous cell carcinoma while lichen simplex chronicus does not.

3. A 57-year-old woman comes to her primary care physician because of severe vaginal itching. She has noticed purple lesions on her vulva for the last 10 months that have progressively worsened. She has a history of HFrEF and knee osteoarthritis. The patient takes metoprolol and occasional acetaminophen for her medical conditions. Physical examination shows purple papules and plaques on the vulva and white reticular lesions on her buccal mucosa. She is hepatitis C negative. Which medication is most likely associated with this patient's current condition?

   - **The medication most likely associated with this patient's current condition is metoprolol.**
   - This patient has pruritic purple papules, plaques on her vulva, and white reticular lesions on her buccal mucosa, consistent with lichen planus.
   - This patient is hepatitis C negative, making infection-induced lichen planus unlikely.
   - Lichen planus can be associated with medications such as beta-blockers and thiazide diuretics.
   - This patient takes metoprolol for her HFrEF. Therefore, metoprolol, a beta-blocker, is this patient's most likely cause of lichen planus.

Gynecology | Section 25: Vulvar Neoplasia

I. Vulvar Intraepithelial Neoplasia
   A. Cellular atypia confined to the epithelium
   B. Risk factors: smoking, immunocompromise
   C. Associated with HPV:
      1. Vulvar LSIL: condylomatous lesions, cytologic atypia
      2. Vulvar HSIL: histologic evidence of dysplasia, loss of maturation
   D. Differentiated VIN: precursor lesion to squamous cell carcinoma

II. Associated with lichen sclerosus and other dermatoses
   A. Clinical presentation
      1. Typically asymptomatic; may present with vulvar itching
      2. Lesions vary in location and appearance
   B. Diagnosis
      1. Lesions that become white or more vascular with acetic acid are suspicious
      2. Biopsy
   C. Treatment
      1. Excision of all high grade lesions
      2. Surgical excision or laser therapy
      3. May consider topical 5-fluorouracil or imiquimod

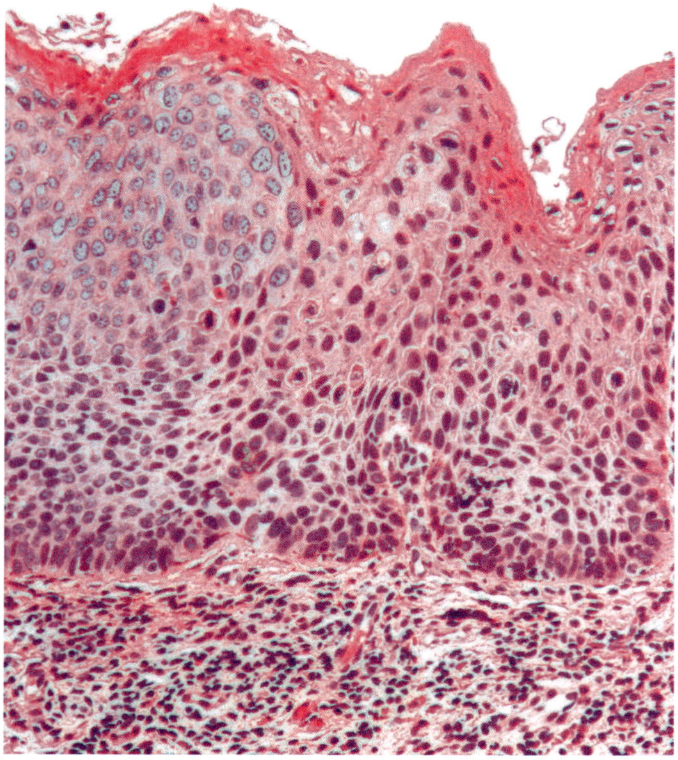

FIGURE 17.2.91 - Light Microscopy: Histopathological Findings of Vulvar High-Grade Squamous Intraepithelial Lesions

III. Vulvar Cancer
   A. Typically squamous cell carcinoma
   B. Usually in postmenopausal women
   C. Risk factors: smoking, HPV 16 and 18, multiple sexual partners
   D. Clinical presentation
      1. Vulvar itching, white lesion, red lesion, ulcer
      2. Lymphatic metastasis
   E. Diagnosis: biopsy
   F. Treatment
      1. Surgical excision ranging from removal of focal lesions to radical vulvectomy
      2. May also include radiation and chemotherapy depending on stage

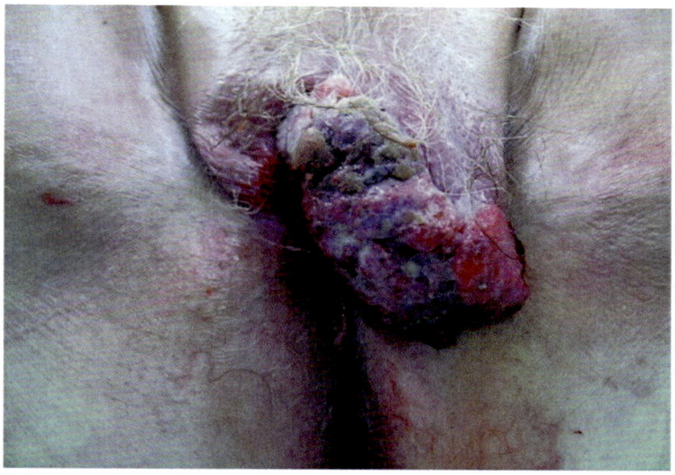

FIGURE 17.2.92 - Ulcerating Lesion of Vulvar Squamous Cell Carcinoma

IV. Vulvar Melanoma
   A. Presents as a pigmented, pruritic lesion
   B. Most often in Caucasian postmenopausal patients
   C. Diagnosis and treatment:
      1. Wide, local excision (like all melanomas)

V. Paget Disease of the Vulva
   A. Also known as extramammary Paget disease
   B. Uncommon apocrine gland neoplasia
   C. Rarely associated with underlying invasive adenocarcinoma
   D. Similar histology to Paget disease of the breast
   E. Bright red lesion with areas of white hyperkeratosis

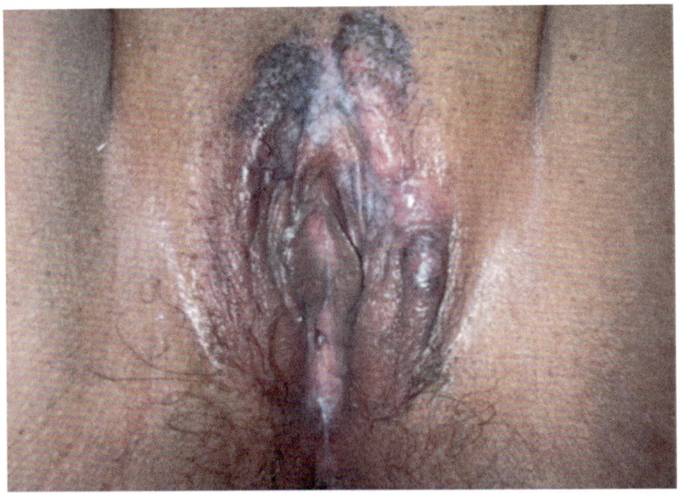

FIGURE 17.2.93 - Lesions of Paget Disease of the Vulva

VI. Bartholin Gland Carcinoma
   A. Rare cancer arising from the Bartholin gland
   B. Can represent a variety of cancers, including squamous cell, adenocarcinoma, and others
   C. Typically presents as a painless vulvar mass
   D. Treatment: radical vulvectomy and lymphadenectomy

Condition	Etiology	Key Features
Vulvar intraepithelial neoplasia	- Cellular atypia of the epithelium	- Associated with HPV - Can progress to squamous cell carcinoma - Excise the lesions or treat with laser therapy
Vulvar cancer	- Typically squamous cell carcinoma	- Associated with HPV and prior VIN - May present with chronic vulvar itching - Surgical excision +/- chemotherapy and radiation
Vulvar melanoma	- Melanoma of the vulvar skin	- Typically postmenopausal Caucasian women - Treat with excision with wide margins
Paget disease of the vulva	- Apocrine gland neoplasia	- Rarely associated with underlying invasive adenocarcinoma - Bright red lesion
Bartholin gland carcinoma	- Can be squamous cell, adenocarcinoma, or other types of cancer	- Painless vulvar mass - Radical vulvectomy and lymphadenectomy

TABLE 17.2.17 - Premalignant and Malignant Vulvar Lesions

REVIEW QUESTIONS

1. A 59-year-old woman comes to her primary care physician because of a vulvar lesion. She first noticed a small papule 7 months ago that has progressively enlarged. She has had 8 sexual partners in the last year and has not used birth control since menopause. Physical examination shows a large white plaque on the right vulva with a central ulcer. Superficial inguinal lymph nodes are enlarged bilaterally. A biopsy of the lesion shows keratin pearls and intercellular bridges. The patient tests positive for human papillomavirus. Which two serotypes of the human papillomavirus are associated the most with the development of her current condition?

   - **Two stereotypes of human papillomavirus that are most strongly associated with vulvar SCC are HPV 16 and 18.**
   - This 59-year-old patient has a large white vulvar plaque with a central ulcer and superficial inguinal lymphadenopathy.
   - Biopsy of her vulvar lesion shows keratin pearls and intercellular bridges, consistent with vulvar squamous cell carcinoma.

2. A 62-year-old woman comes to her primary care physician because of severe vulvar itching for the past 3 days. Her last menstrual period was 10 years ago. She has also noticed pain during sexual intercourse for the last 2 years. She is sexually active with four male partners, and she stopped taking oral contraceptive pills after menopause. Her vital signs include a temperature of 98.6° F (37° C), blood pressure of 140/85 mmHg, heart rate of 86 beats/min, and respiratory rate of 14 breaths/min. Physical examination shows a white plaque of 3 cm in diameter on the right labia majora that bleeds on manipulation. Colposcopy shows atrophic vaginal mucosa. Which of the following is the next best step in the management?

   A. Biopsy of the lesion
   B. Follow-up in one month
   C. Topical estrogen
   D. Topical triamcinolone

   - **The correct answer is option A.**
   - This postmenopausal woman presents with severe vulvar itching and pain during sexual intercourse, that is, dyspareunia.
   - Colposcopy shows atrophic vaginal mucosa.
   - Dyspareunia and atrophic vaginal mucosa indicate genitourinary syndrome of menopause, also known as atrophic vaginitis.
   - She is sexually active with several male partners with no protection. This increases her risk of sexually transmitted infections like human papillomavirus.
   - Physical examination shows a white plaque of 3 cm in diameter on the right labia majora that bleeds on manipulation.
   - Considering itching and her high-risk sexual behavior, this lesion is most consistent with vulvar cancer.
   - The best next step in the management of a patient with suspected vulvar cancer is biopsy of the lesion.
   - Option B is incorrect because this patient is suspected of having vulvar cancer. Follow-up in one month will likely delay diagnosis and treatment.
   - Option C is incorrect because although this patient exhibits signs of atrophic vaginitis, topical estrogen will not have any effect on her white plaque.
   - Option D is incorrect because topical triamcinolone is used in the treatment of lichen sclerosis, not vulvar cancer.

Gynecology | Section 26: Vaginal Neoplasia

I. Vaginal Intraepithelial Neoplasia
   A. 3 primary types based on the degree of epithelial involvement:
      1. VAIN 1: first ⅓ of epithelium
      2. VAIN 2: up to ⅔ epithelium
      3. VAIN 3: more than ⅔ epithelium
      4. Carcinoma in situ: full thickness involvement
   B. Associated with HPV, especially 16 and 18
   C. Usually asymptomatic
   D. Diagnosis
      1. Application of acetic acid reveals acetowhite changes in areas that should be biopsied
      2. Definitive diagnosis is histologic
   E. Treatment
      1. VAIN 1 and some 2: surveillance
      2. VAIN 3 and some 2: surgery, laser ablation, topical treatment

II. Vaginal Cancer
   A. Majority are squamous cell carcinoma
   B. Risk factors
      1. Multiple sexual partners
      2. Smoking
      3. HPV
      4. Previous VAIN
   C. Treatment
      1. Surgical: radical hysterectomy, upper vaginectomy, and pelvic lymph node dissection
      2. Radiation therapy

III. Sarcoma Botryoides
   A. Embryonal rhabdomyosarcoma
   B. Arises from vaginal or bladder wall
   C. Presents as "grape-like" polyps protruding from the vagina of a female infant
   D. Local metastasis, may spread hematologically
   E. Treatment: chemotherapy and surgical removal

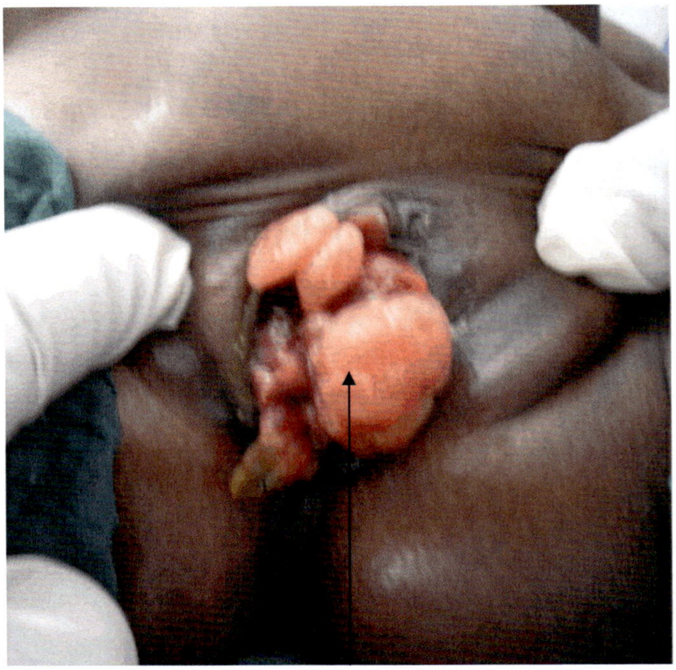

FIGURE 17.2.94 - "Grape-Like" Masses of Sarcoma Botryoides

Condition	Etiology	Key Features
Vaginal intraepithelial neoplasia	- Premalignant lesion with three types based on depth of invasion	- Associated with high risk HPV types - High grade will need treatment to avoid progression to vaginal cancer
Vaginal cancer	- Typically squamous cell carcinoma	- Associated with high risk HPV subtypes -Typically surgical excision +/- radiation
Sarcoma botryoides	- Rare embryonal rhabdomyosarcoma	- "Grape-like" masses from bladder or vagina of female infant - Excision and chemotherapy

TABLE 17.2.18 - Premalignant and Malignant Vaginal Lesions

REVIEW QUESTIONS

1. A 53-year-old woman comes to her primary care physician because of vaginal bleeding for one week. Her last menstrual period was 3 years ago. She has had unprotected sexual intercourse with multiple sexual partners over the 2 years. Physical examination shows an exophytic mass on the lateral vaginal wall. A biopsy of the lesion reveals keratin pearls. What is most likely to have protected this patient from the causative agent of her condition?

   - **Barrier contraception use is most likely to have protected this patient from the causative agent.**
   - This postmenopausal patient presents with vaginal bleeding.
   - She has a history of unprotected sexual intercourse with multiple partners for the past few years
   - Physical examination shows an exophytic vaginal mass, the biopsy of which reveals keratin pearls which is characteristic of vaginal squamous cell carcinoma.
   - The greatest risk factor for vaginal squamous cell carcinoma is infection with human papillomavirus.
   - Barrier contraception use is most likely to have protected this patient from getting HPV infection.

2. A 4-year-old girl is brought to her primary care physician by her mother due to a vaginal mass. The mother first noticed the lesion when bathing her daughter 3 days ago. Physical examination shows a grape-like mass protruding from the vagina. Biopsy of the lesion shows desmin-positive cells with cross-striations. What is the most appropriate treatment for this patient's condition?

   - **The most appropriate treatment for this patient's condition is surgical excision and chemotherapy.**
   - This 4-year-old girl has a grape-like mass protruding from her vagina.
   - Biopsy of the lesion shows desmin-positive cells with cross-striations, consistent with sarcoma botryoides, a subtype of embryonal rhabdomyosarcoma.
   - The most appropriate treatment for sarcoma botryoides is surgical excision and chemotherapy.

3. A 48-year-old woman comes to her primary care physician for a routine examination. She has no specific complaints. She had acute cystitis 6 months ago. She is sexually active with multiple sexual partners, and she takes oral contraceptive pills. Vital signs include a temperature of 98.6° F (37° C), blood pressure of 125/70 mmHg, heart rate of 92 beats/min, and respiratory rate of 14 breaths/min. Genitourinary examination shows acetowhite changes on the left lateral wall upon application of the acetic acid. A biopsy of the suspicious mucosal area shows dysplastic changes in the lower one-third of the vaginal epithelium. Which of the following is the next best step in the management of this patient?

   A. Surveillance
   B. Surgical excision
   C. Laser ablation
   D. Topical chemotherapy

   - **The correct answer is option A.**
   - This 48-year-old sexually active woman has a suspicious mucosal area on the left lateral vaginal wall.
   - Biopsy of the lesion shows dysplastic changes in the lower one-third of the vaginal epithelium.
   - This description is consistent with the diagnosis of vaginal intraepithelial neoplasia 1.
   - The next best step in the management of this patient is active surveillance to monitor dysplasia for further progression.
   - Options B, surgical excision, C, laser ablation, and D, topical chemotherapy, are incorrect because these treatment modalities are used for vaginal intraepithelial neoplasia 2 or 3.

Gynecology | Section 27: Cervical Neoplasia

I. Cervical Neoplasia: Definition
   A. Neoplastic proliferation of cervical epithelial cells

II. Cervical Neoplasia: Pathophysiology
   A. High-risk strains of the human papillomavirus (e.g. HPV 16, HPV 18)
      1. Spread via direct skin-to-skin contact
      2. Invade cervical epithelial cells
      3. Induce oncogenic changes
   B. Cervical intraepithelial neoplasia (CIN)
      1. Premalignant cellular changes in the cervical epithelium
      2. May progress to cervical cancer
   C. Cervical cancer usually originates at the cervical transformation zone
      1. Area of transition between squamous epithelium of the exocervix and columnar epithelium of the endocervix

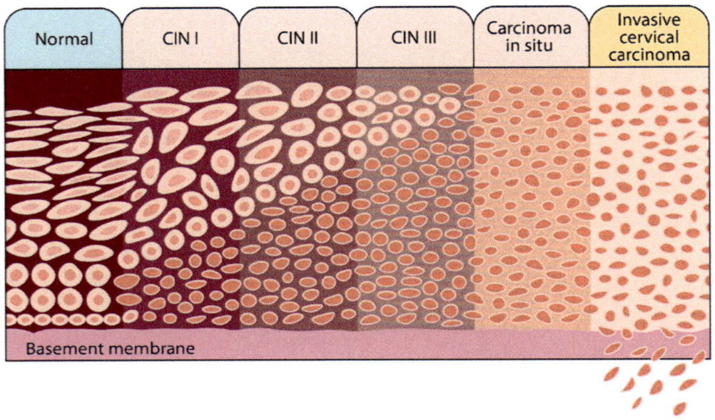

FIGURE 17.2.95 - Cervical Epithelium in Different Stages of Neoplasia

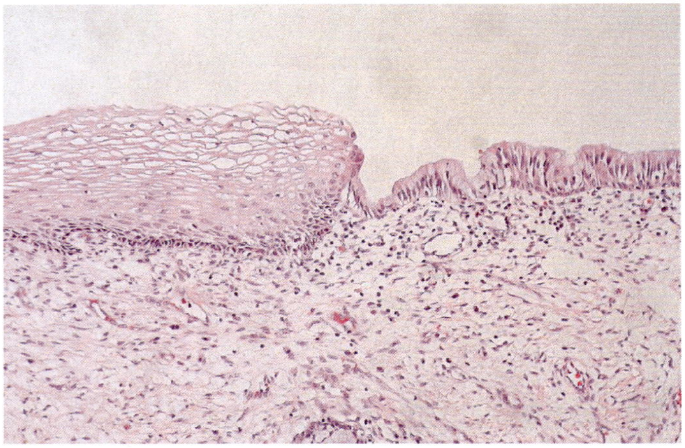

Ed Uthman. https://www.flickr.com/photos/euthman/4796821432

FIGURE 17.2.96 - Light Microscopy: Transformation Zone of the Cervix

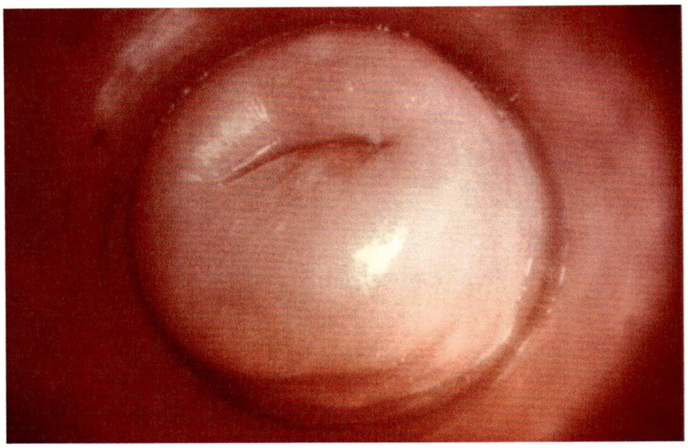

CDC/ N.J. Fiumara, M.D. Public Domain.

FIGURE 17.2.97 - The Cervix

III. Cervical Neoplasia: Risk Factors
   A. High-risk sexual behaviors (e.g. multiple sexual partners)
   B. Early onset of intercourse
   C. Immunosuppression (e.g. AIDS)
   D. Low socioeconomic status
   E. Cigarette smoking
   F. Family history

IV. Cervical Neoplasia: Clinical Features
   A. Early disease (e.g. CIN) is asymptomatic
   B. Late disease may present with:
      1. Postcoital bleeding (most common symptom)
      2. Pelvic pain
      3. Vaginal discharge
      4. Urinary symptoms (e.g. dysuria)
      5. Rectal symptoms (e.g. dyschezia)

V. Cervical Neoplasia: Diagnosis
   A. Screening options
      1. Pap smear
      2. HPV testing
      3. Cotesting (pap smear + HPV testing)
   B. Definitive diagnosis
      1. Colposcopy with cervical biopsy
      2. Endocervical curettage
   C. Pap smear results:
      1. Negative
      2. ASC-US: atypical squamous cells of undetermined significance
      3. ASC-H: atypical squamous cells, cannot rule out high-grade lesion
      4. LSIL: low-grade squamous intraepithelial lesion
      5. HSIL: high-grade squamous intraepithelial lesion
      6. AGC: atypical glandular cells
      7. SCC: squamous cell carcinoma

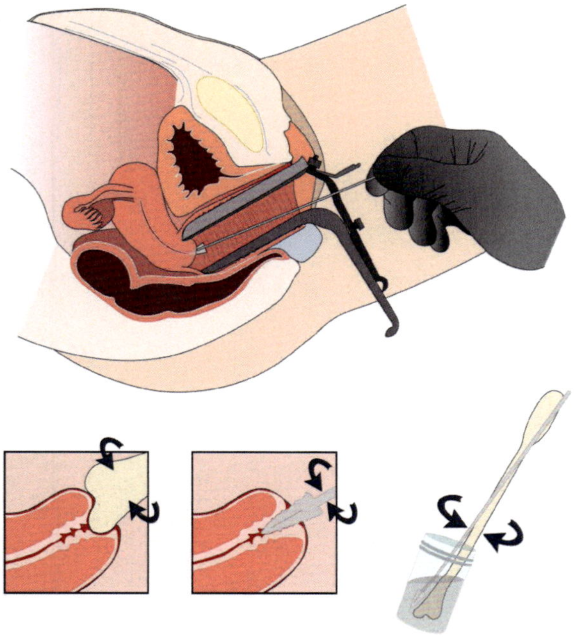

FIGURE 17.2.98 - Obtaining Pap Smear

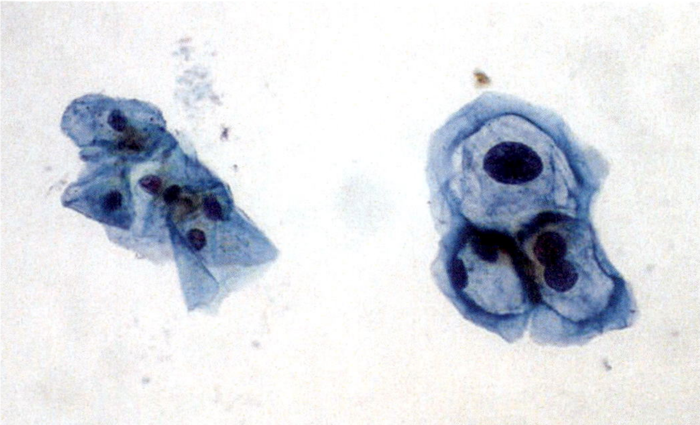

Photomicrograph by Ed Uthman, MD. 20 July 2006 Euthman 20:24, 29 November 2006 (UTC) / Public domain

FIGURE 17.2.99 - Normal Cervical Cells vs. Koilocytes

General Population	Cervical Cancer Screening Recommendations
< 21 years old	- No screening (unless HIV-positive)
21 - 29 years old	- Pap smear every 3 years
30 - 64 years old	- Pap smear every 3 years - Primary HPV testing every 5 years - Pap smear with HPV cotesting every 5 years
≥ 65 years old	- Stop screening if screening for the past 10 years has been negative

TABLE 17.2.19 - Cervical Cancer Screening Recommendations in the General Population

Special Population	Cervical Cancer Screening Recommendations
- HIV-positive	- Age < 21: pap smear within 1 year of onset of sexual activity - Age ≥ 21: pap smear at the time of HIV diagnosis - Pap smear obtained annually until three consecutive negative results - Regular screening thereafter
- Immunocompromised	- Pap smear within 1 year of onset of sexual activity - Pap smear with HPV cotesting annually thereafter
- Total hysterectomy	- No screening if no history of CIN II, CIN III, or carcinoma in situ in the last 20 years
- In-utero DES exposure	- Pap smear annually for the rest of the patient's life

TABLE 17.2.20 - Cervical Cancer Screening Recommendations in Special Populations

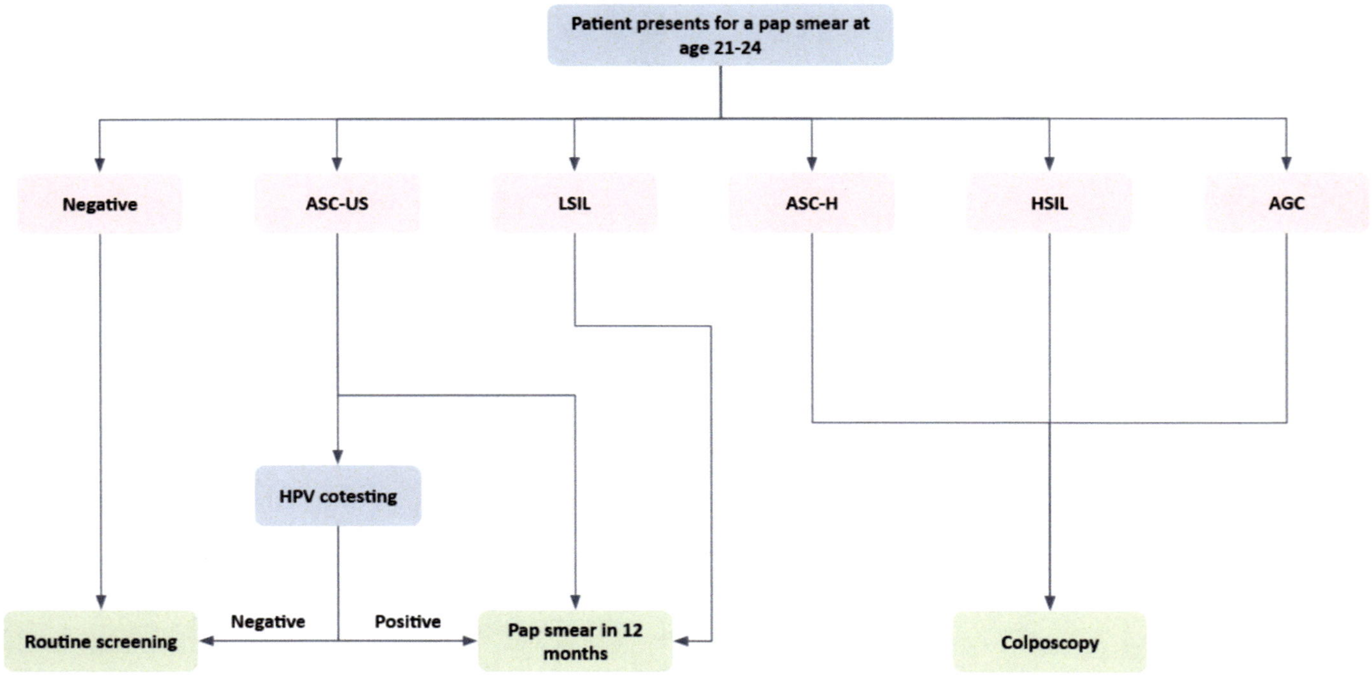

FIGURE 17.2.100 - Evaluation of Pap Smear Findings for Patients at Age 21 - 24 Years

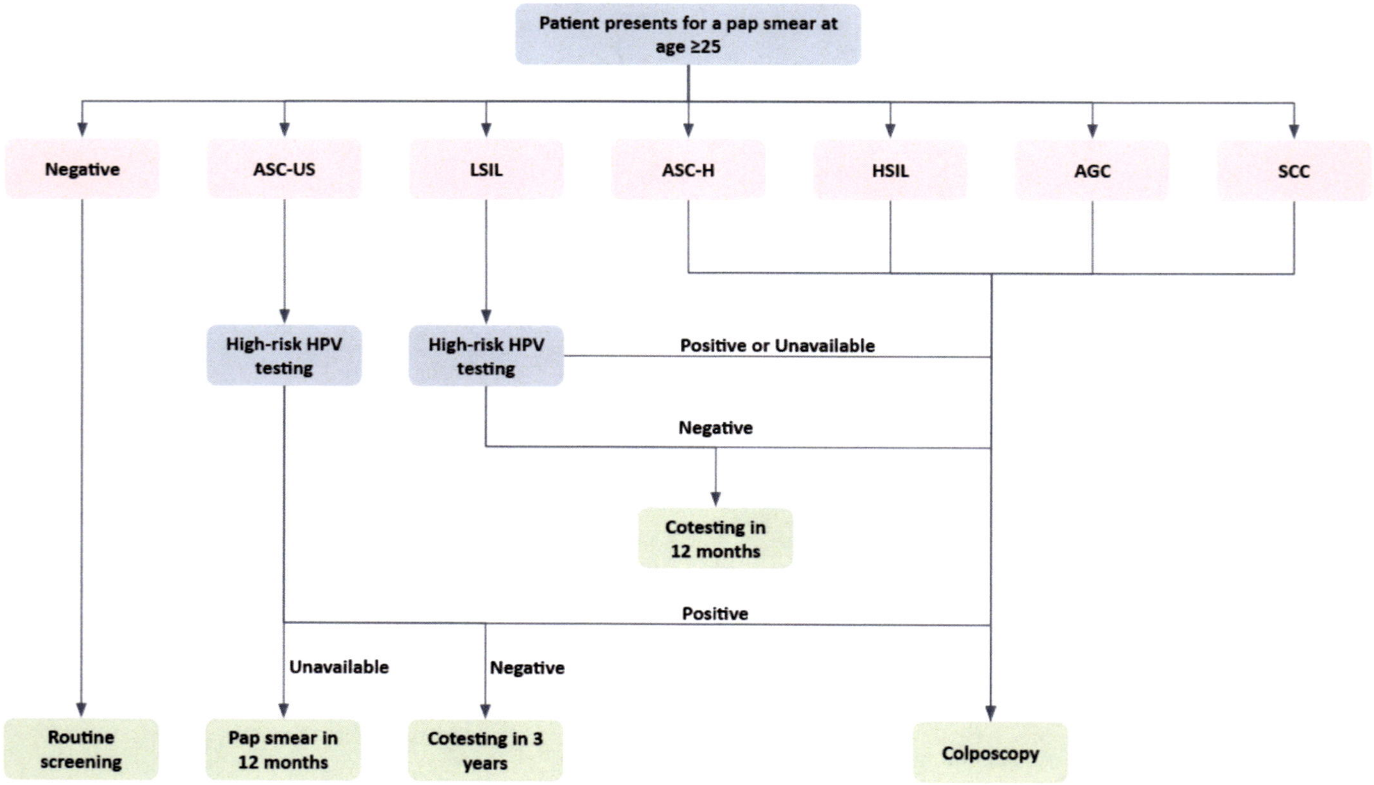

FIGURE 17.2.101 - Evaluation of Pap Smear Findings for Patients at Age ≥ 25 Years

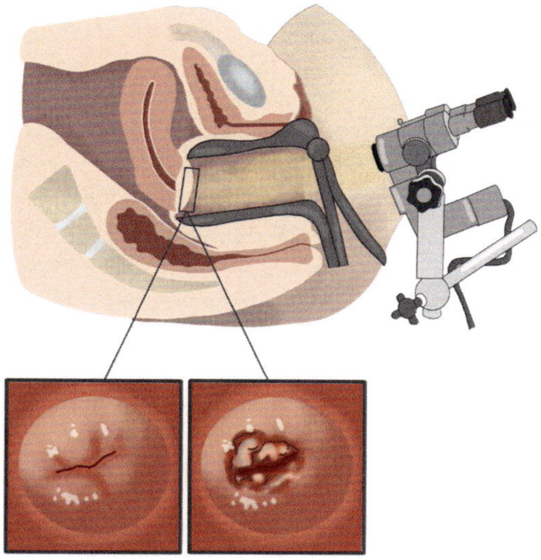

FIGURE 17.2.102 - Colposcopy

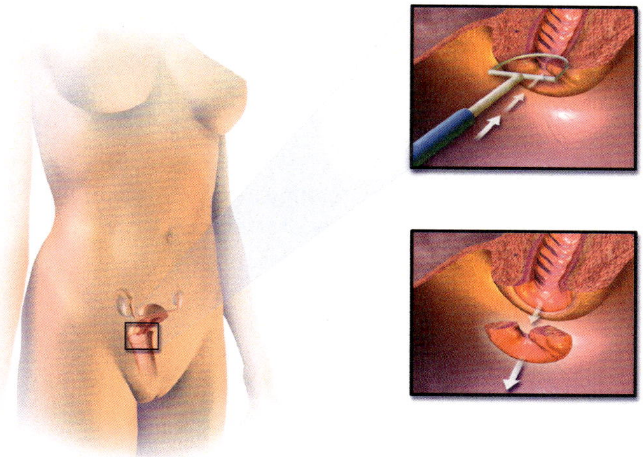

FIGURE 17.2.104 - Loop Electrosurgical Excision Procedure

VI. Cervical Neoplasia: Management
   A. Prevention
      1. HPV vaccination (e.g. Gardasil) for males and females ages 9 - 45
      2. Safe sex practices (e.g. consistent use of condoms)
   B. CIN I (LSIL)
      1. Observation and follow-up testing
   C. CIN II (HSIL)
      1. Observation in young women
      2. Ablation of the transformation zone (e.g. cryotherapy)
      3. Cold knife or laser conization
   D. CIN III (HSIL)
      1. Ablation of the transformation zone
      2. Cold knife or laser conization
      3. Loop electrosurgical excision procedure (LEEP)
   E. Invasive cervical cancer (e.g. SCC)
      1. Clinical staging based on extent of spread
      2. Surgery (e.g. hysterectomy)
      3. Radiation therapy
      4. Chemotherapy

VII. Cervical Neoplasia: Complications
   A. Cervical cancer invades surrounding structures (e.g. bladder)
   B. Most common cause of death is postrenal failure due to hydronephrosis

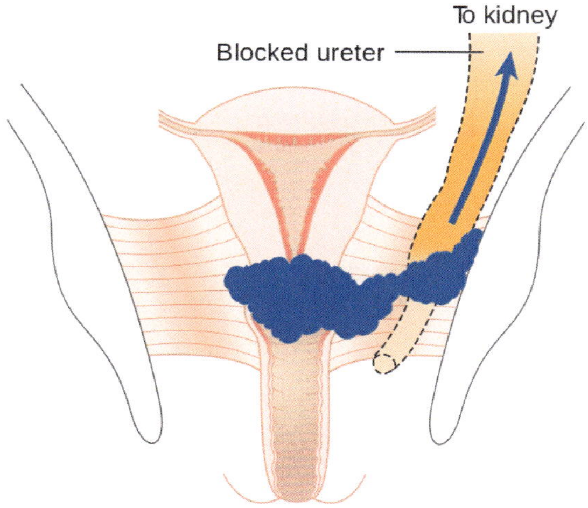

FIGURE 17.2.105 - Cervical Cancer

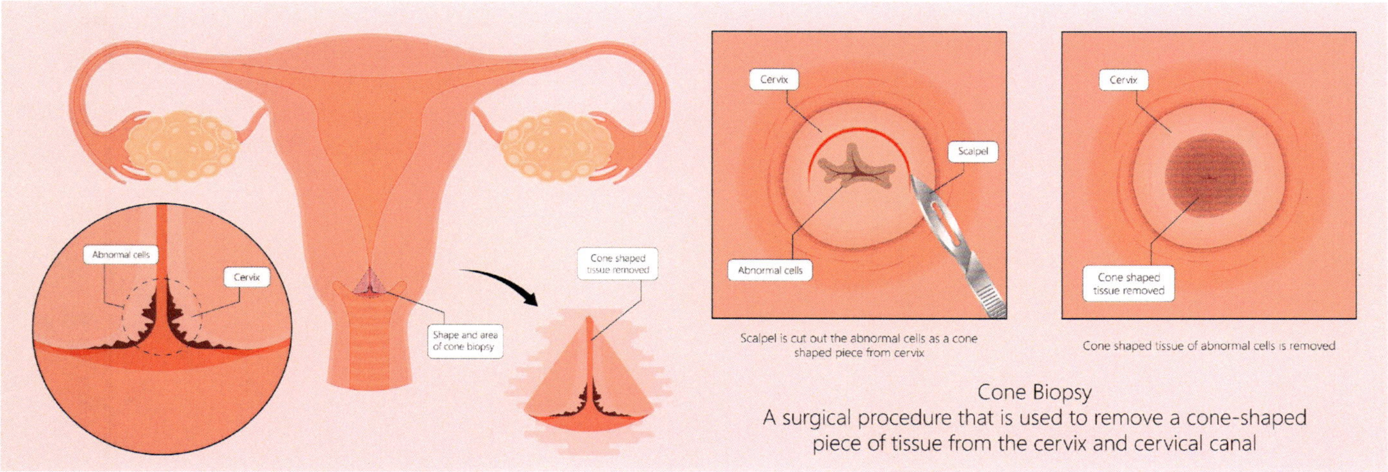

FIGURE 17.2.103 - Cold Knife Conization

REVIEW QUESTIONS

1. In what patient populations may cervical cancer screening be necessary at an age younger than 21?
    - **The only two patient populations that may need cervical cancer screening at ages younger than 21 are either patients with HIV or patients who are otherwise immunocompromised.**

2. A pap smear obtained from a 37-year-old woman shows atypical glandular cells (AGC). In addition to colposcopy with endocervical curettage, which additional diagnostic procedure should the patient undergo?
    - **This patient should also undergo an endometrial biopsy.**
    - Endometrial biopsy is indicated for all women aged 35 or older if their pap smear shows atypical glandular cells.
    - Atypical glandular cells can be a product of either cervical cancer or endometrial cancer, which is why it is important to assess the patient for both possibilities.
    - A colposcopy with endocervical curettage will assess for cervical cancer, and an endometrial biopsy will assess for endometrial cancer.

3. What is the primary contraindication to endocervical curettage?
    - **The primary contraindication to endocervical curettage is pregnancy.**
    - Endocervical curettage is often performed during colposcopy to sample the cells from the endocervical canal and minimize the likelihood of missing an insidious malignancy.
    - However, endocervical curettage is contraindicated during pregnancy. This is because disrupting the integrity of the cervix may interfere with the normal course of the pregnancy and lead to complications.

4. What complications may develop following cervical conization?
    - **Following cervical conization, complications that may develop include second-trimester pregnancy loss, preterm birth, preterm premature rupture of membranes, and cervical stenosis.**
    - All of these complications occur because cervical conization disrupts the integrity of a healthy cervix, which may interfere with its normal function.

5. A 23-year-old woman comes to her primary care physician for a scheduled pap smear. Her past medical history is unremarkable. She takes oral contraceptive pills for birth control. She denies alcohol use but smokes one pack of cigarettes daily. She says she's had four male sexual partners in the last six months. She describes her use of condoms as inconsistent. Blood pressure is 123/77 mmHg, pulse is 72 beats/minute, temperature is 98.8° F (37.1° C). A pap smear is obtained, and the preliminary analysis is consistent with atypical glandular cells. Which of the following is the next best step in management?

    A. Colposcopy with endocervical curettage
    B. Colposcopy with endometrial biopsy
    C. HPV co-testing
    D. Follow-up pap smear in one year
    E. Cold knife conization

    - **The correct answer is option A.**
    - This 23-year-old female comes to her primary care physician for a scheduled pap smear.
    - The preliminary analysis is consistent with atypical glandular cells.
    - If a patient between the ages of 21 and 24 has atypical glandular cells or AGC on her pap smear, the next best step in management is colposcopy.
    - Option B, colposcopy with endometrial biopsy, is incorrect because this patient does not need an endometrial biopsy. An endometrial biopsy would be indicated if atypical glandular cells were detected in a woman aged 35 years or older.
    - Option C, HPV co-testing, is incorrect because it wouldn't change the management. This patient would need a colposcopy whether HPV testing comes back negative or positive.
    - Option D, a follow-up pap smear in one year, is incorrect because this patient needs a colposcopy now to assess her risk of cervical cancer better.
    - Option E, cold knife conization, is incorrect because this patient first needs colposcopy with appropriate biopsies to determine the extent of her cervical intraepithelial neoplasia. As such, it is too early to know whether this patient would benefit from cold knife conization.

Gynecology | Section 28: Endometrial Cancer

I. Endometrial Cancer: Introduction
   A. Cancer of lining of the uterus
   B. Most common gynecological malignancy in developed countries
   C. Peak incidence in postmenopausal age group

II. Endometrial Cancer: Classification
   A. Endometrioid
      1. Most common type; estrogen-dependent
      2. Loss of PTEN or mismatch repair proteins → cell growth
   B. Serous
      1. Arises in atrophic endometrium in postmenopausal women
      2. Aggressive; poor prognosis

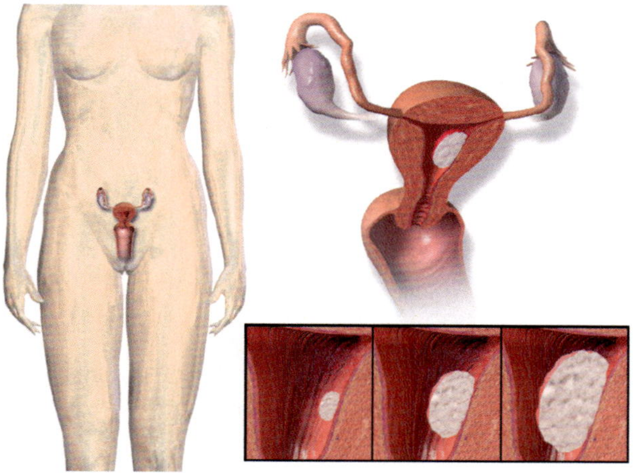

FIGURE 17.2.106 - Endometrial Cancer

III. Endometrial Cancer: Risk Factors
   A. Endometrioid carcinoma
      1. Mostly due to excess estrogen exposure
      2. Nulliparity
      3. Polycystic ovary syndrome
      4. Early menarche and late menopause
      5. Others: diabetes, obesity, tamoxifen therapy
      6. Lynch syndrome

IV. Endometrial Cancer: Protective Factors
   A. Combination oral contraceptive pills
   B. Multiparity
   C. Late menarche and early menopause

V. Endometrial Cancer: Clinical Features
   A. Abnormal vaginal bleeding in postmenopausal women
   B. Heavy and prolonged menstrual/intermenstrual bleeding in premenopausal women
   C. Sense of pelvic mass; pelvic pain; weight loss
   D. Pelvic examination: enlarged/fixed uterus in advanced cases

VI. Endometrial Cancer: Diagnosis
   A. Transvaginal ultrasound
      1. Endometrial thickness: > 20 mm (high risk); < 4 mm (low risk)
   B. Endometrial tissue sampling: gold standard
      1. Blind biopsy; dilation and curettage; hysteroscopy
      2. Endometrioid: abnormal glandular proliferation, atypical cells with mitosis
      3. Serous: papillary structures and psammoma bodies
   C. Imaging
      1. CT/MRI: assess for metastasis

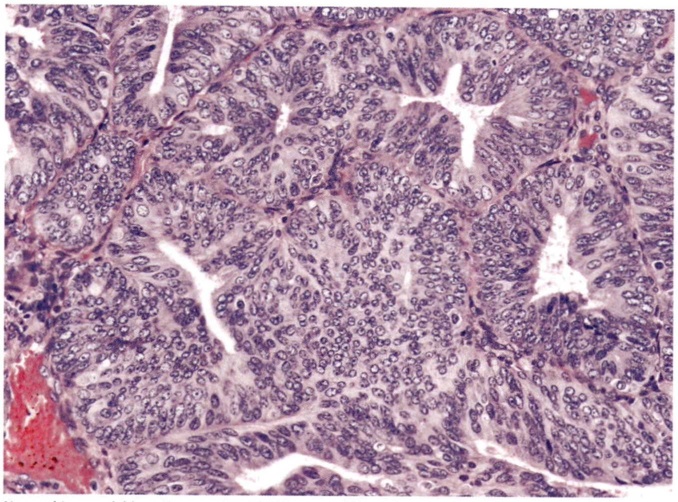

FIGURE 17.2.107 - Light Microscopy: Endometrioid Endometrial Carcinoma

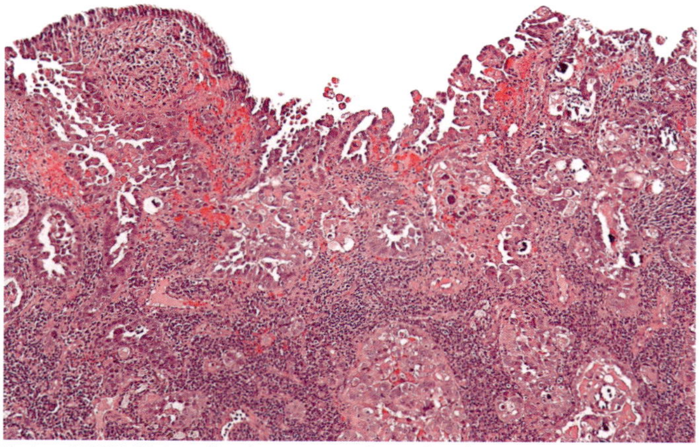

FIGURE 17.2.108 - Light Microscopy: Papillae and Psammoma Bodies in Uterine Serous Carcinoma

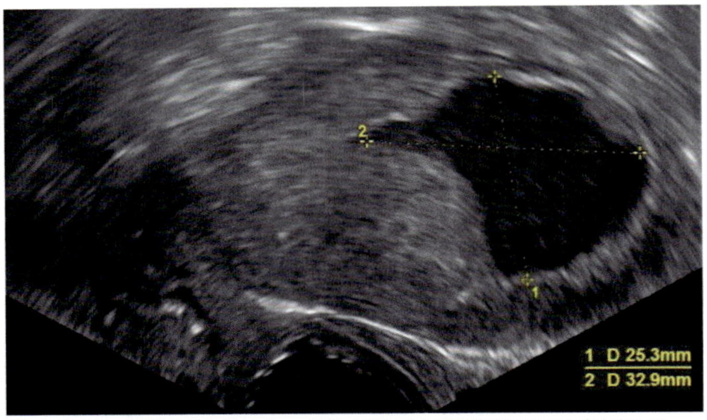

Häggström, Mikael (2014). "Medical gallery of Mikael Häggström 2014". WikiJournal of Medicine 1 (2). DOI:10.15347/wjm/2014.008. ISSN 2002-4436. Public Domain.orBy Mikael Häggström, used with permission., CC0, via Wikimedia Commons

FIGURE 17.2.109 - Transvaginal Ultrasound: Uterine Fluid Accumulation

VII. Endometrial Cancer: Management
   A. Surgical procedures
      1. Necessary for staging; recommended for most patients
      2. Hysterectomy, bilateral salpingo-oophorectomy, lymphadenectomy
   B. Radiotherapy and chemotherapy for adjunctive or palliative care

REVIEW QUESTIONS

1. A 37-year-old G3P3 woman comes to the physician for an annual check-up. She has no specific complaints. Her mother has been recently diagnosed with endometrial cancer at the age of 58. She is anxious and asks about how she can reduce her risk of developing endometrial cancer. The physician notes that multiparity is a protective factor. What is the most likely rationale behind the physician's statement?

- **The most likely rationale behind the physician's statement is that multiparity means higher cumulative exposure to progesterone, which opposes estrogen-induced endometrial proliferation, decreasing the risk of endometrial cancer.**
- During pregnancy, both estrogen and progesterone are increased. Progesterone opposes the proliferative effect of estrogen on the endometrium.
- Multiparity → high cumulative exposure to progesterone → opposition of estrogen-induced endometrial proliferation.

REVIEW QUESTIONS

2. A 55-year-old obese G0P0 woman comes to her primary care provider because of intermittent vaginal bleeding for the past 3 months. Her last menstrual period was 2 years ago. She complains of a pulling sensation in her lower abdomen. Her last Pap smear was negative 2 months ago. Vital signs include a temperature of 37° C (98.6° F), a blood pressure of 135/80 mmHg, a heart rate of 88 beats/min, and a respiratory rate of 15 breaths/min. Genitourinary examination shows poorly rugated, pale vaginal mucosa. Cervix is unremarkable. Transvaginal ultrasound shows an endometrial thickness of 25 mm (Normal is < 4 mm). An endometrial biopsy is performed and shows histological findings of abnormal glandular proliferation with atypical cells. Which of the following is the best next step in management?

   A. CT scan of chest, abdomen, and pelvis
   B. Radiotherapy
   C. Chemotherapy
   D. Plasma estrogen concentration

- **The correct answer is option A.**
- This nulliparous postmenopausal obese woman presents with intermittent vaginal bleeding for the past 3 months.
- Since she is postmenopausal, her recent bleeding most likely suggests an underlying pathology rather than a normal process.
- She also complains of a pulling sensation in her lower abdomen.
- Speculum examination shows poorly rugated, pale vaginal mucosa, which is a normal finding in postmenopausal women; however, TVUS shows severely thickened endometrial lining.
- Endometrial biopsy reveals abnormal glandular proliferation and atypical cells, which are the classic histological findings of endometrioid endometrial carcinoma
- Before the appropriate therapy is chosen, one needs to evaluate for the presence of any metastasis therefore, the correct answer is option A, CT of C/Abd/Pelvis
- Options B and C are incorrect because evaluating for the presence of metastasis is essential before the patient is started on either radiotherapy or chemotherapy.
- Option D is incorrect because although unopposed estrogen predisposes women to endometrial cancer, determining the plasma estrogen concentration will not help in further management of the patient.

Gynecology | Section 29: Ovarian Cyst and Torsion

I. Ovarian Cysts: Definition
  A. Fluid-filled ovarian sacs

II. Ovarian Cysts: Pathophysiology
  A. Follicular cysts: form if follicles do not rupture during ovulation
  B. Corpus luteal cysts: form during pregnancy
  C. Theca lutein cysts: form due to overstimulation with hCG
  D. Neoplastic cysts: form due to abnormal growth of ovarian cells
    1. Can be benign or malignant

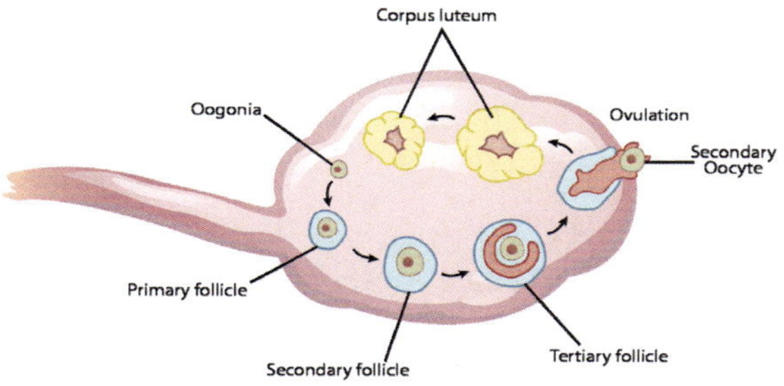

FIGURE 17.2.110 - Ovarian Ovulation Cycle

III. Ovarian Cysts: Risk Factors
  A. Females of reproductive age
  B. Pregnancy
  C. History of infertility treatment (e.g. ovulation induction)

IV. Ovarian Cysts: Clinical Features
  A. Asymptomatic
  B. Unilateral pelvic pain or pressure that can be intermittent or constant
  C. Physical examination may reveal an adnexal mass
  D. Complications
    1. Cyst rupture
    2. Ovarian torsion

V. Ovarian Cysts: Ovarian Cyst Rupture
  A. Tends to occur following strenuous activity or intercourse
  B. Sudden, severe, unilateral pelvic pain
  C. Peritoneal signs (e.g. guarding, rebound tenderness)
  D. Hemodynamic instability (e.g. hypotension, tachycardia)
  E. Referred pain to the shoulder (due to phrenic nerve irritation)

VI. Ovarian Cysts: Diagnosis
  A. Clinical diagnosis
  B. Pregnancy test
  C. Ultrasound
    1. Ovarian cyst: homogenous mass with a thin wall
    2. Ruptured ovarian cyst: free fluid in the pelvis +/- ovarian cyst

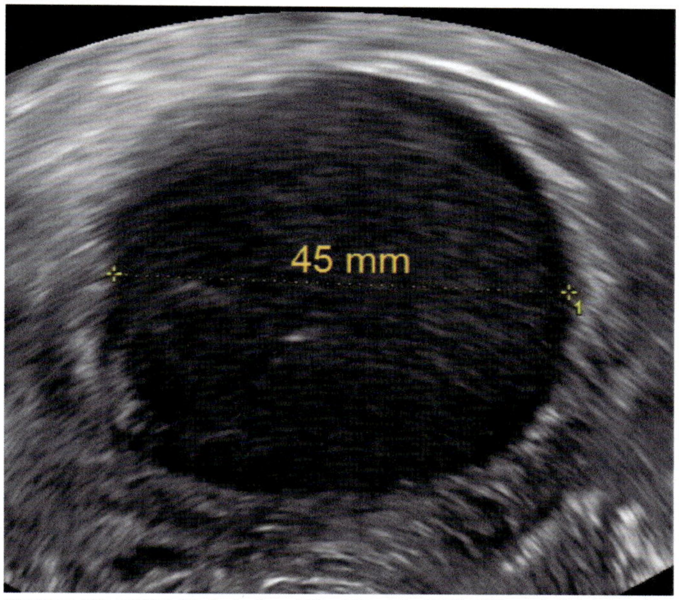

FIGURE 17.2.111 - Ultrasonogram: Ovarian Cyst

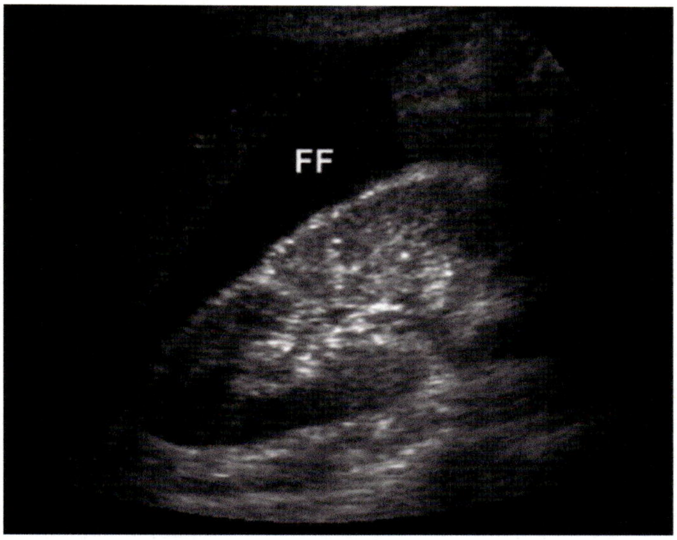

FIGURE 17.2.112 - Abdominal Ultrasound: Ruptured Ectopic Pregnancy

VII. Ovarian Cysts: Management
  A. Ovarian cysts
    1. Observation for asymptomatic cysts
    2. Needle aspiration to drain simple cysts
    3. Surgical excision of large cysts
  B. Ovarian cyst rupture, patient stable and without signs of infection
    1. Conservative management (e.g. pain medications)
  C. Ovarian cyst rupture, patient unstable (e.g. hypotension, peritonitis)
    1. Surgery

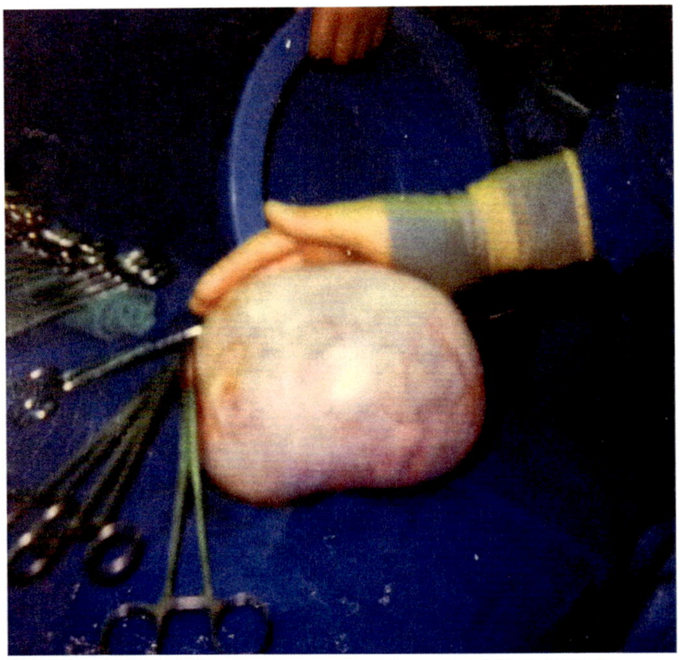

FIGURE 17.2.113 - Ovarian Cyst

VIII. Ovarian Torsion: Definition
   A. Twisting of the ovary around its ligaments cuts off the blood supply to the organ, leading to ischemia
   B. Also known as adnexal torsion

IX. Ovarian Torsion: Pathophysiology
   A. The ovary has a dual blood supply:
      1. Ovarian vessels (suspensory/infundibulopelvic ligament)
      2. Uterine vessels (utero-ovarian ligament)
   B. Twisting of the ligaments occludes the arteries that feed the ovary and the veins that drain it
      1. Ischemia
      2. Necrosis

X. Ovarian Torsion: Risk Factors
   A. Females of reproductive age
   B. History of an ovarian mass (e.g. cyst, tumor)
   C. Strenuous exercise
   D. Pregnancy
   E. History of infertility treatment (e.g. ovulation induction)

XI. Ovarian Torsion: Clinical Features
   A. Partial ovarian torsion: intermittent abdominal pain, often with activity
   B. Complete ovarian torsion: sudden onset of severe, unilateral pelvic pain with accompanying nausea and vomiting
      1. Physical examination: painful, unilateral adnexal mass
      2. Fever may develop if the ovary becomes necrotic

XII. Ovarian Torsion: Diagnosis
   A. Clinical diagnosis
   B. Rule out pregnancy
   C. Ultrasound of the pelvis with doppler velocimetry
      1. Large, edematous ovary
      2. Diminished or absent blood flow to the ovary
      3. Negative ultrasound does not rule out ovarian torsion
   D. Consider diagnostic laparoscopy

XIII. Ovarian Torsion: Management
   A. Complete ovarian torsion is a surgical emergency
      1. Laparoscopic detorsion
      2. Removal of the ovarian mass or cyst (e.g. cystectomy)
   B. Consider oophorectomy if there's intraoperative evidence of malignancy or necrosis

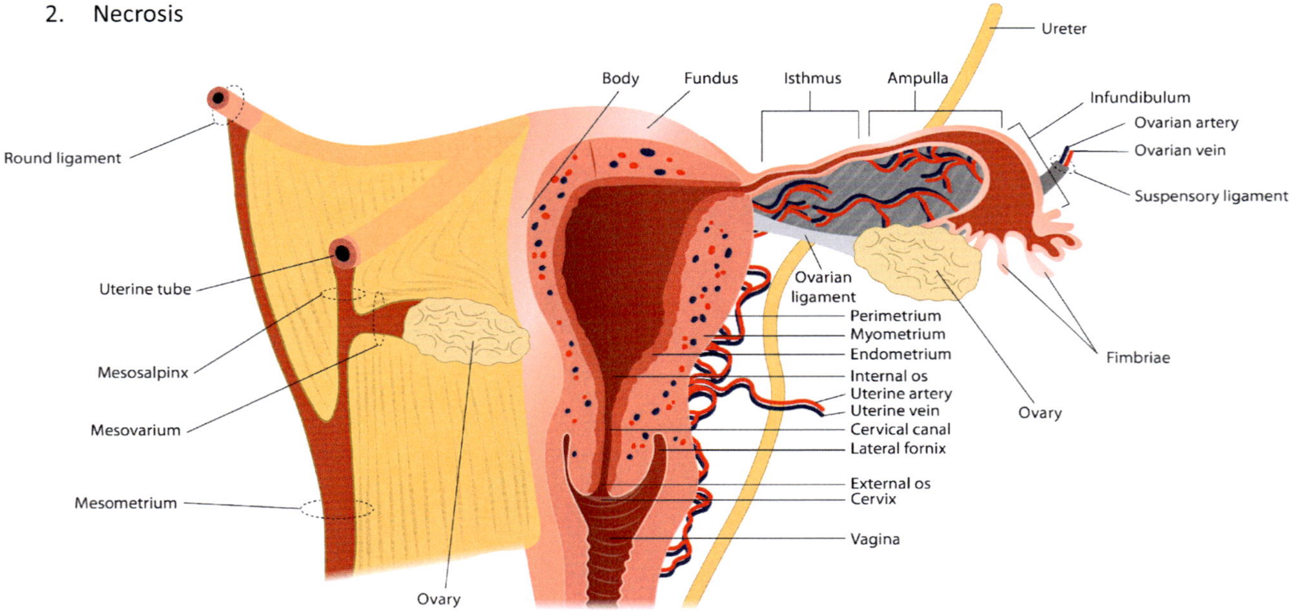

FIGURE 17.2.114 - Female Genital Tract

REVIEW QUESTIONS

?

1. What type of ovarian cyst is most likely to develop in a woman with a hydatidiform mole?
   - **The type of ovarian cyst most likely to develop in a woman with a hydatidiform mole is a theca lutein cyst.**
   - Hydatidiform moles are essentially "false pregnancies" which are associated with extremely high levels of human chorionic gonadotropin (hCG).
   - Theca lutein cysts arise in response to overstimulation by hCG.
   - Since hCG overstimulation affects both ovaries, theca lutein cysts tend to develop in both ovaries rather than one.

2. How can you distinguish a ruptured ovarian cyst from a ruptured ectopic pregnancy?
   - **A pregnancy test can distinguish a ruptured ovarian cyst from a ruptured pregnancy.**
   - Both a ruptured ovarian cyst and a ruptured ectopic pregnancy may present with severe abdominal pain, hemodynamic instability, and peritonitis, which clinically makes it difficult to distinguish.
   - Fortunately, these conditions are easily distinguished by performing a pregnancy test, which will be negative in patients with a ruptured ovarian cyst and positive in a patient with a ruptured ectopic pregnancy.

3. A 26-year-old woman is brought to the emergency room by her roommate because of severe lower abdominal pain. They were working out when suddenly, the patient had severe pain. The pain is most severe in the right pelvis and lower abdomen. She is given medication for pain relief with dose help. An ultrasound is performed and shows an edematous ovary, on Doppler there is minimal blood flow. What is the most likely diagnosis?
   - **The most likely diagnosis is ovarian torsion**
   - This young woman presents with severe sudden onset right-sided pelvic and abdominal pain which started during her workout.
   - Ultrasound shows an edematous ovary with minimal blood flow, which is characteristic of ovarian torsion.
   - In ovarian torsion the ovary and fallopian tube twist around the ligaments with contain the ovarian veins and lympathics. This compression leads to decreased venous and lymphatic drainage.
   - As the ovary becomes more edematous from poor venous and lymphatic drainage the ovarian artery becomes compressed causing ischemia.

	Ovarian Torsion	Ovarian Cyst Rupture
Similarities	- Sudden, severe unilateral pelvic pain - Tends to occur after strenuous physical activity	
Physical examination	- Adnexal mass	- No adnexal mass
Ultrasound	- Edematous ovary - No blood flow	- Free fluid

TABLE 17.2.21 - Ovarian Torsion vs. Ovarian Cyst Rupture

Gynecology | Section 30: Neoplasms - Germ Cell and Sex Sord-Stromal Tumors

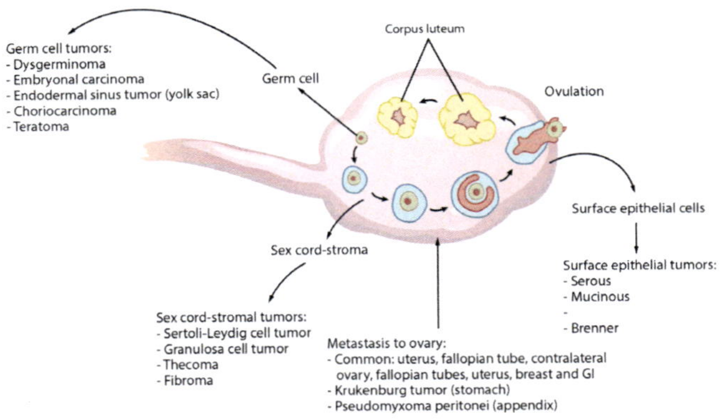

FIGURE 17.2.115 - Ovarian Neoplasms

I. Germ Cell Tumors
   A. Most germ cell tumors are benign
      1. Most common subtype: cystic mature teratoma (dermoid cyst)
   B. Present mostly in younger women (age < 20)
   C. Tumors grow rapidly, causing symptoms early in the disease course
   D. Surgery is the mainstay of treatment, often with adjuvant chemotherapy
   E. Tumor markers are used to monitor response to treatment

II. Germ Cell Tumors: Mature Cystic Teratoma (Dermoid Cyst)
   A. Cystic mass containing mature cells from all three germ layers (e.g. hair, bones, liver tissue)
   B. May differentiate into thyroid tissue, producing thyroid hormone
      1. This variant of teratomas is known as struma ovarii
      2. Patients will exhibit signs of hyperthyroidism (e.g. tachycardia)
   C. Ultrasound: complex cyst +/- calcifications
   D. Definitive diagnosis occurs following surgical excision

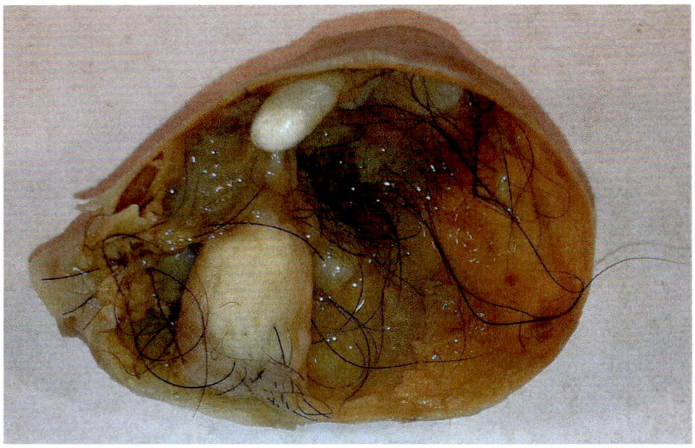

FIGURE 17.2.116 - Mature Cystic Teratoma

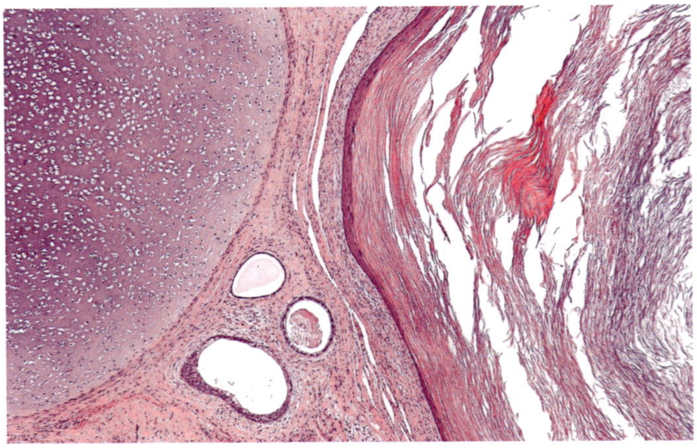

FIGURE 17.2.117 - Light Microscopy: Mature Cystic Teratoma

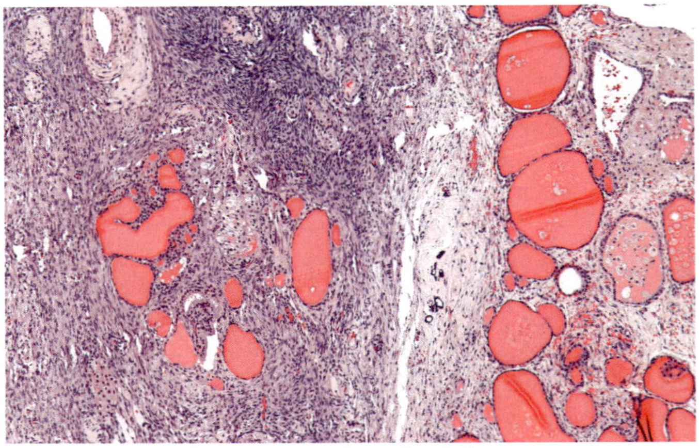

FIGURE 17.2.118 - Light Microscopy: Struma Ovarii

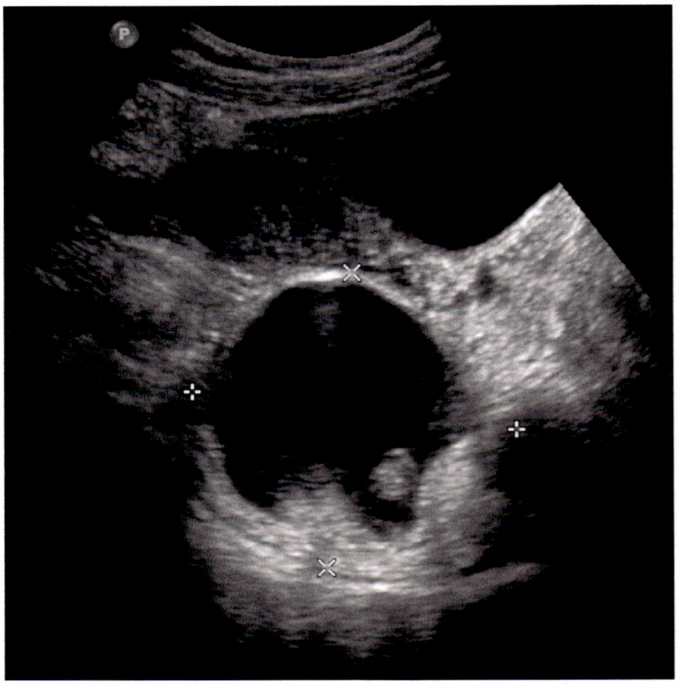

FIGURE 17.2.119 - Ultrasonogram: Mature Cystic Teratoma

III. Germ Cell Tumors: Choriocarcinoma
   A. Arises from malignant proliferation of placental trophoblastic tissue
      1. Frequently develops following a hydatidiform mole
      2. May develop following normal gestation or a miscarriage
   B. Presentation: abnormal vaginal bleeding, pelvic pain
   C. Ultrasound: enlarged uterus, uterine mass
   D. Spreads hematogenously
      1. Frequently metastasizes to lungs ("cannonball lesions" on CXR)
      2. May metastasize to the vagina and present as a friable mass
   E. Tumor marker: β-hCG (markedly elevated)
   F. Treatment: chemotherapy

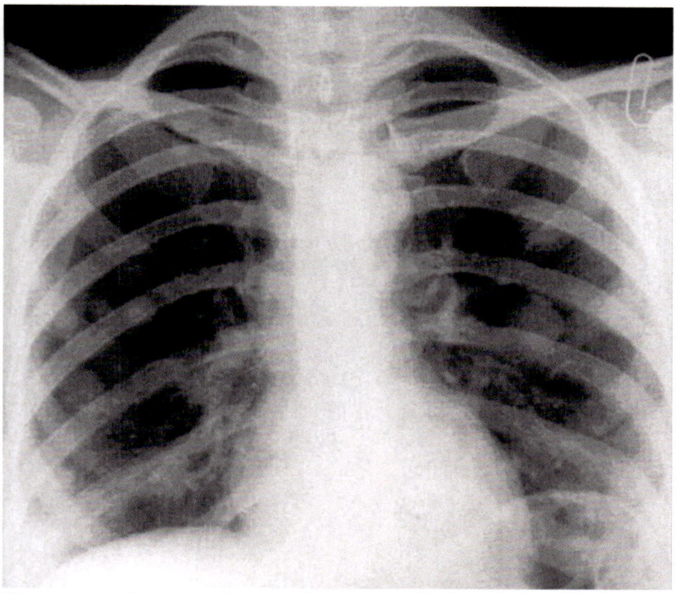

"The appearance of lung metastasis in patient that was reported" by Ghaemmaghami F, Zarchi MK, Early Onset of Metastatic Gestational Trophoblastic Disease after Full-Term Pregnancy, International Journal of Biomedical Science, licensed under CC BY 2.5. Modifications: removed yellow arrow.

FIGURE 17.2.120 - Chest X-ray: Cannonball Lesions in Metastasized Choriocarcinoma

Germ Cell Tumor	Key Feature(s)	Tumor Marker(s)
Dysgerminoma	- Most common malignant germ cell tumor - Testicular counterpart: seminoma	- ↑ LDH
Endodermal sinus tumor (a.k.a. yolk sac tumor)	- Most common germ cell tumor in children - Resembles the yolk sac	- ↑ AFP
Embryonal carcinoma	- Rare - Malignant	- ↑ AFP - ↑ hCG

TABLE 17.2.22 - Overview of Other Germ Cell Tumors

IV. Sex Cord-Stromal Tumors
   A. Arise from cells surrounding the oocyte or from the ovarian stroma
      1. Granulosa cell tumors are the most common subtype
   B. Present in women of all ages
   C. Most are treated with surgery
      1. Fertility desired: unilateral salpingo-oophorectomy
      2. Fertility not desired: hysterectomy with bilateral salpingo-oophorectomy

V. Sex Cord-Stromal Tumors: Granulosa Cell Tumor
   A. Presents as an adnexal mass and signs of high estrogen
      1. Children and teenagers: precocious puberty
      2. Older women: abnormal uterine bleeding and breast tenderness
   B. Tumor markers: inhibin and estradiol
   C. Histology: Call-Exner bodies (pathognomonic)
   D. Ultrasound: complex ovarian mass +/- irregular endometrial stripe
   E. Endometrial biopsy: hyperplasia or intraepithelial neoplasia

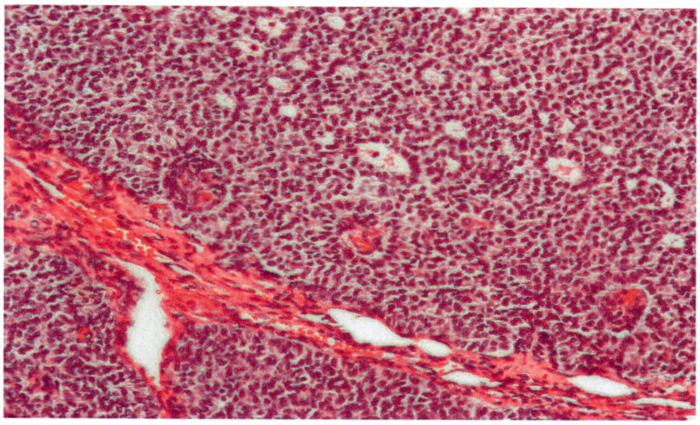

Nephron, CC BY-SA 3.0 <https://creativecommons.org/licenses/by-sa/3.0>,

FIGURE 17.2.121 - Light Microscopy: Call-Exner Bodies in Granulosa Cell Tumor

VI. Sex Cord-Stromal Tumors: Sertoi-Leydig Cell Tumor
   A. Patients present with an adnexal mass, menstrual irregularities, and rapid-onset virilization:
      1. Increased musculature
      2. Deepened voice, receding hairline
      3. Clitoromegaly
   B. Patients may develop signs of estrogen deficiency (e.g. breast atrophy)
   C. Tumor marker: testosterone

VII. Sex Cord-Stromal Tumors: Fibroma
   A. Arises from mature fibroblasts
   B. Does not secrete any hormones
   C. Associated with Meigs syndrome
   D. Ovarian tumor (fibroma)
   E. Ascites
   F. Right-sided hydrothorax

REVIEW QUESTIONS

1. A 22-year-old woman comes to her primary care physician because of severe anxiety and paranoia. She started feeling this way about two weeks ago after she recovered from the flu. She says she's never felt this way in the past and considers herself healthy. A review of records shows a recent diagnosis of ovarian teratoma, and the patient is scheduled for surgical resection in three weeks. Physical examination shows rigidity in the upper extremities and brisk deep tendon reflexes. The patient seems to be whispering to herself during the examination. What is the most likely underlying cause of her neuropsychiatric symptoms?

   - **The most likely underlying cause of her neuropsychiatric symptoms is anti-NMDA receptor encephalitis.**
   - This is a case of a young woman who presents to the clinic with new-onset anxiety and paranoia after recovering from the flu several weeks ago.
   - Several neurologic signs, such as rigidity in the upper extremities and brisk deep tendon reflexes, accompany her psychiatric symptoms.
   - The woman is also whispering to herself during the examination.
   - She had a recent diagnosis of ovarian fibroma.
   - All of these neuropsychiatric symptoms in the context of a flu-like prodrome and a known ovarian teratoma point to the diagnosis of anti-NMDA receptor encephalitis, which is a type of autoimmune encephalitis.

2. What is the difference between hirsutism and virilization?

   - **The clinical features of hirsutism include excessive growth of dark or coarse hair on the face, back, or chest.**
   - **The clinical features of virilization include increased musculature, deepened voice, receding hairline, and clitoromegaly.**
   - Both terms describe clinical features stemming from excess testosterone in females.
   - Notably, hirsutism may be a component of virilization, but virilization is never a component of hirsutism.
   - Hirsutism alone usually points to conditions like polycystic ovarian syndrome or Cushing disease.
   - Virilization, on the other hand, is almost always due to sertoli-leydig cell tumors or androgen-producing adrenal tumors.

3. What is the key way of distinguishing Sertoli-Leydig cell tumors from polycystic ovarian syndrome?

   - **Sertoli-leydig cell tumors will cause markedly elevated testosterone levels, whereas polycystic ovarian syndrome leads to only mildly elevated testosterone levels.**
   - **Sertoli-leydig cell tumors will cause rapid-onset virilization, usually within a year of onset, whereas polycystic ovarian syndrome will not cause virilization at all.**
   - Both sertoli-leydig cell tumors and polycystic ovarian syndrome may lead to hirsutism in affected women.

REVIEW QUESTIONS

4. A 63-year-old woman comes to her primary care physician because of abnormal menstrual bleeding for the past 2 weeks. She says she underwent menopause in her early 50s. Review of systems shows bloating and early satiety. Abdominal examination shows a mass in the right adnexa and a positive fluid wave test. Pelvic ultrasound shows a 7 cm adnexal mass and ascites. Laboratory evaluation is as follows:

   A. Estradiol
   41 pg/mL (< 10 pg/mL)
   B. Testosterone
   20 ng/dL (15 - 70 ng/dL)
   C. LDH
   65 IU/L (48 - 115 IU/L)
   D. hCG
   0 ng/mL (0 ng/mL)
   E. AFP
   3 ng/mL (< 15 ng/mL)
   F. CA-125
   G. 21 U/mL (0 - 35 U/mL)

   Which of the following is the most likely diagnosis?

   H. Granulosa cell tumor
   I. Sertoli-Leydig cell tumor
   J. Mature cystic teratoma
   K. Choriocarcinoma
   L. Dysgerminoma
   M. Serous cystadenocarcinoma

- **The correct answer is option A.**
- This 63-year-old postmenopausal woman presents with abnormal menstrual bleeding and abdominal bloating associated with early satiety.
- Abdominal examination shows a mass in the right adnexa and a positive fluid wave test.
- Pelvic ultrasound shows a 7 cm adnexal mass and confirms the presence of ascites, which, along with her symptoms, is suspicious for ovarian cancer.
- Looking through the labs, estradiol is the only lab value that stands out as abnormal, elevated above its reference range in this postmenopausal woman.
- Therefore, the most likely diagnosis is a granulosa cell tumor which secretes estrogen. Note that levels of inhibin would also be high as its secreted by granulosa cells and is a marker for this type of tumor.
- Option B is incorrect because sertoli-leydig cell tumors present with signs of virilization and markedly elevated testosterone levels, neither of which is the case in this patient.
- Option C is incorrect because mature cystic teratomas do not cause elevations of estradiol or any other tumor markers. Typically, these tumors are recognized by their characteristic appearance on ultrasound, which usually reveals a complex cyst with internal calcifications.
- Option D is incorrect because choriocarcinoma causes elevated levels of hCG, not estradiol. Additionally, it occurs more commonly following hydatidiform moles, spontaneous abortions, or normal pregnancies. This woman doesn't have a recent history of any of those events.
- Option E is incorrect because dysgerminomas cause elevated levels of LDH, not estradiol.
- Option F is incorrect because serous cystadenocarcinoma is a type of surface epithelial tumor that leads to elevated levels of CA-125, not estradiol.

Gynecology | Section 31: Ovarian Neoplasms - Introduction and Surface Epithelial Tumors

I. Ovarian Neoplasms: Definition
   A. Neoplastic ovarian growths that arise from one of these components:
      1. Surface epithelium (most common)
      2. Germ cells
      3. Sex cord-stroma
   B. Most ovarian neoplasms are benign

II. Ovarian Neoplasms: Risk Factors
   A. Long-term uninterrupted ovulation (e.g. old age, nulliparity, infertility)
   B. Obesity (BMI > 30)
   C. Endometriosis
   D. Hormone replacement therapy
   E. Genetic syndromes (e.g. BRCA1/2 mutations, Lynch syndrome)
   F. Family history of breast and/or ovarian cancer
   G. Personal history of breast cancer

III. Ovarian Neoplasms: Protective Factors
   A. OCPs (> 5 years)
   B. Multiparity
   C. Breastfeeding
   D. Tubal ligation
   E. Hysterectomy

IV. Ovarian Neoplasms: Clinical Features
   A. Early disease is mostly asymptomatic
   B. As the disease progresses, patients progressively develop:
      1. Nonspecific gastrointestinal symptoms (e.g. bloating, early satiety)
      2. Urinary symptoms (e.g. dysuria, pelvic pressure)
      3. Menstrual changes
      4. Ascites
   C. Pelvic mass may or may not be present on physical examination

V. Ovarian Neoplasms: Diagnosis
   A. There are no effective screening modalities
   B. History and physical examination
   C. Ultrasound is the first-line imaging modality
      1. Benign features: small, cystic mass with no solid components or septations
      2. Malignant features: large mass with solid components or septations
   D. Tumor markers (e.g. CA-125, AFP)
   E. Advanced imaging (e.g. CT, MRI)
   F. Surgical staging (e.g. exploratory laparotomy)
   G. Avoid ovarian cyst aspiration or paracentesis of ascites

VI. Ovarian Neoplasms: Management
   A. Surgical excision
   B. Chemotherapy
   C. Radiation therapy

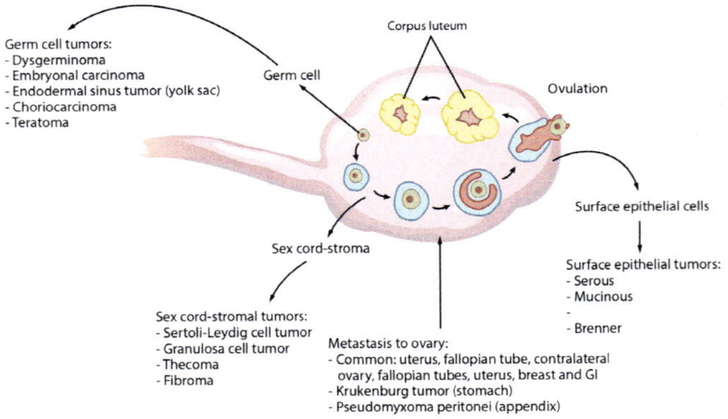

FIGURE 17.2.115 - Ovarian Neoplasms

VII. Surface Epithelial Tumors
   A. Neoplastic growth of epithelial cells within ovaries or fallopian tubes
   B. Most common type of ovarian neoplasms
      1. Serous cystadenocarcinomas are the most common subtype
   C. Present mostly in older women
   D. Notable findings on histopathologic examination
      1. Serous epithelial tumors: psammoma bodies
      2. Brenner tumors: urothelium, coffee bean nuclei
   E. Surgery is the mainstay of treatment, often with adjuvant chemotherapy
   F. Track treatment response and monitor for recurrence using CA-125 and CT scans

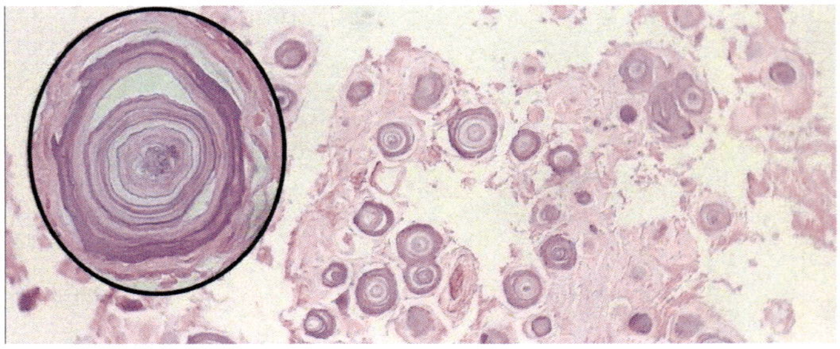

FIGURE 17.2.122 - Light Microscopy: Psammoma Bodies in Serous Epithelial Tumors

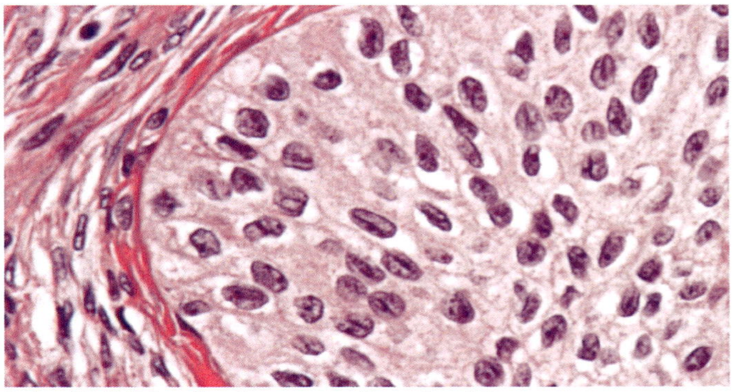

FIGURE 17.2.123 - Light Microscopy: Coffee Bean Nuclei in Brenner Tumors

REVIEW QUESTIONS

1. A 78-yar-old G4P4 woman comes to her primary care physician because of bloating and abdominal enlargement, as well as a 10 kg weight loss over the last 2 months. Her last menstrual period was at the age of 60. Before the birth of her children, she was on birth control. She breastfed all of her children. Her vital signs include a temperature of 96.8° F (36° C), blood pressure of 130/80 mmHg, heart rate of 82 beats/min, and respiratory rate of 16 breaths/min. Physical examination shows left lower quadrant tenderness. Pelvic ultrasound shows a large left ovarian mass with internal septations and solid components. Which of the following most likely predisposed this patient to her current condition?

    A. Multiparity
    B. Breastfeeding
    C. Oral contraceptive use
    D. Age at menopause

- **The correct answer is option D.**
- This multiparous woman presents with bloating, abdominal enlargement, and 10 kg weight loss over the last 2 months.
- Pelvic ultrasound shows a large left ovarian mass with internal septations and solid components.
- This description is consistent with surface epithelial ovarian tumor.
- Her last menstrual period was at the age of 60.
- This can be considered late menopause because women typically undergo menopause around the age of 50.
- Late menopause increases the total amount of ovulation cycles in her lifetime, predisposing her ovarian epithelium to abnormal repair and malignancy.
- Therefore, age at menopause most likely predisposed this patient to ovarian cancer.
- Option A is incorrect because multiparity is a protective factor against ovarian cancer. Multiple pregnancies decrease the overall amount of ovulation cycles.
- Option B is incorrect because breastfeeding is another protective factor against ovarian cancer. Increased prolactin during breastfeeding inhibits ovulation.
- Option C is incorrect because oral contraceptive use is also a protective factor as it inhibits ovulation.

Gynecology | Section 32: Cancer of the Fallopian Tubes

I. Cancer of the Fallopian Tubes: Definition
   A. Neoplastic proliferation of cells within the fallopian tubes of the uterus
   B. Extremely rare

II. Cancer of the Fallopian Tubes: Pathophysiology
   A. Adenocarcinomas are the most common type Cancer of the Fallopian Tubes: Risk Factors
   B. Caucasian women
   C. Nulliparity
   D. Infertility
   E. Genetic syndromes (e.g. BRCA1/2 mutations)

III. Cancer of the Fallopian Tubes: Clinical Features
   A. Asymptomatic
   B. Latzko triad (pathognomonic)
      1. Pelvic mass
      2. Pelvic pain
      3. Profuse watery discharge
   C. Hydrops tubae profluens (pathognomonic)
      1. Colicky abdominal pain due to intermittent hydrosalpinx

IV. Cancer of the Fallopian Tubes: Diagnosis
   A. Most cases are diagnosed incidentally during surgery for other purposes
   B. Ultrasound: complex adnexal mass, ascites
   C. Elevated CA-125

V. Cancer of the Fallopian Tubes: Management
   A. Surgery (e.g. hysterectomy)
   B. Adjuvant chemotherapy

REVIEW QUESTIONS ?

1. A 57-year-old woman comes to her primary care physician because of left lower abdominal pain for the last 2 weeks. Physical examination shows abdominal ascites. A pelvic ultrasound is performed and shows a complex mass in the left fallopian tube. She is later diagnosed with fallopian tube cancer. What is the most common histological type of this patient's malignancy?

- **The most common histological type of this patient's malignancy is adenocarcinoma.**
- This woman presents with left lower abdominal pain and is found to have abdominal ascites.
- Pelvic ultrasound shows a complex mass in the left fallopian tube.
- She is eventually diagnosed with fallopian tube cancer.
- The most common histological type of fallopian tube cancer is adenocarcinoma.

REVIEW QUESTIONS ?

2. A 75-year-old G0P0 Caucasian woman comes to her primary care physician because of intermittent, colicky left abdominal pain for the past 2 weeks. She has bowel movements every other day. She noticed a left lower abdominal mass and also mentions she has had intermittent watery vaginal discharge. Vital signs include a temperature of (98.6° F (37° C), blood pressure of 145/90 mmHg, heart rate of 86 beats/min, and respiratory rate of 15 breaths/min. Physical examination shows abdominal ascites and a left adnexal mass. Laboratory findings are significant for elevated CA-125. Which of the following is the next best step in the diagnosis of this patient?

   A. Pelvic ultrasound
   B. Pelvic ultrasound with biopsy
   C. Abdominal X-ray
   D. Complete blood count

- **The correct answer is option A.**
- This nulliparous Caucasian woman presents with intermittent, colicky left abdominal pain, intermittent watery discharge and is found to have a left adnexal mass.
- These three findings constitute the Latzko triad, pathognomonic for fallopian tube cancer.
- Intermittent colicky abdominal pain is most likely due to hydrops tubae profluens, that is, episodic hydrosalpinx due to fallopian tube cancer.
- Elevated CA-125 further suggests fallopian tube cancer.
- The best next step in the diagnosis is pelvic ultrasound to further characterize the mas.
- Option B, pelvic ultrasound with biopsy, is incorrect because biopsy is avoided in reproductive tract malignancies as the risk of peritoneal seeding and metastasis is high with percutaneous biopsy.
- Option C is incorrect because abdominal X-ray is not sensitive enough to detect fallopian tube cancer.
- Option D is incorrect because complete blood count is too general of a test and will ultimately not help much with the diagnosis of fallopian tube cancer.

Gynecology | Section 33: Benign Trophoblastic Disease

I. Complete Molar Pregnancy: Definition
   A. Abnormal proliferation of syncytiotrophoblasts
   B. Replacement of normal placental tissue with trophoblastic tissue by hydropic placental villi
   C. Also known as a complete hydatidiform mole

II. Complete Molar Pregnancy: Pathophysiology
   A. Fertilization of empty ovum
      1. One haploid sperm that duplicates
      2. Two sperm (rare)
   B. Karyotype: 46 chromosomes, typically XX
   C. Trophoblastic proliferation associated with swelling of chorionic villi

III. Complete Molar Pregnancy: Risk Factors
   A. Extremes of age (young teens or advanced maternal age)
   B. Prior history of GTD
   C. History of spontaneous abortion
   D. Infertility
   E. Nulliparity
   F. Smoking
   G. Nutritional deficiencies: folate, beta carotene, animal fat

IV. Complete Molar Pregnancy: Clinical Presentation
   A. Vaginal bleeding in early pregnancy
   B. Uterus larger than expected for dates
   C. Excessive nausea/vomiting (hyperemesis gravidarum)
   D. Preeclampsia prior to 20 weeks
   E. Hyperthyroidism
   F. Theca lutein cysts
   G. Many clinical features secondary to the structure of β-hCG
      1. Moles associated with increased β-hCG due to proliferation of syncytiotrophoblasts
      2. β-hCG beta subunit is analogous to subunits in LH, FSH, TSH
      3. Results in hyperthyroidism, theca lutein cysts, hyperemesis

V. Complete Molar Pregnancy: Diagnosis
   A. Quantitative β-hCG
      1. Typically > 100,000 mIU/mL
   B. Ultrasound
      1. "Snowstorm appearance"
      2. No fetal parts or heart tones
      3. No amniotic fluid
      4. May see bilateral theca lutein cysts
   C. If presenting late, may see passage of grape-like molar clusters
   D. CBC, type and screen, coagulation studies
   E. TSH, CMP (for liver and renal function)
   F. CXR if patient complains of any pulmonary symptoms
   G. Pathologic examination after tissue removal
   H. Immunohistochemical stain: p57 negative

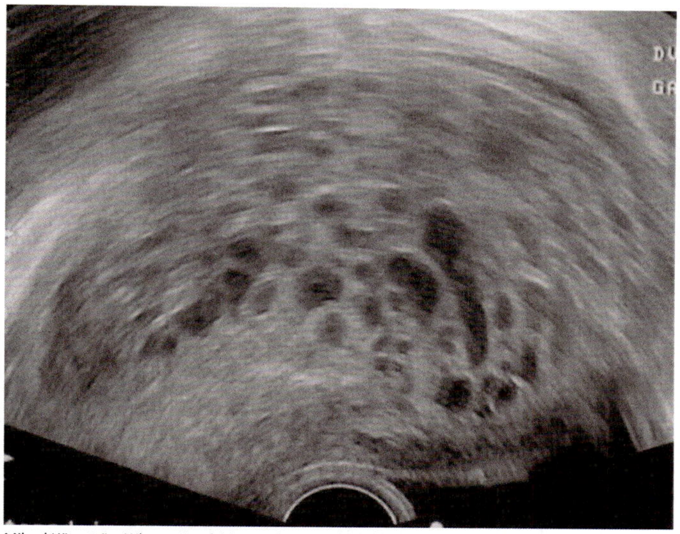

FIGURE 17.2.124 - Ultrasonogram: "Snowstorm" or "Swiss Cheese" Appearance in Complete Hydatidiform Mole

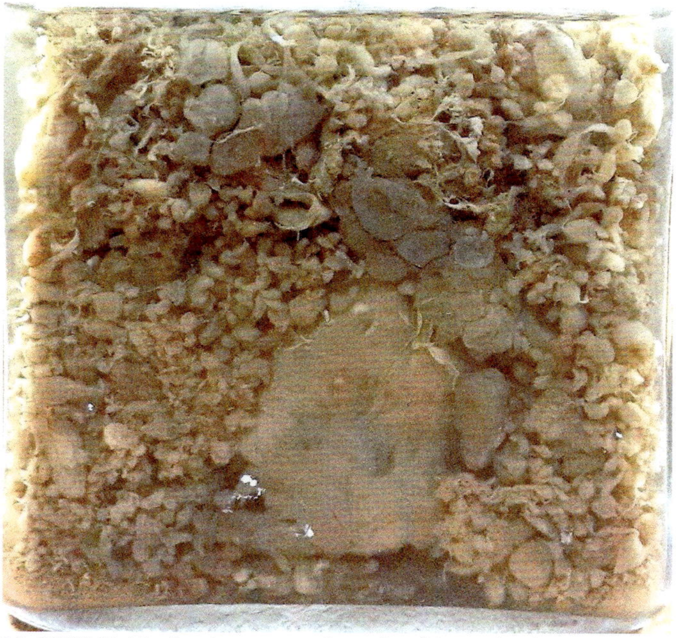

FIGURE 17.2.125 - Hydropic Villi in Complete Hydatidiform Mole

VI. Complete Molar Pregnancy: Management
   A. Dilation and suction curettage
      1. Uterotonic after evacuation
      2. Blood transfusion if needed
      3. RhoGAM if Rh-
   B. Hysterectomy if patient is done with childbearing
   C. Theca lutein cysts typically regress after D&C
   D. Treat medical complications of the molar pregnancy
      1. Antihypertensives

2. Beta-blockers if patient is hyperthyroid

E. Monitor serial β-hCGs

1. Weekly until negative for three weeks, then monthly for three months

F. Prevent pregnancy with reliable contraception

VII. Partial Molar Pregnancy: Definition

A. Abnormal chorionic villi with trophoblastic hyperplasia following aberrant fertilization

B. Also known as partial hydatidiform mole

VIII. Partial Molar Pregnancy: Pathophysiology

A. Fertilization of normal ovum by 2 sperm

B. Karyotype: triploid (69 chromosomes)

C. Hyperplasia of trophoblastic tissue

1. Primarily cytotrophoblasts

IX. Partial Molar Pregnancy: Risk Factors

A. Extremes of maternal age

B. Prior molar pregnancy

C. Prior spontaneous abortion

D. Infertility

X. Partial Molar Pregnancy: Clinical Presentation

A. Delayed menses and pregnancy diagnosis

B. Vaginal bleeding in early pregnancy

C. Uterus small or appropriate for gestational age

D. May result in spontaneous abortion

E. Symptoms related to excessive β-hCG are rare

1. Theca lutein cysts, early preeclampsia, hyperthyroidism

XI. Partial Molar Pregnancy: Diagnosis

A. Quantitative β-hCG (may be normal)

B. Ultrasound

1. Abnormally formed fetus or fetal parts

2. May have heart tones

3. IUGR

C. Pathologic examination of tissue after removal

D. Immunohistochemical staining: p57 positive

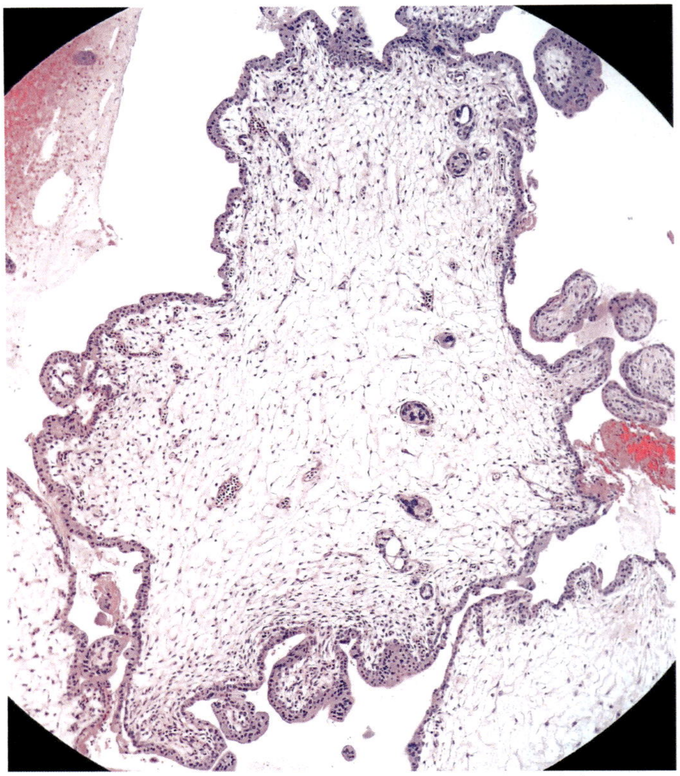

FIGURE 17.2.126 - Light Microscopy: Hydropic Villi in Partial Hydatidiform Mole

XII. Partial Molar Pregnancy: Management

A. Monitor β-hCG levels and ultrasound until normal pregnancy can be ruled out

B. Dilation and suction curettage

C. Monitor serial hCGs

1. Weekly until negative for three weeks, then monthly for three months

D. Provide reliable contraception

Condition	Etiology	Key Features
Complete mole	- Aberrant fertilization of an empty ovum by a sperm that duplicates, or by two sperm	- 46 chromosomes - Vaginal bleeding, uterus large for expected dates - Symptoms related to elevated b-hCG: hyperemesis, early preeclampsia, theca lutein cysts, hyperthyroidism
Partial mole	- Aberrant fertilization of a normal ovum by two sperm	- Triploid karyotype (69 chromosomes) - May have fetal parts or fetal heart tones on ultrasound - May present as a spontaneous abortion

TABLE 17.2.23 - Benign Trophoblastic Disease

REVIEW QUESTIONS

1. A 15-year-old G1P0 girl comes to her primary care physician at 7 weeks of gestation because of severe nausea and vomiting for the last 5 weeks. She has not been able to tolerate keeping anything down. She used to weigh 154 lbs before pregnancy and now weighs 127 lbs. She has also experienced intermittent vaginal bleeding recently. Physical examination shows a fundal height of 15 cm, and transabdominal ultrasound reveals the absence of a fetus. What additional finding(s) will be found on ultrasound assessment?
   - **The ultrasound assessment of this will show a "snowstorm" appearance.**
   - This 15-year-old girl presents with severe nausea and vomiting associated with significant weight loss.
   - This is consistent with hyperemesis gravidarum.
   - She also has had intermittent vaginal bleeding, and physical examination shows a fundal height inappropriately large for gestational age.
   - Transabdominal ultrasound reveals the absence of a fetus.
   - All of these findings should raise suspicion for a complete mole.
   - An additional ultrasound finding in a complete mole is the "snowstorm" appearance caused by cystic swelling of the chorionic villi.

2. A 21-year-old G3P0 woman comes to her primary care physician at 5 weeks of gestation because of intermittent vaginal bleeding. She has had two prior spontaneous abortions. Her beta-hCG is 50,000 mIU/mL (18 - 7,340 mIU/mL). A transabdominal ultrasound shows a fetal trunk but no head or extremities. Some villi look normal, while others look swollen. What is the best next step in management?
   - **The best next step in management is dilation and suction curettage.**
   - This patient presents with intermittent vaginal bleeding and extremely high beta-hCG concerning for a mole.
   - A transabdominal ultrasound shows a fetal trunk without other extremities. On US some villi look normal while others look swollen, which is a classic presentation of a partial mole.
   - Dilation and suction curettage is performed to to remove the abnormal tissue responsible for all of the clinical manifestations.

Gynecology | Section 34: Malignant Trophoblastic Disease

I. Invasive Molar Pregnancy: Definition
- A. Presence of large hydropic villi and trophoblast proliferation invading the myometrium

II. Invasive Molar Pregnancy: Pathophysiology
- A. Usually follows evacuation of molar pregnancy
- B. Appears similar on histology to molar pregnancy

III. Invasive Molar Pregnancy: Risk Factors
- A. Prior molar pregnancy (especially complete mole)
- B. Advanced maternal age (> 40)
- C. Asian, African, or American Indian ancestry

IV. Invasive Molar Pregnancy: Clinical Presentation
- A. Plateauing or rising β-hCG during serial monitoring after evacuation of a molar pregnancy
- B. Usually asymptomatic
- C. May have abnormal uterine bleeding
- D. Large uterus for gestational age
- E. Theca lutein cysts
- F. Rarely metastasize and may spontaneously regress

V. Invasive Molar Pregnancy: Diagnosis
- A. Quantitative β-hCG
- B. Ultrasound
  1. Intrauterine masses with potential invasion of myometrium
  2. Doppler: high vascular flow

VI. Invasive Molar Pregnancy: Management
- A. Repeat dilation and suction curettage
  1. If β-hCG plateauing and no evidence of metastasis
- B. Responds well to single-agent chemotherapy
  1. Methotrexate
  2. Actinomycin D
- C. Monitor serial β-hCGs
- D. Provide reliable contraception

VII. Gestational Choriocarcinoma: Definition
- A. Malignant necrotizing tumor consisting of invasive, anaplastic trophoblastic tissue
- B. Can arise weeks to years after any type of pregnancy

VIII. Gestational Choriocarcinoma: Pathophysiology
- A. Pure epithelial tumor
- B. Invades uterine wall and vasculature
  1. Destroys uterine tissue
  2. May lead to necrosis and hemorrhage
- C. Hematogenous spread
- D. Histology: sheets of anaplastic cytotrophoblasts and syncytiotrophoblasts without chorionic villi

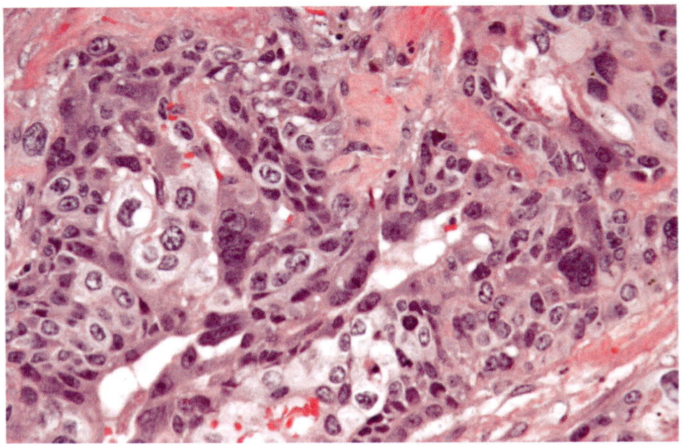

FIGURE 17.2.127 - Light Microscopy: Anaplastic Cytotrophoblasts and Syncytiotrophoblasts in Choriocarcinoma

IX. Gestational Choriocarcinoma: Risk Factors
- A. Prior molar pregnancy
- B. Advanced maternal age (> 40)
- C. More common in those of Asian, African, or American Indian ancestry

X. Gestational Choriocarcinoma: Clinical Presentation
- A. Can follow normal, molar, or ectopic pregnancy
- B. Late postpartum bleeding or AUB years after pregnancy
- C. Rapid hematogenous metastasis
- D. Symptoms of metastatic disease:
  1. Lungs: cough, dyspnea, hemoptysis, respiratory distress
  2. CNS: headache, dizziness, syncope
  3. Vaginal bleeding

XI. Gestational Choriocarcinoma: Diagnosis
- A. Quantitative β-hCG
- B. Ultrasound
  1. Uterine mass with hemorrhage and necrosis
  2. Doppler: highly vascular
- C. Chest X-ray or CT
- D. Abdomen and pelvis CT or MRI
- E. CT or MRI brain if lung or vaginal metastases present

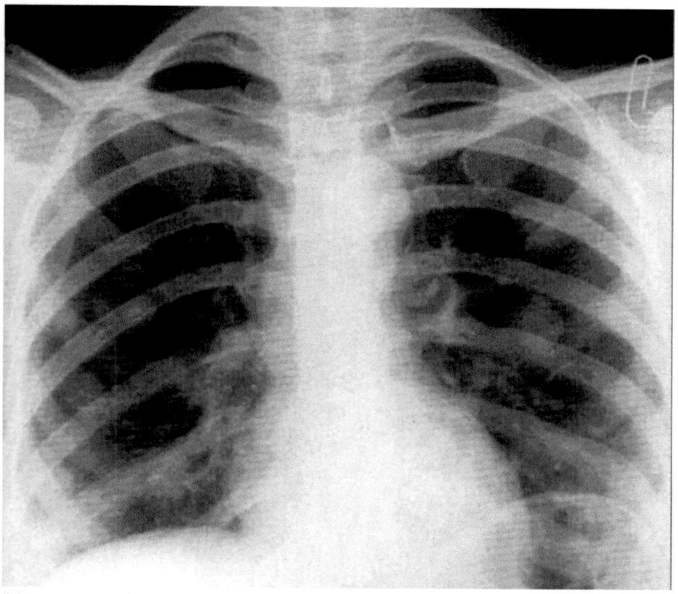

FIGURE 17.2.128 - Chest X-ray: "Cannonball" Lesions in Metastatic Choriocarcinoma

XII. Gestational Choriocarcinoma: Management
- A. Highly sensitive to chemotherapy
- B. Nonmetastatic disease
  - 1. Single-agent chemotherapy: methotrexate or actinomycin D
- C. Metastatic disease
  - 1. Combined chemotherapy
- D. Radiotherapy if there are brain metastases
- E. Serial β-hCG monitoring and reliable contraception

XIII. Placental Site Trophoblastic Tumors: Definition
- A. Intermediate cytotrophoblastic cells that invade locally at site of placental implantation
- B. Infiltrates the myometrium and invades blood vessels

XIV. Placental Site Trophoblastic Tumors: Pathophysiology
- A. Produces human placental lactogen
- B. Histology
  - 1. Absence of villi
  - 2. Proliferation of intermediate trophoblasts

XV. Placental Site Trophoblastic Tumors: Risk Factors
- A. Prior molar pregnancy
- B. Advanced maternal age (> 40)
- C. More common in those of Asian, African, or American Indian ancestry

XVI. Placental Site Trophoblastic Tumors: Clinical Presentation
- A. Irregular vaginal bleeding
- B. May have an enlarged uterus

XVII. Placental Site Trophoblastic Tumors: Diagnosis
- A. Serum human placental lactogen
- B. Ultrasound
  - 1. May see a mass with solid and cystic components
  - 2. Tumor can invade wall and surrounding tissues

XVIII. Placental Site Trophoblastic Tumors: Management
- A. Resistant to standard chemotherapy
- B. Hysterectomy is often curative

Condition	Etiology	Key Features
Invasive mole	- Trophoblastic proliferation that invades into the myometrium	- Typically follows evacuation of a molar pregnancy - Plateauing or rising b-hCG during serial monitoring - Responds well to chemotherapy
Choriocarcinoma	- Malignant necrotizing tumor of invasive, anaplastic trophoblastic tissue	- Can follow any type of pregnancy - Metastasizes quickly via a hematogenous route - Nonmetastatic responds well to single-agent chemotherapy
Placental site trophoblastic tumor	- Intermediate cytotrophoblastic cells that invade at the site of placental implantation	- Elevated human placental lactogen - Does not respond well to chemotherapy - Hysterectomy typically curative

TABLE 17.2.24 - Malignant Trophoblastic Disease

REVIEW QUESTIONS

1. A 40-year-old G3P3 woman comes to her primary care physician because of a cough and shortness of breath for the past month. She gave birth to a healthy baby girl 3 months ago. She also complains of intermittent vaginal bleeding. The patient has not resumed sexual activity. Her serum b-hCG level is 120,000 mIU/mL. What is the most likely diagnosis of this patient?

   - **The most likely diagnosis is metastatic choriocarcinoma.**
   - This patient presents with a cough and shortness of breath for the past month.
   - She gave birth to a healthy baby girl 3 months ago and now has been having intermittent vaginal bleeding.
   - Although she has not resumed sexual activity, making another pregnancy unlikely; she still has very high serum beta-hCG levels.
   - All of these findings are consistent with choriocarcinoma.
   - Cough and shortness of breath are highly concerning for pulmonary metastases of choriocarcinoma.

2. A 17-year-old G1P0 girl comes to her primary care physician at 9 weeks gestation because of intermittent vaginal bleeding. She has been experiencing excessive nausea and vomiting, heat intolerance, and a mild hand tremor. Vital signs include a temperature of 96.8° F (36° C), blood pressure of 155/100 mmHg, heart rate of 110 beats/min, and respiratory rate of 16 breaths/min. Physical examination shows a fundal height of 16 cm. Urinalysis shows 4+ proteinuria. A transabdominal ultrasound is significant for alternating regions of hyper and hypoechogenicity with no fetus. She is diagnosed with a complete molar pregnancy, and she undergoes dilation and suction curettage. What is the next best step in the management?

   A. Serial hCG monitoring
   B. Serial hCG monitoring with reliable contraception
   C. Single-agent chemotherapy
   D. Combined chemotherapy

   - **The correct answer is option B.**
   - This woman presents at 9 weeks gestation with intermittent vaginal bleeding and excessive nausea and vomiting concerning for hyperemesis gravidarum.
   - She also complains of heat intolerance and a mild hand tremor concerning for hyperthyroidism.
   - Her blood pressure is elevated, and she has significant proteinuria, consistent with preeclampsia.
   - Ultrasound shows hyper and hypoechogenity with no fetus diagnostic for a molar pregnancy.
   - She undergoes dilation and suction curettage. After this procedure, she should undergo serial hCG monitoring to monitor for the potential development of choriocarcinoma, and she should start a reliable contraception method to prevent pregnancy-induced hCG elevation.
   - Option A is incorrect because although serial hCG monitoring should be performed, the patient should also start a reliable contraception method to prevent hCG elevation by normal pregnancy.
   - Option C, single-agent chemotherapy, and option D, combined chemotherapy, are incorrect because they are used to treat choriocarcinoma, not the complete molar pregnancy.

Gynecology | Section 35: Benign Breast Diseases - Cysts, Fibrocystic Change & Mastitis

I. Cysts: Definition
   A. A closed fluid-filled sac
   B. Common, usually benign

II. Cysts: Types
   A. Simple cyst
      1. Has thin and regular lining
      2. Completely fluid-filled
   B. Complex cyst
      1. Has thick and irregular lining
      2. May contain solid content or debris

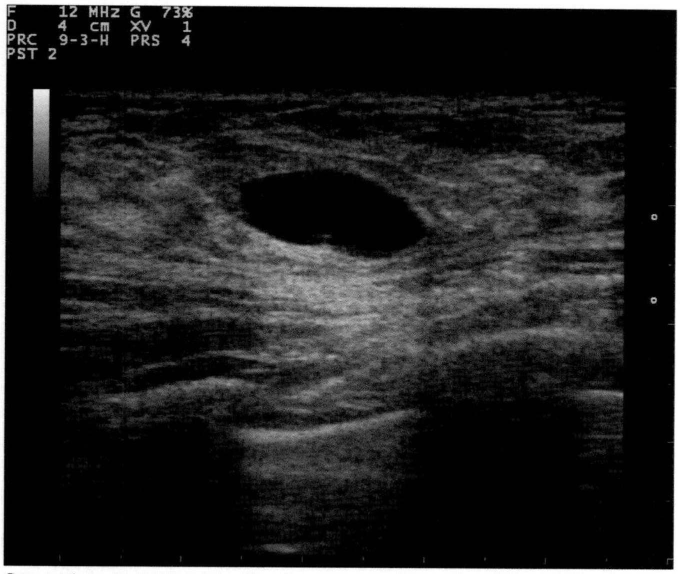

FIGURE 17.2.129 - Ultrasonogram: Simple Breast Cyst

III. Cysts: Clinical Features
   A. Asymptomatic
   B. Round, mobile mass; may be tender

IV. Fibrocystic Change: Definition
   A. Benign breast change characterized by fibrotic and cystic changes
   B. Most common benign lesion of the breast
   C. Unknown etiology
   D. Women age 20 - 50
   E. No increased risk of cancer

V. Fibrocystic Change: Clinical Features
   A. Cyclic, premenstrual, bilateral breast pain; improves after menstruation
   B. Breast nodules: multiple and diffuse; irregular breast consistency
   C. Nipple discharge

VI. Fibrocystic Change: Diagnosis
   A. Clinical diagnosis
   B. History and physical exam
      1. Bumpy, irregular breast
   C. Ultrasound and mammography are first line
      1. Ultrasound: women < 30 years; focal thickening +/- cysts
      2. Mammography: women ≥ 30 years
   D. Fine needle aspiration
      1. Indicated in case cysts are present on imaging, in symptomatic patients, and upon patients' request
      2. Relieves symptoms
   E. Biopsy: if the diagnosis is still not clear

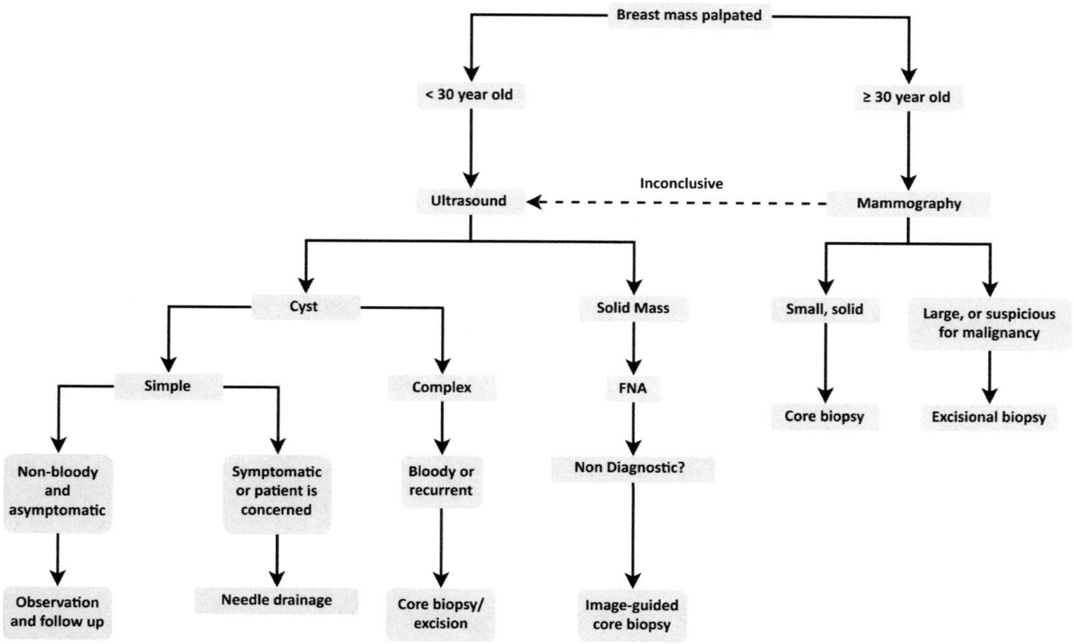

FIGURE 17.2.130 - Evaluation of Palpated Breast Mass

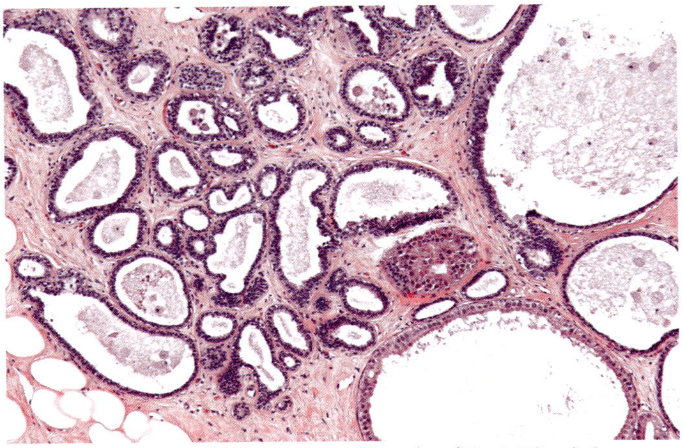

FIGURE 17.2.131 - Light Microscopy: Cystic Ducts and Fibrosis in Fibrocystic Breast Change

VII. Fibrocystic Change: Management
- A. Symptomatic treatment: NSAIDs, OCPs
- B. Cyst drainage (if present): fine needle aspiration
- C. Warm compresses may help
- D. Supportive bra
- E. Follow-up in 4 - 6 weeks

VIII. Mastitis: Definition
- A. Inflammation of the breast

IX. Mastitis: Pathophysiology
- A. Skin breakage and fissures allow entry of skin bacterial flora (most commonly *Staphylococcus aureus*) or from the mouth and nose of a breastfeeding infant → bacteria multiply → inflammation of milk ducts → decreased drainage and breast engorgement

X. Mastitis: Risk Factors
- A. History of mastitis
- B. Factors that impede milk drainage and/or increase breast engorgement (e.g. weaning, tight-fitting bra)

XI. Mastitis: Clinical Features
- A. Inflamed breast: tender, swollen, erythematous breast; usually unilateral
- B. Pain with breastfeeding
- C. Associated symptoms: fever, myalgias, chills, malaise
- D. Complications: breast abscess
- E. Breast abscess occurs as a result of severe or untreated mastitis
- F. Symptoms of breast abscess
    1. Mastitis symptoms (e.g. fever, tender and enlarged breast) in addition to a soft fluctuant breast mass
    2. Purulent nipple discharge

XII. Mastitis: Diagnosis
- A. Mastitis
    1. Clinical diagnosis
    2. Culture if treatment-resistant
- B. Breast abscess
    1. Clinical diagnosis; suspect in patients with mastitis that do not get better with treatment
    2. Ultrasound can also be used

XIII. Mastitis: Management
- A. Pain management (e.g. ibuprofen)
- B. Adequate and frequent breast draining
    1. Direct breastfeeding every 2 - 3 hours
    2. Use both breasts and alternate between them
    3. Breast pumps can be used as an alternative, although less effective
    4. Prevents progression to abscess
- C. Antibiotics
    1. Dicloxacillin or cephalexin (methicillin-sensitive *S. aureus*)
    2. Clindamycin, vancomycin, or TMP-SMX (methicillin-resistant *S. aureus*)
- D. Abscess
    1. Fine needle aspiration and antibiotics: dicloxacillin, cephalexin (first line)
    2. Incision and drainage: non-responsive, large (> 5 cm) abscess

XIV. Mastitis: Differential Diagnosis
- A. Normal breast engorgement
    1. Due to milk accumulation without adequate drainage
    2. During postpartum and early breastfeeding period (or anytime during breastfeeding): ↑ milk production
    3. Clinical diagnosis: tender, warm, enlarged breasts; usually bilaterally; no erythema or fever
    4. Management
        - a) Ensure proper nursing techniques
        - b) Frequent breastfeeding or pumping
        - c) Cool breast compresses
        - d) Analgesics (e.g. acetaminophen, NSAIDs)
        - e) Symptoms should improve after breast drainage

Condition	Key Features
Cysts	- Asymptomatic; round, mobile mass; may be tender
Fibrocystic changes	- Premenstrual cyclic bilateral breast pain; improves after menstruation - Breast nodules: multiple and diffuse; irregular breast consistency; nipple discharge
Mastitis	- Tender, swollen, erythematous breast; usually unilateral - Pain with breastfeeding, fever, myalgias, chills, malaise

TABLE 17.2.25 - Overview of Benign Breast Diseases

REVIEW QUESTIONS

1. A 28-year-old woman comes to her primary care physician because of a painful left breast mass she noticed one month ago. She appears well and has no fever, or chills. Breast examination shows a tender, well-circumscribed, mobile mass in the upper left quadrant. What is the next best step in management?
   - **The next best step in management is breast ultrasound.**
   - This 28-year-old woman presents with a palpable, tender, well-circumscribed, mobile mass in her left breast.
   - The next step in management depends on her age.
   - Since she is less than 30 years old, an ultrasound examination is indicated. A mammogram would be the answer if she were 30 years or older.

2. A 35-year-old woman comes to her primary care physician because of a painful, swollen right breast for the 3 days. She also reports having fevers and feeling tired over the past 2-days. She gave birth two weeks ago and is currently breastfeeding. Physical examination shows a tender, swollen, erythematous right breast. The left breast appears normal. What is the next best step in management?
   - **The next best step in management is antibiotics, adequate and frequent breast drainage, and NSAIDs.**
   - This breastfeeding woman comes in with a painful, swollen, and erythematous breast.
   - Breast engorgement and mastitis should be on the differential.
   - Because this patient is having a fever and feeling tired and only one breast is affected, mastitis is the most likely diagnosis.
   - In breast engorgement, no fever is present, and both breasts are usually affected.
   - The best next step for mastitis is prescribing an antibiotic such as dicloxacillin or cephalexin and advising the patient to continue breastfeeding from the affected breast to maintain proper breast drainage. NSAIDs can also be prescribed for pain management.

3. A 28-year-old woman comes to her primary care physician because of a breast mass that she palpated yesterday. She is otherwise asymptomatic and prefers non-invasive measures. She does not smoke or drink alcohol and has no history of serious illness. Physical examination shows a non-tender, mobile mass is palpated in the right upper quadrant of the right breast. There are no overlying skin changes. Her temperature is 99° F (37.3° C), pulse is 80/min, and blood pressure is 128/70 mmHg. An ultrasound of the mass shows a well-circumscribed, hypoechoic mass with a thin lining. Which of the following is the next best step in the management of this patient?

   A. Fine needle aspiration
   B. Reassurance and follow-up
   C. Core needle biopsy
   D. Excisional biopsy

   - **The correct answer is option B.**
   - This 28-year-old patient is presenting with a breast mass that she palpated yesterday.
   - Physical examination shows a non-tender, mobile mass is palpated in the right upper quadrant of the right breast.
   - On ultrasound, the mass appears well-circumscribed and hypoechoic with a thin lining consistent with a simple cyst.
   - Patients should be informed that this is a benign condition with no malignant potential, and therefore, the most appropriate management is reassurance and follow-up to monitor patients' symptoms.
   - If the patient is asymptomatic, only reassurance and follow-up are needed.
   - If, on the other hand, the patient remains concerned after counseling or is experiencing pain, fine needle aspiration could be performed.
   - Option A is incorrect because this patient is asymptomatic, is reassured, and wants no further treatment.
   - Option C, core needle biopsy, and option D, excisional biopsy, are incorrect because they are required in patients with masses that raise concern for malignancy. This patient is asymptomatic, with ultrasound findings showing a simple breast cyst.

Gynecology | Section 36: Benign Breast Diseases - Fat Necrosis, Galactocele & Mammary Duct Ectasia

I. Fat Necrosis: Definition
   A. Necrosis of fat tissue of the breast as a result of trauma or surgery
   B. Positive history is not always present
   C. No associated increased risk of carcinoma

II. Fat Necrosis: Clinical Features
   A. Presents as a fixed, irregular mass
   B. Associated skin changes: skin or nipple retraction, ecchymosis, erythema

III. Fat Necrosis: Diagnosis
   A. Ultrasound and mammography: hyperechoic mass; calcifications
   B. Biopsy
      1. Necrotic fat cells
      2. Foam cells and multinucleated giant cells

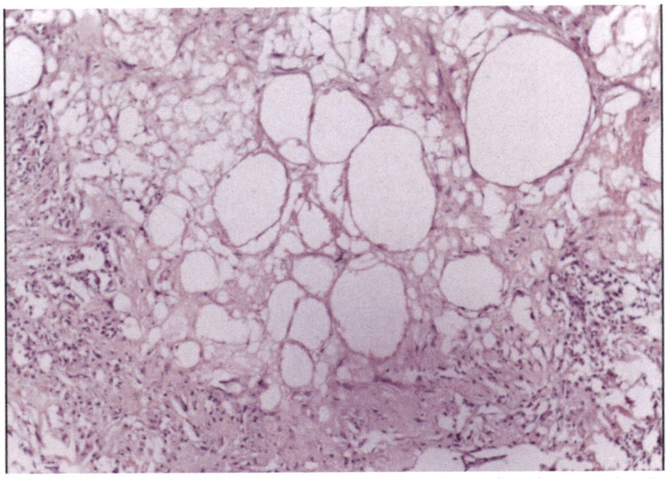

FIGURE 17.2.132 - Light Microscopy: Fat Necrosis of the Breast

IV. Fat Necrosis: Management
   A. Does not require treatment

V. Galactocele: Definition
   A. A cyst composed of accumulated breast milk
   B. During or after lactation
   C. No increased risk of carcinoma

VI. Galactocele: Pathophysiology
   A. Occurs as a result of obstruction of lactiferous ducts which causes stagnant milk accumulation and cyst formation

VII. Galactocele: Clinical Features
   A. Well-circumscribed mass; non-tender
   B. In the subareolar region
   C. If it gets infected will become painful

VIII. Galactocele: Diagnosis
   A. Clinical diagnosis
   B. Fine needle aspiration: milky
   C. Ultrasound: complex lesion

IX. Galactocele: Management
   A. Not needed
   B. Usually resolves spontaneously

X. Mammary Duct Ectasia: Definition
   A. Dilated mammary ducts causing inflammation and leading to clogged ducts
   B. Perimenopausal women (40 - 50 years)

XI. Mammary Duct Ectasia: Clinical Features
   A. Noncyclic breast pain
   B. Greenish-bloody nipple discharge; usually unilateral
   C. Other findings: nipple retraction, subareolar mass

XII. Mammry Duct Ectasia: Diagnosis
   A. Ultrasound or mammogram
   B. Excisional biopsy
      1. Rule out malignancy
      2. Obstruction of ducts and ductal inflammation

XIII. Mammary Duct Ectasia: Management
   A. Usually not required: improves without treatment
   B. Warm compresses and antibiotics: if it progresses to mastitis
   C. Local excision: definitive treatment; for persistent symptoms

Condition	Key Features
Fat necrosis	- Fixed, irregular mass - Nipple retraction, ecchymosis, erythema
Galactocele	- Well-circumscribed non-tender mass in the subareolar region
Mammary duct ectasia	- Noncyclic breast pain - Greenish-bloody nipple discharge

TABLE 17.2.26 - Overview of Benign Breast Diseases

REVIEW QUESTIONS

1. A 53-year-old woman comes to her primary care physician because of a mass that she felt in her breast. Physical examination shows a hard, non-tender mass in the upper outer quadrant of the right breast. She does not recall any trauma to the breast. She is a lifetime smoker and drinks alcohol occasionally. Mammography is ordered and shows an irregular breast mass with microcalcifications. Biopsy of the mass shows multinucleated giant cells and foam cells. What is the most likely diagnosis?

- **The most likely diagnosis is fat necrosis of the breast.**
- This 53-year-old woman presents with a mass in her right breast that is hard, nontender and located in the upper outer quadrant.
- Mammography shows an irregular breast mass with microcalcifications, which should raise suspicion for possible malignancy.
- A biopsy is then performed, showing multinucleated giant cells and foam cells, which is characteristic of fat necrosis and requires reassurance to the patient.
- Patients often do not recall trauma to the breast, but that still doesn't rule out the diagnosis.

2. A 27-year-old woman comes to her primary care physician because of mild discomfort in her left breast. She noticed a subareolar mass while taking a shower 2 days ago. The patient gave birth to a healthy neonate 1 week ago. She breastfeeds the baby every 2 - 3 hours. Vital signs include a temperature of 96.8° F (36° C), blood pressure of 110/70 mmHg, heart rate of 86 beats/min, and respiratory rate of 15 breaths/min. Physical examination shows a non-tender subareolar mass with no erythema or induration. An ultrasound shows a complex mass prompting fine needle aspiration. Aspiration yields white fluid. Which of the following is the best next step in the management?

   A. Mammography
   B. Core needle biopsy
   C. Dicloxacillin
   D. Reassurance

- **The correct answer is option D.**
- This 27-year-old woman presents with a subareolar mass that she noticed recently.
- She gave birth to a healthy neonate 1-week ago and breastfeeds the baby every 2 - 3 hours.
- Lactating women are at risk of developing mastitis or galactocele.
- Her temperature is 96.8° F (36° C), making mastitis unlikely.
- Additionally, the mass is non-tender with no erythema or induration. These clues also make mastitis unlikely.
- The fine needle aspiration yields white fluid. This confirms the diagnosis of a galactocele.
- Galactocele is a cyst with accumulated stagnant milk. It usually resolves spontaneously, so the patient needs reassurance.
- Options A and B are incorrect because mammography and core needle biopsy are necessary when there is high suspicion of breast cancer. This patient is young, and the fine needle aspiration yields white fluid, making breast cancer very unlikely.
- Option C is incorrect because dicloxacillin is used to treat acute mastitis. This patient is afebrile, and her subareolar mass is non-tender with no erythema or induration. This practically excludes mastitis.

Gynecology | Section 37: Gynecomastia

I. Gynecomastia: Definition
   A. Breast glandular tissue proliferation and enlargement
   B. Breast enlargement due to fat deposition alone is termed pseudogynecomastia

II. Gynecomastia: Pathophysiology
   A. Occurs either due to ↑ estrogen production or ↓ androgen production/sensitivity
   B. Imbalance of the net estrogen/testosterone leads to stimulation of breast glandular tissue to proliferate

III. Gynecomastia: Etiology
   A. Physiological causes
      1. Neonatal gynecomastia: transfer of maternal estrogens through the placenta; bilateral breasts; both genders affected; resolves within weeks-months
      2. Pubertal gynecomastia: adolescent boys; resolves by age 17; reassurance only
      3. Senile gynecomastia: age-related testosterone decrease
   B. Pathological causes
      1. ↑ estrogen: tumors (e.g. leydig and sertoli cell tumors), liver cirrhosis, hyperthyroidism/thyrotoxicosis, obesity
      2. ↓ testosterone: Klinefelter's, chronic kidney disease, hyperprolactinemia
      3. Drugs: spironolactone, ketoconazole, exogenous androgen use
   C. Idiopathic

IV. Gynecomastia: Clinical Features
   A. Concentric, rubbery mass under the nipple/areola
   B. May be tender; mostly in adolescents
   C. Symptoms of the underlying disease (e.g. liver or kidney disease)

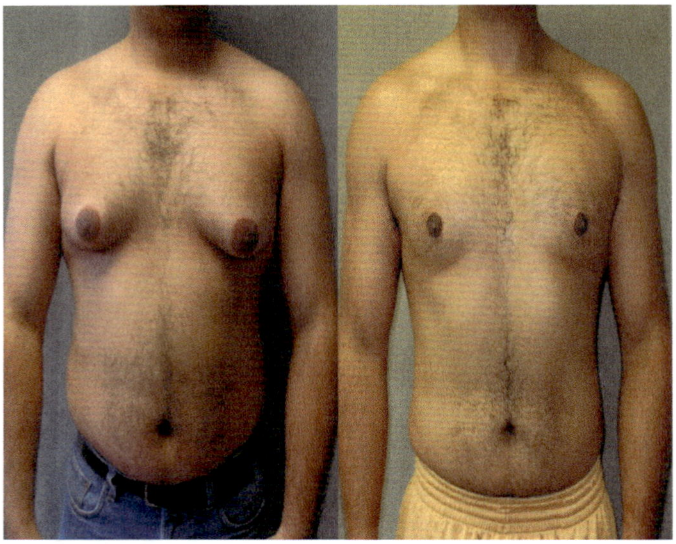

FIGURE 17.2.133 - Gynecomastia

V. Gynecomastia: Diagnosis
   A. History and physical exam
   B. Labs
      1. Serum testosterone, LH, hCG, estradiol
      2. Liver, kidney, and thyroid function tests
      3. Prolactin
   C. Imaging: ultrasound, mammography, and ultrasound-guided biopsy
   D. Look for underlying cause

VI. Gynecomastia: Management
   A. Patient discomfort and psychological distress must be minimized.
   B. Physiological gynecomastia: observation and follow-up
   C. Pathological gynecomastia: treatment of underlying cause (e.g. treat hyperthyroidism, stop the inducing drug)
   D. Estrogen-receptor modulators (SERMs)
   E. Testosterone replacement
   F. Mastectomy surgery

REVIEW QUESTIONS

?

1. A 25-year-old G1 P1 woman gave birth to a baby boy via spontaneous vaginal delivery 2 hours ago. Apgar scores were 8 and 10 at 1 and 5 minutes, respectively. She had regular prenatal care without any prenatal complications. Vital signs of the neonate include a temperature of 98.6° F (37° C), blood pressure of 70/50 mmHg, heart rate of 145 beats/min, and respiratory rate of 50 breaths/min. Physical examination shows bilateral breast enlargement. His mother is concerned about breast enlargement and asks if medical or surgical intervention is appropriate. Which of the following is the next best step in the management?

    A. Tamoxifen
    B. Anastrozole
    C. Surgery in 6 months
    D. Parental reassurance

- **The correct answer is option D.**
- This 2-hour-old infant had normal Apgar scores of 8 and 10 at 1 and 5 minutes, respectively.
- Vital signs are appropriate for a neonate.
- Physical examination of the infant reveals bilateral breast enlargement.
- His mother is concerned about breast enlargement and asks if medical or surgical intervention is appropriate.
- Neonatal gynecomastia is common in both genders and is caused by transplacental transfer of maternal estrogen during pregnancy. It is temporary because the neonate is no longer exposed to maternal estrogen after birth. Therefore, neonatal gynecomastia does not require any medical or surgical intervention. Only parental reassurance is indicated here.
- Options A, B, and C are incorrect because neither anti-estrogen therapy nor surgery is appropriate for neonatal gynecomastia.

Gynecology | Section 38: Breast Cancer Generalities

I. Breast Cancer: Clinical Features
   A. Depends on the stage
   B. Palpable non-tender lump; most common in upper outer quadrant
   C. Lymphadenopathy
   D. Associated skin changes: nipple inversion, skin dimpling/retraction

II. Breast Cancer: Workup
   A. Additional tests on diagnosed breast cancer
      1. Receptors: estrogen receptor (ER), progesterone receptor (PR), human epidermal growth factor receptor 2 (HER2/neu)
      2. Tumor markers: CEA
   B. Metastasis
      1. Imaging: chest X-ray, CT scan, brain MRI
      2. Lab: ↑ ALP, ↑ calcium

III. Breast Cancer: Management
   A. General approach
      1. Management depends on the TNM stage
      2. Treatment includes surgery, chemotherapy, radiotherapy, targeted therapy, and hormone treatment
   B. Surgery
      1. Breast conserving surgery: only cancerous breast tissue is removed
      2. Mastectomy (e.g. radical, double, total mastectomies)
   C. Radiation: post-surgery for patients at high risk of recurrence
   D. Chemotherapy
   E. Hormone therapy
      1. ER+ and PR+ tumors
      2. Tamoxifen, aromatase inhibitors, and raloxifene
   F. Targeted therapy
      1. Against HER2 receptors
      2. Trastuzumab
   G. Regarding contraception
      1. Hormonal contraception contraindicated; copper IUD is the contraceptive method of choice
   H. Prognostic factors: most important factor is nodal involvement
      1. Good prognostic factors: ER+ and PR+ tumors
      2. Poor prognostic factors: high tumor grade (poorly differentiated), HER2 overexpression

IV. Breast Cancer: Screening
   A. No family history of breast cancer: mammography starting ≥ 50 years
      1. 50 - 74 years: every 2 year
   B. Patients at high risk (e.g. BRCA gene, chest irradiation): start at 40
      1. First-degree relative: begin screening 10 years before the earliest diagnosis in the family

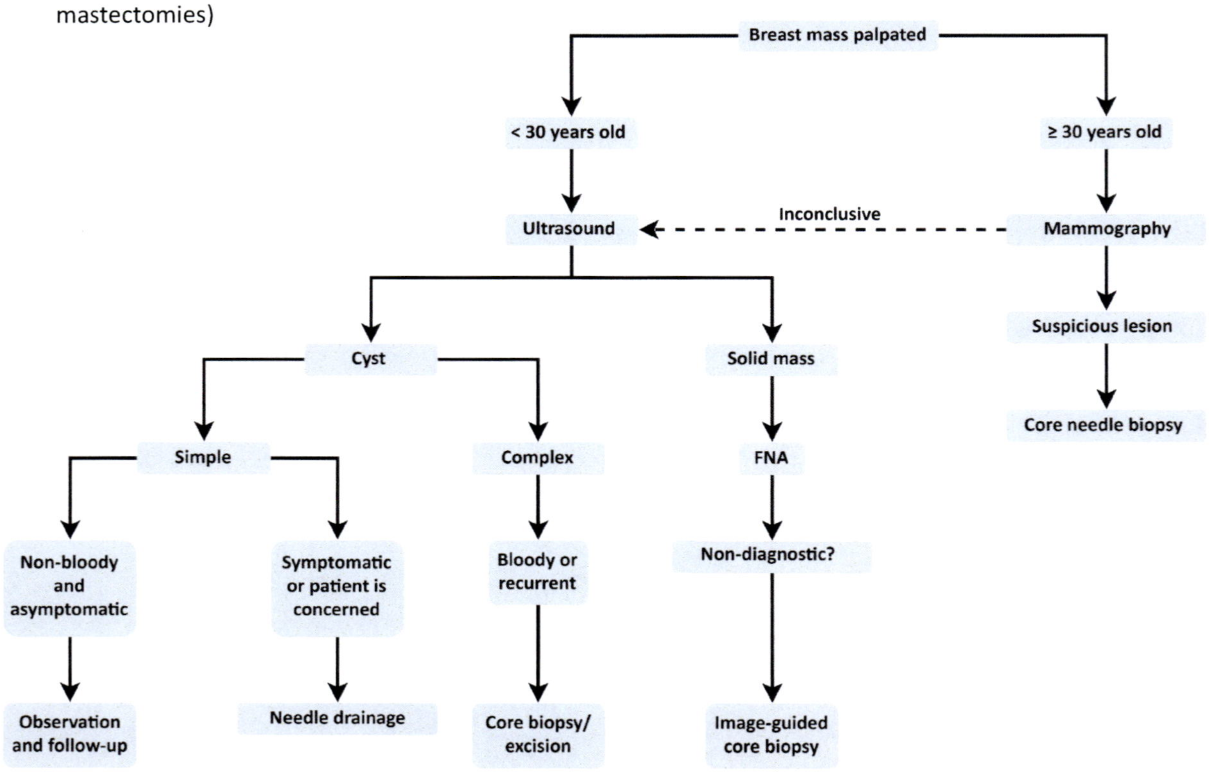

FIGURE 17.2.134 - Evaluation of Palpable Breast Mass

REVIEW QUESTIONS

1. A 54-year-old woman comes to the clinic for a routine screening mammogram. Mammography results show a suspicious 2.5 cm lesion in the right breast. Physical examination of the breast shows a hard, non-tender mass. There are no associated skin or nipple changes, and no lymphadenopathy is present. What is the best next step in the diagnosis?
    - **The best next step in the diagnosis of this patient is an ultrasound-guided core needle biopsy.**
    - This 54-year-old woman has a hard, non-tender mass in her right breast that appears suspicious on mammography.
    - The next best step is to perform an ultrasound-guided core needle biopsy to evaluate the mass histology to determine the diagnosis and determine its receptor profile for further management.
    - In this case, an excisional biopsy would be too invasive. It can be used if the core needle biopsy results are inconclusive.

2. A 2 cm suspicious lesion is detected on routine mammogram screening of a 47-year-old woman. Histology reveals poorly differentiated cells that show HER2 receptor overexpression. Sentinel lymph node biopsy reveals tumor infiltration. What factor has the most effect on the prognosis of this patient?
    - **The factor that has the most effect on the prognosis of this patient is lymph node involvement.**
    - This question presents multiple prognostic factors, including a high tumor grade, HER2 receptor overexpression, and sentinel node biopsy revealing tumor infiltration.
    - Even though a high tumor grade and HER2 receptor overexpression constitute a poor prognosis for this patient, axillary lymph node status is the most important prognostic factor as it makes metastatic spread much more likely.

Gynecology | Section 39: Benign Breast Neoplasms

I. Fibroadenoma: Definition
   A. Most common benign breast tumor in women, especially < 35 years
   B. Made of fibrous and glandular breast tissue

II. Fibroadenoma: Clinical Features
   A. Well-circumscribed, mobile breast mass
   B. Usually unilateral and solitary
   C. Hormone-sensitive tumor
      1. Cyclic premenstrual pain
      2. ↑ in size before menses

III. Fibroadenoma: Diagnosis
   A. History: ↑ in size prior to menses, during pregnancy, with OCP use
   B. Physical examination: rubbery, well-defined, mobile, non-tender mass
   C. Ultrasound/mammogram
   D. Fine needle aspiration

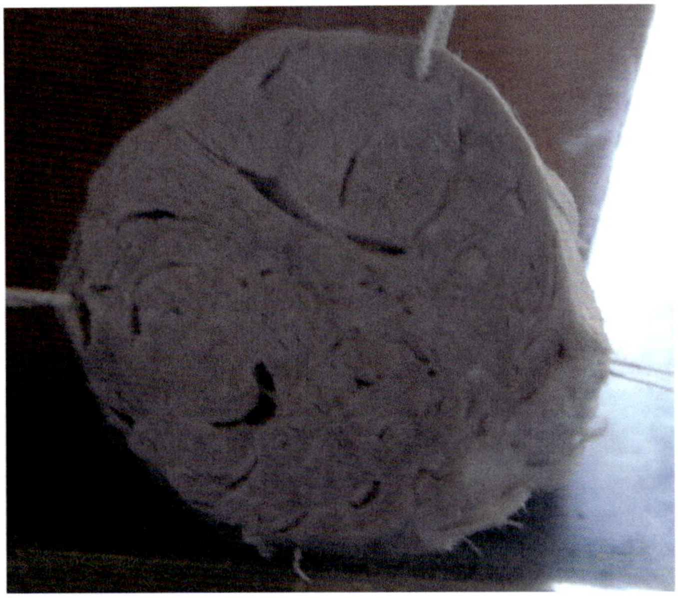

FIGURE 17.2.135 - Mammary Fibroadenoma

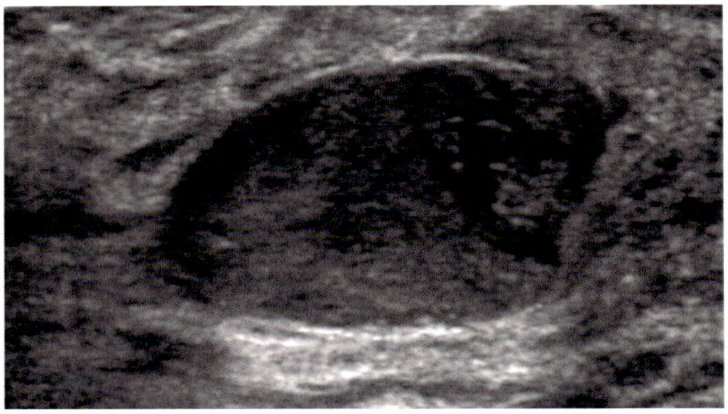

FIGURE 17.2.136 - Breast Ultrasound: Fibroadenoma 1

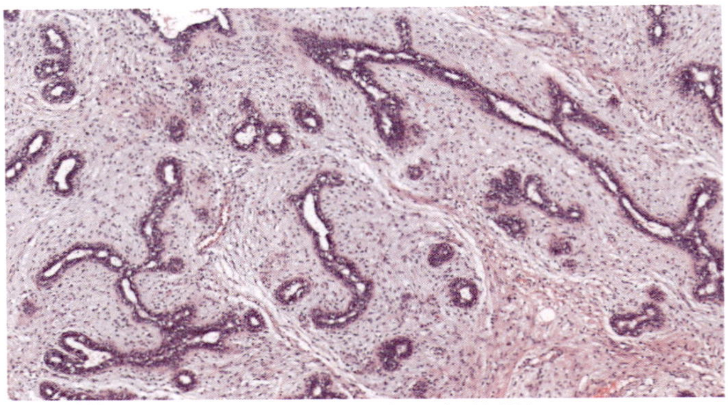

FIGURE 17.2.137 - Light Microscopy: "Slit-Like" Appearance in Fibroadenoma

IV. Fibroadenoma: Management
   A. Patients < 30 with classical presentation and no family history of breast cancer: observation and follow-up
   B. All other cases: fine needle aspiration to confirm fibroadenoma
      1. Asymptomatic patients: observation
      2. Symptomatic patients with large fibroadenoma or ↑ in size: excision

V. Phyllodes Tumor: Definition
   A. Rare variant of fibroadenoma with stromal and epithelial proliferations
   B. Also called "cystosarcoma phyllodes"
   C. Most commonly benign; small percentage malignant
   D. Premenopausal women

VI. Phyllodes Tumor: Clinical Features
   A. Lump: large, painless, smooth or multinodular, mobile; grows rapidly
   B. Overlying skin changes: erythematous, warm, shiny
   C. Engorged breast

VII. Phyllodes Tumor: Diagnosis
   A. Considered as "low-grade malignant" tumor
   B. Ultrasound/mammogram: similar to fibroadenoma, but larger, and rapidly growing
   C. Core-needle biopsy: pathological diagnosis must be established
      1. Stromal and epithelial proliferations
      2. Leaf-like papillary projections

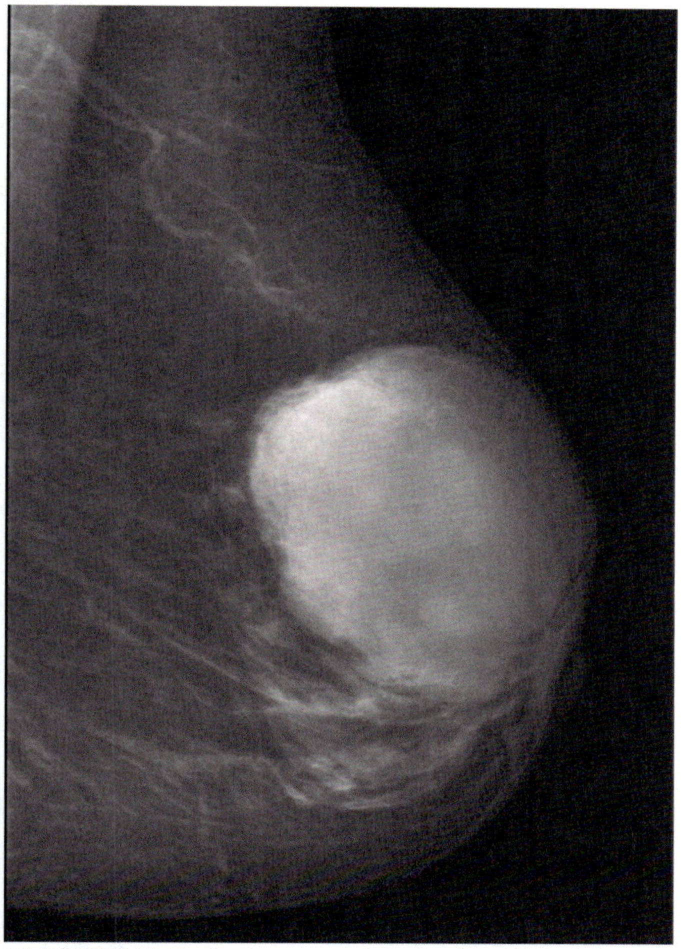

FIGURE 17.2.138 - Mammogram: Phyllodes Tumor

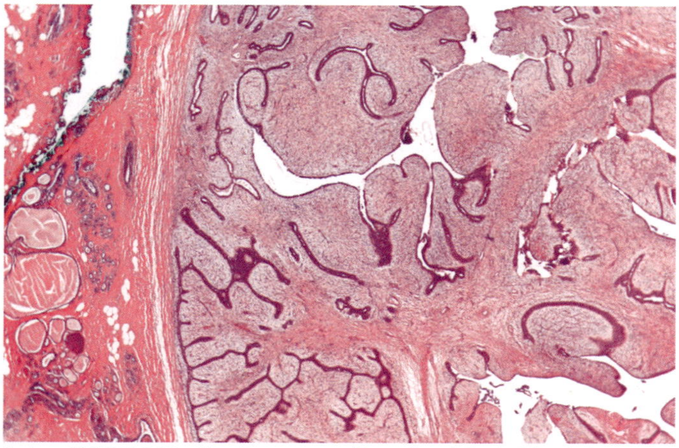

FIGURE 17.2.139 - Light Microscopy: "Leaf-Like" Papillary Projections in Phyllodes Tumor

VIII. Phyllodes Tumor: Management
- A. High rate of recurrence
- B. Allo tumors: local excision with wide margins
- C. Recurrent tumor: mastectomy
- D. Follow-up

IX. Intraductal Papilloma: Definition
- A. Benign epithelial growth from the lining of breast ducts
- B. Women in 40 - 50s

X. Intraductal Papilloma: Clinical Features
- A. Unilateral bloody nipple discharge
- B. Does not form a mass
- C. No associated lymphadenopathy

XI. Intraductal Papilloma: Diagnosis
- A. Cytology of bloody discharge: rule out malignancy
- B. Ultrasound and mammography: normal breast tissue, dilated breast duct
- C. Ductogram: visualizes ducts using contrast; detects small lesions
- D. Core-needle biopsy: if lesion is large or palpable; confirms the diagnosis

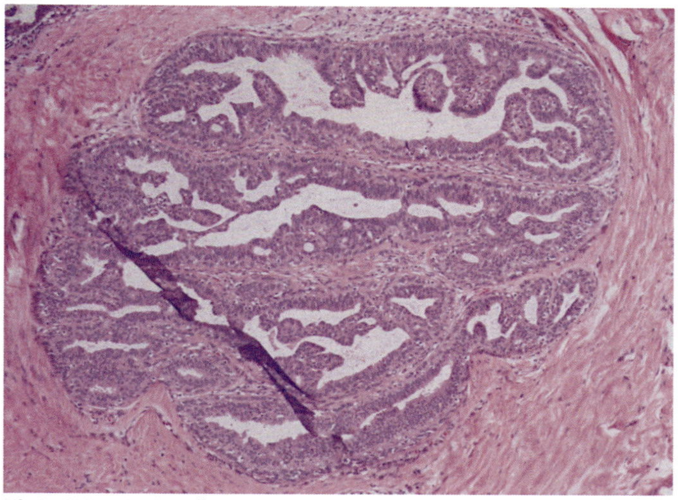

FIGURE 17.2.140 - Light Microscopy: "Finger-Like" Projections and Fibrovascular Core in Intraductal Papilloma

XII. Intraductal Papilloma: Management
- A. Benign condition
- B. Surgical excision: confirms the diagnosis and treats the condition

XIII. Lobular Carcinoma in Situ
- A. Epithelial cell proliferation in breast lobules without invasion of the wall
- B. Multicentric and bilateral
- C. Usually does not form a mass
- D. Increases the risk of invasive carcinoma; not considered malignant in itself
- E. Treatment
  1. Close observation and follow-up
  2. Prophylactic chemotherapy and SERMs (e.g. tamoxifen, raloxifene)
  3. Bilateral mastectomy

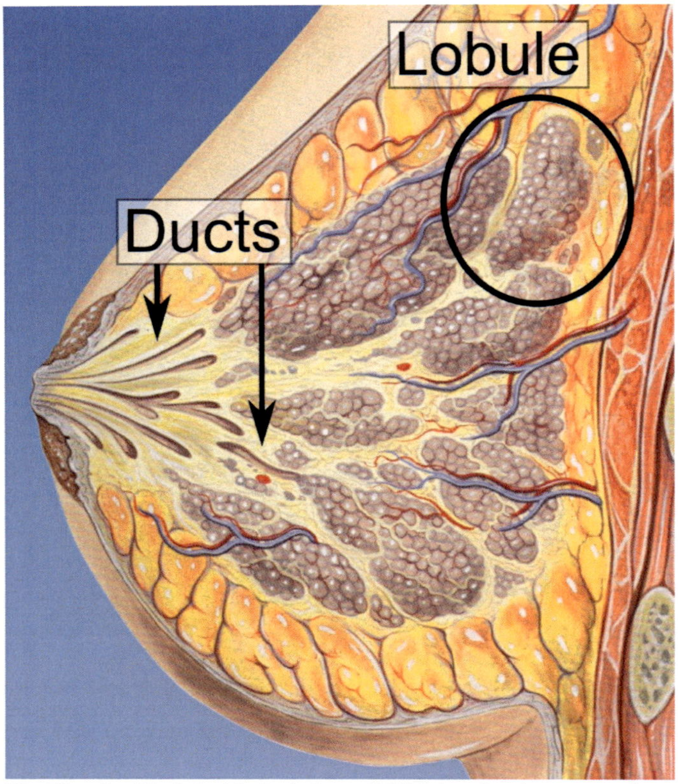

Mikael Häggström, M.D. - Author info - Reusing images, CC BY 2.5 <https://creativecommons.org/licenses/by/2.5>, via Wikimedia Commons

FIGURE 17.2.141 - Breast Ducts and Lobules

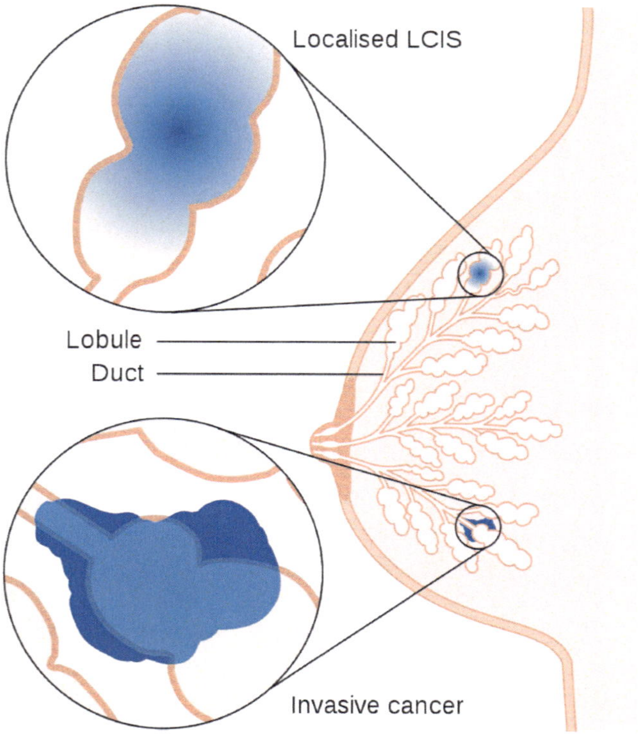

Cancer Research UK, CC BY-SA 4.0 <https://creativecommons.org/licenses/by-sa/4.0>, via Wikimedia Commons

FIGURE 17.2.142 - Lobular Carcinoma in Situ vs. Invasive Carcinoma

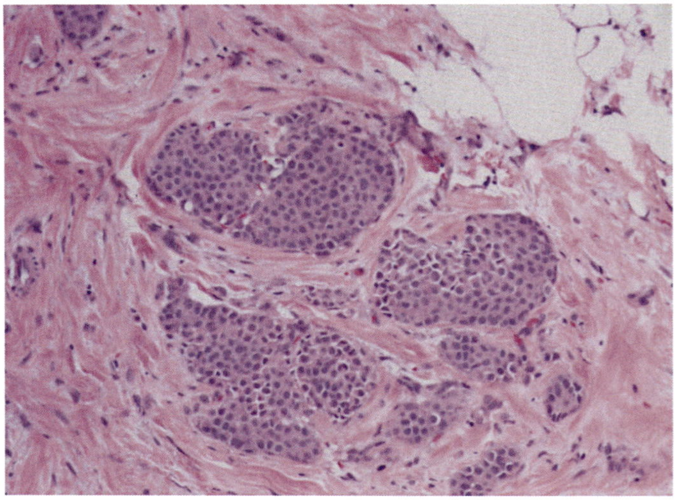

Difu Wu., CC BY-SA 3.0 <https://creativecommons.org/licenses/by-sa/3.0>, via Wikimedia Commons

FIGURE 17.2.143 - Light Microscopy: Lobular Carcinoma in Situ

REVIEW QUESTIONS

1. A 28-year-old woman comes to her primary care physician because of a mass in her left breast. Physical examination shows a non-tender, small (2.5 cm), rubbery, round, mobile mass. There is no lymphadenopathy. What is the best next step in the diagnosis?

   - **The best next step in the diagnosis of this patient is a breast ultrasound.**
   - This 28-year-old woman with a small left breast mass that is well-circumscribed, rubbery, round, mobile, and painless.
   - There is no lymphadenopathy.
   - This is a typical presentation of fibroadenoma, the most common benign tumor in women < 35 years.
   - The next step would be to evaluate the mass using ultrasound, which will likely show a well-defined hypoechogenic mass.
   - In contrast to fibroadenoma, phyllodes tumor is large, grows rapidly, and affects women in their 40s - 50s.

2. A 47-year-old woman comes to the gynecology office because of bloody discharge from her right nipple. She is premenopausal and has regular monthly menstrual cycles with no associated pain or bleeding abnormalities. Breast examination shows no masses bilaterally, but bloody discharge is expressed from the right nipple. Physical examination shows no lymphadenopathy. What is the best next step to rule out malignancy in this patient?

   A. Cytology of discharge
   B. Ultrasound
   C. Mammogram
   D. Serum estrogen level

   - **The correct answer is option A.**
   - This 47-year-old woman presents with a unilateral bloody nipple discharge.
   - Breast examination shows no masses, and the physical exam reveals no lymphadenopathy.
   - Unilateral bloody nipple discharge with no associated masses or lymphadenopathy is highly concerning for an intraductal papilloma.
   - The best way to rule out intraductal malignancies is to perform cytology on the discharge, looking for dysplasia.
   - Options B and C are incorrect because they would not confirm the diagnosis nor rule out malignancy.
   - Option D is incorrect because a serum estrogen level would reveal nothing about the nature of this breast pathology.

Gynecology | Section 40: Malignant Breast Neoplasms

I. Malignant Breast Neoplasms: General Information
  A. Most common malignancy after skin cancer in women
  B. 2nd leading cause of cancer-related death in the US
  C. Females > males
  D. Postmenopausal > premenopausal

II. Malignant Breast Neoplasms: Risk Factors
  A. Increasing age (≥ 65)
  B. Race: ↑ risk for European descent; African Americans (triple negative breast carcinoma)
  C. Family history of breast cancer or gynecological malignancies
  D. Genetic predisposition: BRCA1, BRCA2, Li-Fraumeni syndrome, Peutz-Jeghers syndrome
  E. Smoking, alcohol consumption
  F. Radiation to the chest
  G. Factors ↑ estrogen exposure
    1. Early menarche, late menopause
    2. Nulliparity, increased age at first birth
    3. Lack of breastfeeding
    4. Obesity
    5. Hormone replacement therapy
  H. Protective factors
    1. Breastfeeding
    2. Exercise
  I. OCPs do not decrease the risk of breast carcinoma

III. Malignant Breast Neoplasms: Types
  A. Non-invasive
    1. Ductal carcinoma in situ (DCIS)
    2. Paget's disease of the nipple
  B. Invasive
    1. Invasive ductal carcinoma
    2. Invasive lobular carcinoma
    3. Inflammatory breast cancer

IV. Ductal Carcinoma in Situ
  A. Malignant proliferation of ductal epithelial cells without invasion of the stroma
  B. More common than LCIS; high invasion potential
  C. Usually unilateral
  D. Mammography: clustered microcalcifications
  E. Biopsy
  F. Treatment
    1. Conservative: microcalcifications excision with wide margins
    2. Radical: mastectomy
    3. Radiation therapy

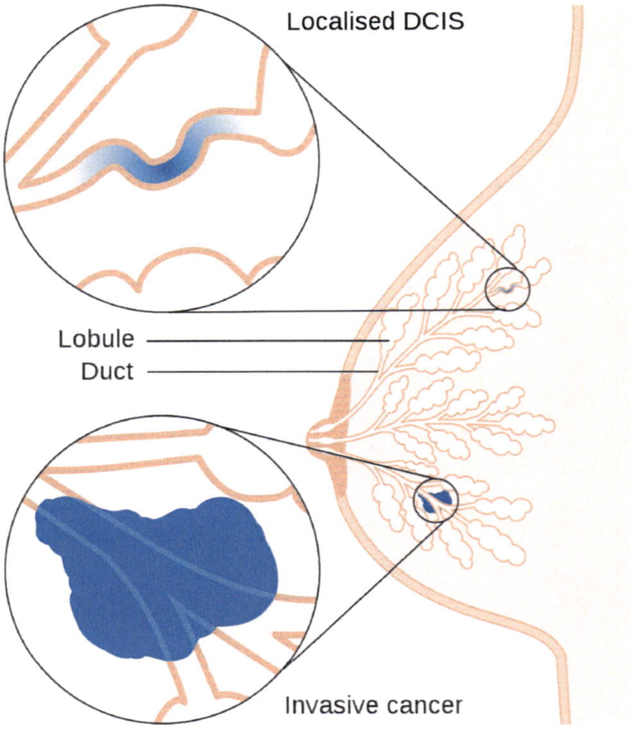

FIGURE 17.2.144 - Localized Ductal Carcinoma in Situ vs. Invasive Carcinoma

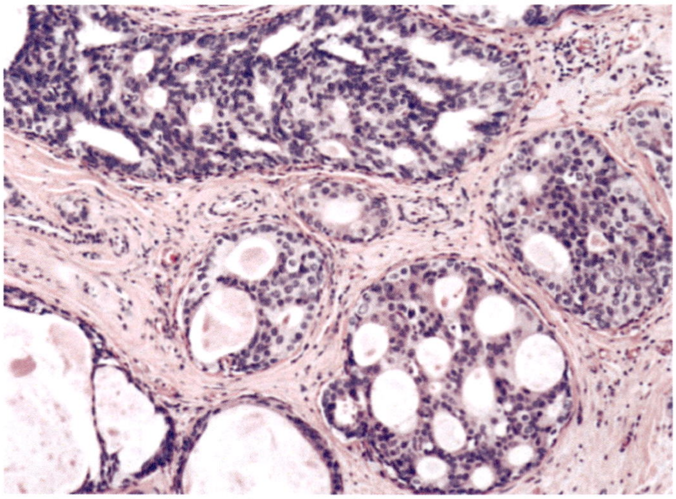

FIGURE 17.2.145 - Light Microscopy: Ductal Carcinoma in Situ

V. Paget Disease of the Nipple
   A. Rare type of breast cancer involving the skin of the nipple and areola
   B. Appears as eczematous lesion: scaling, erythema, crusting, erosions
   C. Associated with itching, bloody nipple discharge
   D. Most commonly associated with underlying breast cancer (DCIS, invasive carcinoma)
   E. Full thickness biopsy (punch biopsy)
      1. Adenocarcinoma
      2. Paget's cells
      3. Signs of infiltration
   F. Imaging: underlying breast carcinoma

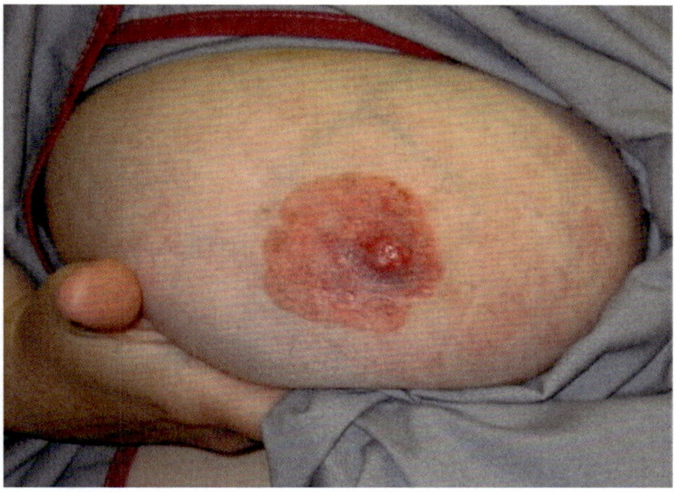

FIGURE 17.2.146 - Paget's Disease of the Nipple

VI. Invasive Ductal Carcinoma
   A. Malignant proliferation of ductal epithelial cells with stromal infiltration
   B. Most common malignancy of the breast
   C. Unifocal and unilateral

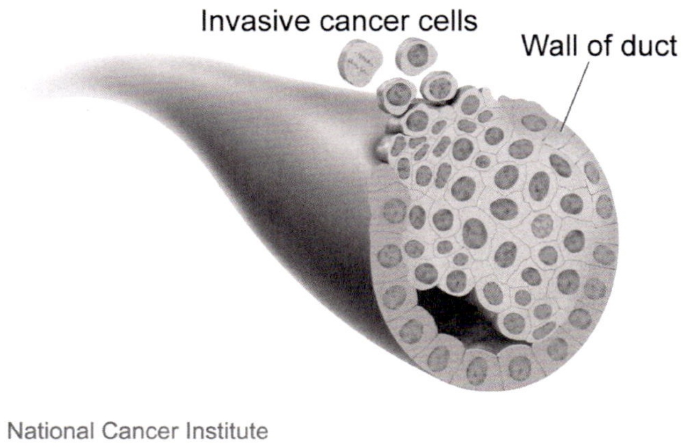

FIGURE 17.2.147 - Invasive Ductal Carcinoma

VII. Invasive Lobular Carcinoma
   A. Malignant proliferation of lobular epithelial cells with stromal infiltration
   B. Usually multifocal and bilateral
   C. Less aggressive than invasive ductal carcinoma

VIII. Inflammatory Breast Cancer
   A. Rare and aggressive malignant tumor of the breast
   B. Poorly differentiated; invasion of breast and dermal lymphatics
   C. Clinical features
      1. Peau d'orange: edematous, erythematous, indurated skin resembling an orange peel
      2. Tender breast and lymphadenopathy
   D. Can be misdiagnosed for mastitis; non-responsive to antibiotics
   E. Full thickness biopsy (punch biopsy) should be performed
   F. Aggressive treatment with mastectomy, chemo and radiotherapy
   G. Poor prognosis

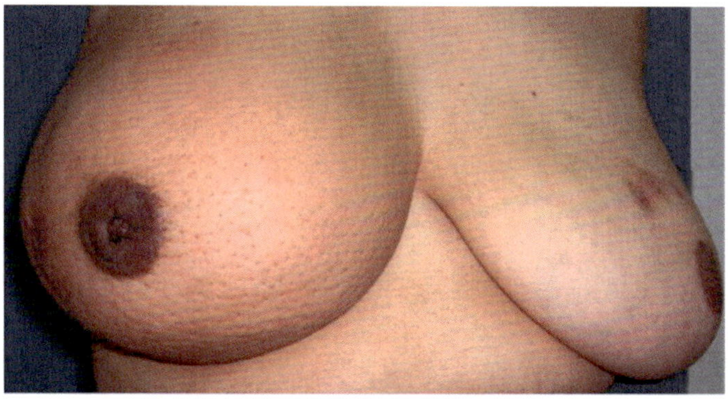

FIGURE 17.2.148 - Inflammatory Breast Cancer

REVIEW QUESTIONS

1. A 43-year-old woman comes to her primary care physician because of a red lesion on her right nipple that she noticed 3 weeks ago. She has a past medical history of asthma. Physical examination shows an erythematous, scaly, ulcerated lesion with erosions involving the right nipple and areola. What is likely to be seen on biopsy of this lesion?

   - **A biopsy of this lesion will likely show intraepithelial adenocarcinoma cells and Paget's cells with infiltration of the epidermis.**
   - This patient is presenting with an erythematous lesion on the right nipple.
   - Physical examination shows a scaly, ulcerated lesion involving the right nipple and areola.
   - This is a classical presentation of Paget's disease of the nipple.
   - On biopsy, intraepithelial adenocarcinoma cells and Paget's cells with infiltration of the epidermis will be evident.
   - Paget's disease of the nipple is most commonly associated with underlying breast cancer such as DCIS or invasive carcinoma. This is due to the migration of neoplastic cells of the underlying carcinoma to the surface of the nipple.

2. A 33-year-old woman comes to her primary care physician for consultation on a contraceptive choice. She was diagnosed with breast cancer a year ago and is undergoing therapy. She is otherwise healthy. She does not smoke or drink alcohol. She is sexually active again and is looking for the most effective contraceptive method. Which of the following is the best contraceptive choice for this patient?

   A. Combined oral contraceptive pills
   B. Hormonal intrauterine device
   C. Barrier contraception
   D. Copper intrauterine device

   - **The correct answer is option D.**
   - This 33-year-old woman is requesting an effective contraception method.
   - She was diagnosed with breast cancer a year ago and is undergoing therapy.
   - The most effective and best contraceptive method for this patient with breast cancer is a copper intrauterine device.
   - Hormonal contraception is contraindicated in patients with breast cancer.
   - Options A, combined oral contraceptive pills, and B, hormonal intrauterine device, are incorrect because they are both hormonal contraceptive methods and are not suitable for this patient with breast cancer.
   - Option C, barrier contraception, is incorrect because it is considered less effective than copper IUDs.

TABLES & FIGURES

Made in United States
Orlando, FL
04 November 2026

90201371R00117